Thyroid Cancer
A Guide for Patients

Editors

Douglas Van Nostrand, M.D., F.A.C.P., F.A.C.N.P.
Director, Division of Nuclear Medicine
Washington Hospital Center

Gary Bloom
Chair, Board of Directors and Co-Founder
ThyCa: Thyroid Cancer Survivors' Association, Inc.

Leonard Wartofsky, M.D., M.A.C.P.
Chair, Department of Medicine
Washington Hospital Center
Professor of Medicine, Georgetown University
Professor of Medicine, Uniformed Services
University of the Health Sciences

■ ■ ■
Keystone Press, Inc.
Baltimore, Maryland

Thyroid Cancer
A Guide for Patients

Published by Keystone Press, Inc.
380 Hickory Point Road
Pasadena, Maryland 21122
Please e-mail comments, suggestions or corrections to
KeystonePress@aol.com

Library of Congress Control Number: 2003115197
ISBN 0-9746239-0-3
Printed in the United States of America by Victor Graphics, Inc.,
        Baltimore, Maryland
Text editing by Jennifer Andes
Cover design by Diana Buell
Illustrations by Shaun Dellar

DISCLAIMER

The authors, editors, and publisher have used their best efforts in the preparation of this book. However, the information in this book is solely the opinions of the authors, and the authors, editors, and publisher make no representations or warranties with respect to the accuracy or completeness of this book for any reason or purpose. In addition, the authors, editors, and publisher assume no legal liability for the accuracy, completeness, appropriateness or usefulness of any information contained in this book.

The information contained in this book is for general informational purposes only, and the information contained within is not guaranteed or warranted to produce any particular result. In addition, the information may not be suitable for every individual. In no situation should any information contained in this book be used without the specific approval of the physician who knows the patient's medical history, has examined the patient and is managing the patient's medical care and treatment.

Dedications

To our patients and staff who give us purpose.

DVN and LW

My thanks and dedication to my family and to the volunteers of ThyCa: Thyroid Cancer Survivors' Association.

GB

Table of Contents

■ v ■

Contributors

Editors

DOUGLAS VAN NOSTRAND, M.D., is the Director of Nuclear Medicine at Washington Hospital Center. His specialty is nuclear medicine, and his primary area of interest and expertise is the nuclear medicine diagnosis and treatment of thyroid cancer. He has held numerous academic and medical society positions including Clinical Professor of Radiology and Nuclear Medicine, Uniformed Services University of Health Sciences; past President, Mid-Eastern Society of Nuclear Medicine; and Director of Continuing Medical Education Department and other elected positions of the Medical Staff of Good Samaritan Hospital. He has published over 50 articles and has been the editor of five medical books.

GARY BLOOM is a co-founder and the Board Chair of ThyCa: Thyroid Cancer Survivors' Association, Inc. (www.thyca.org). ThyCa is an all-volunteer, non-profit organization of thyroid cancer survivors, family members, and health care professionals advised by nationally recognized leaders in the field of thyroid cancer and dedicated to education, communication and support for thyroid cancer survivors, families and friends. Gary Bloom is a thyroid cancer survivor and is involved in the association as a volunteer.

LEONARD WARTOFSKY, M.D., is the Chairman of the Department of Medicine at Washington Hospital Center. His specialty is endocrinology, and his primary area of interest and expertise is thyroid disease in general and thyroid cancer in particular, for which he is world-renowned. He has held numerous academic and medical society positions including Professor of Medicine, Georgetown University, Professor of Medicine, Uniformed Services University of Health Sciences, and past President of the American Thyroid Association. He also received the Distinguished Educator Award of the Endocrine Society in 2001. He has published over 300 articles and is the editor of the medical textbook entitled *Thyroid Cancer, A Comprehensive Guide to Clinical Management*.

Authors

Jeanne F. Allegra, Ph.D.
Psychologist
Silver Spring, Maryland
Washington Hospital Center
Washington, D.C.

Frank Atkins, Ph.D.
Nuclear Medicine Physicist
Washington Hospital Center
Washington, D.C.

Andrew J. Bauer, M.D.
Major, MC, USA
Pediatric Endocrinology, Walter Reed Army Medical Center
Washington, D.C.
Assistant Professor of Pediatrics
Uniformed Services University of the Health Sciences
Bethesda, Maryland

Gary Bloom
Chair, Board of Directors
ThyCa: Thyroid Cancer Survivors' Association, Inc.

Lisa Boyle, M.D.
Director, Thyroid Cancer Surgery
Washington Hospital Center
Washington, D.C.

Robert Birdwell, M.D.
Nuclear Medicine
Walter Reed Army Medical Center
Washington, D.C.

James D. Brierley, BSc, M.B., M.R.C.P., F.R.C.R., F.R.C.P.C.
Associate Professor
Department of Radiation Oncology
Princess Margaret Hospital
University of Toronto
Toronto, Canada

Kenneth D. Burman, M.D.
Chief, Endocrine Section
Washington Hospital Center
Professor, Department of Medicine
Uniformed Services University of the Health Sciences
Clinical Professor, Department of Medicine
Georgetown and George Washington Universities
Washington, D.C.

Dianne Dodd, Ph.D.
Historian, Parks Canada
Past President
Canadian Thyroid Cancer Support Group (Thry'vors), Inc.

James John Figge, M.D., M.B.A., F.A.C.P
Adjunct Associate Professor
Department of Biomedical Sciences School of
    Public Health
State University of New York
Albany, New York

Gary L. Francis, M.D., Ph.D.
Col, MC, USA
Professor of Pediatrics
Director of Pediatric Endocrinology and
    Metabolism Fellowship
Associate Chair of Research Operations
Uniformed Services University of the Health Sciences
Bethesda, Maryland

John E. Glenn, Ph.D.
Director of Radiation Safety
Georgetown University Hospital
Former Chief, Radiation Protection and Health Effects Branch
    of the Nuclear Regulatory Commission
Washington, D.C.

James Jelinek, M.D., F.A.C.R.
Chair, Department of Radiology
Washington Hospital Center
Washington, D.C.

Alexander Mark, M.D.
Director, NeuroRadiology
Department of Radiology
Washington Hospital Center
Washington, D.C.

Ernest L. Mazzaferri, M.D., M.A.C.P
Emeritus Professor and Chair of Internal Medicine,
    Ohio State University, Ohio
Adjunct Professor of Medicine, University of Florida
Gainesville, Florida

Yolanda C. Oertel, M.D.
Director, Fine Needle Aspiration Service
Washington Hospital Center.
Professor Emerita of Pathology
The George Washington University School of Medicine
    and Health Sciences
Washington, D.C.
Adjunct Professor of Pathology and Laboratory Medicine,
MCP Hahnemann University School of Medicine
Philadelphia, P.A.

Yasser H. Ousman, M.D.
Associate Director, Diabetes Team
Section of Endocrinology
Washington Hospital Center
Washington, D.C.

Diane Patching
Director, Canadian Thyroid Cancer Support Group, (Thry'vors) Inc.
Member, Thyroid Foundation of Canada
Dundalk, Ontario

Stephen Peterson, M.D.
Chair, Department of Psychiatry
Washington Hospital Center
Preceptor, Consultation—Liaison for St.Elizabeths Hospital.
Washington, D.C.

Howard M. Richard, III, M.D.
Interventional Radiologist
Washington Hospital Center
Washington, D.C.

Matthew D. Ringel, M.D.
Associate Professor of Medicine
Divisions of Endocrinology and Hematology/Oncology
Ohio State University
Columbus, Ohio

Ron Sall, C.P.A.
Area Director
Professional Recruiting Group
Spherion Corporation
Washington, D.C.

Lalitha Shankar, M.D.
Program Director
National Cancer Institute
Bethesda, Maryland

Joan Shey
President and Founder, The Light of Life Foundation
Englishtown, New Jersey

Nikolaos Stathatos, M.D.
Division of Endocrinology
Washington Hospital Center
Georgetown University Hospital
Washington, D.C.

Shari Thomas, C.R.C.
Nuclear Medicine Research Coordinator
Washington Hospital Center
Washington, D.C.

Douglas Van Nostrand, M.D., F.A.C.P., F.A.C.N.P.
Director, Division of Nuclear Medicine
Washington Hospital Center
Washington, D.C.

Leonard Wartofsky, M.D., M.A.C.P.
Chair, Department of Medicine
Washington Hospital Center
Washington, D.C.
Professor of Medicine, Georgetown University
Professor of Medicine, Anatomy, Physiology and Genetics
Uniformed Services University of Health Sciences

Foreword

When you hear that you have cancer, your world starts spinning, not for a moment or two, but for what feels like an eternity. Then in a short time, it often comes crashing down around you, as well as upon those who love you and care for you, leaving you depressed, frightened, and in deep anguish. The questions are almost always the same. How do I deal with this? Will I see my kids grow up? Will I live long enough to see my daughter get married? Will my grandchildren ever know me? Or if it is your child who has cancer, the first response is "NOT MY CHILD!" Then after a bit, more questions come. Children don't get thyroid cancer, do they? What did I do *wrong*?

I have told hundreds of patients the same thing at this moment: "live one day at a time. If it's a good day, don't ruin it with anxiety about the future or regrets about the past. To the extent that you can, let the sun shine in today." After you think about this for more than a heart beat the question is always, "how do I deal with this bad news right now?" The answer is astonishingly simple for most people. You need reliable information about your problem. This is not to mean a pat on the head and the trite words, "Don't worry, this is a good cancer." It always breaks my heart to hear this. There is no good cancer—at least not according to any patient or family that I ever met. If it's your cancer, how on earth could it be "good"?

It became clear to me early in my career that long explanations in the office usually don't penetrate the wall of fear and anxiety and often go unheard by even the most sophisticated patients when the subject is their life and the words "thyroid cancer" come into the conversation. Many times I have had to give a person the bad news that the fine-needle aspiration results show thyroid cancer. Then, after answering a barrage of questions as clearly as I know how to do, the patient often leaves the office shook up and looking stunned. An hour later I get a call from the patient with the following question, "But Doc, do I have *cancer*? It's OK, you can tell me straight out, I want to know." It usually takes several visits to communicate this information in a way that makes sense to the patient. Even so, this is often less than satisfactory. It takes time to absorb all the information that you need to care for yourself, and unfortunately the particulars of this subject are rife with misinformation.

This book is long overdue. It will provide thyroid cancer patients with a strong set of tools: information from experts, access to Web sites, books, and friendly people who have been there and want to help, and much more. It tells you what your doctor knows about this disease. It should help you to understand and to fight back. Reliable information is a powerful weapon against cancer. It not only puts the problem in perspective, but it gives options and choices that might not be readily apparent to a person. This book might at first glance look intimidating, containing more than you want to know about thyroid cancer and a bit daunting to a person who has no medical background. Reading it like you would a novel is probably not the right approach for most people. I never read textbooks from cover to cover—I can't remember what I am reading when I take this approach. Instead I hunt and peck for information that I want. When one of my questions is answered a barrage of new ones comes to mind. If you do this, you will find the book a rich source of information, treasures, and nuggets—what doctors have for years called "pearls."

So, this is a book of "pearls" for patients. I have no doubt that my patients will find the answers for many questions that they just don't remember to ask when they are in the office. You will find that this book has answers from experts and truly dedicated people who want to make your life or that of someone dear to you better. My guess is that your doctor will provide further clarification and tailoring of the answers to your personal problem, but you will have a better grasp of the information about your thyroid cancer when the doctor does this.

Physicians must respect the wishes of our patients. To make your own choices and decisions you need information. This book will give you that knowledge. It will give you options and will help you define your own personal choices. This is necessary if you want to help your doctor find the best routes for your recovery. It's your body and your choices that count!

ERNEST L. MAZZAFERRI, M.D., M.A.C.P.
Emeritus Professor and Chair of Internal Medicine,
    Ohio State University
Adjunct Professor of Medicine, University of Florida

Preface

The Purpose of the Book

I believe it is self–evident that the more the patient understands his or her disease, the better the care the patient will receive. I also believe that the more the family members and friends understand the disease, the more support they can give to their loved one or friend. Accordingly, the goals of this book are (1) to offer an additional source of information to educate the patient and the patient's family and friends and (2) to improve not only the patient's quality of medical care, but also the patient's support from family and friends.

How to Use the Book

Although you could read this book from cover to cover, I recommend that you read the sections related to your specific question or situation. In these sections, you will find valuable "nuggets of information," which physicians often call "pearls." The table of contents and index will help you find these "pearls."

I believe that everyone should read chapter 26 entitled "Living with Thyroid Cancer." This chapter shares the experiences and insights of not only several individuals who have had or have thyroid cancer, but also a family member, a psychologist, and a psychiatrist. I believe this chapter will be valuable to every reader.

Challenges of the Book

At first glance, one may have the perception that writing a book such as this is easy and perhaps easier than writing a medical textbook. That is not necessarily true. A book such as this presents unique and different challenges.

The first challenge is expressing the information as clearly as possible to you—the reader. In fact, one of our primary responsibilities as authors and editors is to make the book as clear and as easy to read as possible. To this end, a significant amount of time and effort have been contributed to write, rewrite, and edit this book. From the initial drafts of the chapters by the authors, to revisions by the authors, medical editors, text editors, and several lay reviewers, the chapters have been revised many times. I believe we have been successful in our responsibilities to you. Nevertheless and despite these efforts, I am confident that sections could be more clearly written and that errors remain. With new research and changing medical practices, we anticipate future editions, and thus we welcome comments, suggestions, identification of errors, and identification of confusing sections. Please e-mail these to Keystonepress@aol.com or mail to Attention: Douglas Van Nostrand, Director, Division of Nuclear Medicine, Washington Hospital Center, 110 Irving Street, N.W., Washington D.C. 20010. Because neither Keystone Press, Inc. nor the editors have the people resources to answer questions or to clarify sections on an individual basis, you will not receive a response. However, in advance, we appreciate your input.

A second challenge is how detailed should the book be? Some readers may believe we have not gone far enough and others may believe that we have gone too far. We have tried to design the book with as much detail as we believed was reasonable such that the patient or the patient's family members and friends could decide how far to go. However, for those who wish to go further, additional references are in appendix C (Additional Sources of Information) and appendix D (Books and Manuals).

Another challenge in the development of this book is whether information should be repeated in different sections, and if so, how much? Many books, and certainly scientific books, typically try to avoid repeating information. We, the editors, chose to repeat selected information in order to facilitate access to some of the information. To avoid repeating too much information, a glossary is present, and in the text we have liberally referred the reader to appropriate chapters for further reading. Of course, an index is also available.

The final challenges are presenting the latest information about thyroid cancer as well as the different approaches and opinions among physicians regarding the management of thyroid cancer. Again, this book represents the best efforts of the authors and editors to achieve these two goals. Nevertheless, it is literally impossible to include all the latest information and to discuss all the potential opinions regarding the management of thyroid cancer. Your team of physicians including your primary care physician, endocrinologist, nuclear medicine physician, nuclear radiologist, surgeon, radiation therapist, and cytologist, will be valuable resources for this information.

Warning

In our modern world, many books are published as "self-help" books or "do-it-yourself" books. This book is neither! This book is only a source of information, and the information contained herein may not be appropriate for you or a loved one who has thyroid cancer. Each person's situation is unique, and other factors may affect the individual's care. In no situation should an individual use any information contained in this book without the specific approval of the individual's physician who knows his or her medical history, has examined him or her, and is directly managing his or her medical care. Nevertheless, we hope that this book will be a valuable resource to educate and through education to help assure that the person with thyroid cancer gets the best possible medical care and the needed support from family and friends.

DOUGLAS VAN NOSTRAND, M.D.

Acknowledgements

Recognition of Grants

To write, edit, illustrate, format, print, store, and distribute a book is an expensive process, and a large number of copies of a book have to be sold to pay for those expenses. Because a book such as this will never sell a large number of copies, most publishers will either set the price per copy very high or not publish the book at all—usually the latter. Fortunately, this book has been published and is available at a reasonable cost because of four generous educational grants from:

Genzyme Corporation

MDS Nordion

Abbott Laboratories

Eastern Isotopes

First and foremost, we are very grateful to the Genzyme Corporation, Cambridge, Massachusetts (developer, manufacturer, and distributor of Thyrogen®), not only for its financial support but also for its commitment to patient education. Without this grant, this book would not have been published. Second, I would like to thank MDS Nordion, Canada (manufacturer of ^{123}I and ^{131}I). Their grant also helped underwrite a major portion of the cost of publication and distribution of this book. Finally, I would like to thank Abbott Laboratories, Chicago, Illinois (manufacturer of Synthroid®) and Eastern Isotopes, Sterling, Virginia (manufacturer and distributor of many radiopharmaceuticals) for additional educational grants.

Recognition of Contributions

In addition to the large number of dollars that are needed to publish this book, a large number of people are needed. It is amazing how many—38 to be exact! And that doesn't count all the individuals at the printing company. Although I cannot acknowledge every one of these individuals, I would like to recognize several.

First, I thank all of the authors. They gathered the information. They first put pencil to paper. They responded to suggestions, modification, and in some cases even "badgering" from me. In addition, they tolerated my errors, deficiencies, and even forgetfulness.

Second, I thank Jennifer Andes. Jennifer was the quiet, behind-the-scene professional editor, who edited every word, corrected the grammar, and asked questions of clarification. In addition, she did this while carrying and delivering her first child. However, if any word is "mispeled" and if the grammar "ain't" perfect, it is not because of her. It is because we—the authors and editors—failed to make the change or because our "writer's ego" got in the way of allowing the change.

Third, I thank Shaun Dellar. Shaun was the artist amongst us, and he did an excellent job in communicating concepts through illustrations. He also tolerated my redo after redo after redo.

Next, I thank Diana Buell, who was the graphic designer. Initially, she designed our hospital's thyroid cancer information manual, which helped inspire this book, and she designed the front and back cover of this book. She did a great job.

To help improve the readability of the book, two non-medical readers also proofed all or part of the book. I would like to thank Cherry Wunderlich and Julian Clarke, Jr., who made excellent suggestions that improved the book.

The final major step of the publication of a book is the printing. Because of a combination of factors such as (1) the difficulty in finding a publisher to take the risk of doing a book such as this, (2) the loss of control to facilitate distribution of the book at the sacrifice of profits, and (3) the loss of control of how we would like to see the book developed, I assumed the role of publisher. As I ventured into the problems of publishing, I was confronted with many new questions and challenges. I could not have successfully managed these without the help of Greg Davis, sales representative for Victor Graphics; Kim Flannery, account representative; and Tom Hicks, CEO and owner of Victor Graphics. Victor Graphics is a large printing company in Baltimore, Maryland, that prints books for such medical publishing companies as Lippincott-Williams & Wilkins, The Endocrine Society, and others. From page layout to "never-heard-of-before" terms such as "EAN bar width reduction," they walked me through the process. Thank you for your patience and help.

No acknowledgement would be complete without mentioning my two co-editors. Because of his thyroid cancer, Gary Bloom co-founded an outstanding resource and excellent support group for patients with thyroid cancer, which as noted elsewhere is ThyCa: Thyroid Cancer Survivors' Association." It is in part because of his inspiration that I was also motivated to publish this book. From my initial idea to the final book off the press, I have appreciated his ideas and suggestions—and most importantly his encouragement. As most writers and editors know, there is a period when the writer or editor wonders "Why am I doing this?" Perhaps this is more vividly expressed by Joyce Carol, who stated, "Getting the first draft finished is like pushing a peanut with your nose across a very dirty floor." It was Gary's e-mails of encouragement that helped me "move that peanut across the floor" while managing my own doubts of the usefulness of the project. Thanks. And now that the book is done, would someone please pass me a tissue?

Finally, I especially would like to thank Dr. Leonard Wartofsky. His combination of expertise, wisdom, and grace are rare, and it has been a pleasure to have had a professional relationship with him for the better part of 25 years. Indeed, it is an honor to call him boss, colleague, and friend.

DOUGLAS VAN NOSTRAND, M.D.

CHAPTER 1

The Thyroid Gland: The Basics

Leonard Wartofsky, M.D.

What is the thyroid gland?

The thyroid gland is one of several endocrine glands of the body. These endocrine glands produce hormones that circulate in the blood and have effects in various tissues and cells of the body. What distinguishes endocrine glands from other glands such as sweat glands or lymph glands is that the endocrine glands do not have any ducts or channels that carry the product of the gland away from the gland itself to the rest of the body. For example, a sweat gland has a channel or pore that carries the sweat to the surface of the skin. In contrast, endocrine glands release their product, in this case hormones, directly into the blood. The blood then carries the endocrine hormone throughout the body to various tissues where it binds to specific cell proteins *(receptors)* that serve to initiate some action of the hormone in that tissue.

The thyroid gland then is a typical endocrine gland, and in its case, thyroid hormones are released into the blood and circulate throughout the body, ultimately binding to thyroid hormone receptors in virtually every cell of the body. After binding to the cells, the effect of thyroid hormones varies depending on the particular tissue. A principal effect of thyroid hormones is to regulate your metabolism, that is, the rate at which your body burns up calories to produce energy. Too much thyroid hormone, as produced in conditions causing *hyper*thyroidism, will drive these metabolic processes too fast and can cause adverse effects. For example, normal thyroid hormone levels in the blood are important to regulate heart rate and heart function. An excessive amount of thyroid hormone will cause the heart to beat more rapidly and pump blood inefficiently. If left untreated, this condition may result in cardiac rhythm abnormalities and heart failure. On the other hand, conditions marked by an under-active thyroid gland, or *hypo*thyroidism, result in low circulating levels of thyroid hormone, a situation that also irritates body function and well-being. Like hyperthyroidism, hypothyroidism also can cause impaired heart function that could result in heart failure, although of a different

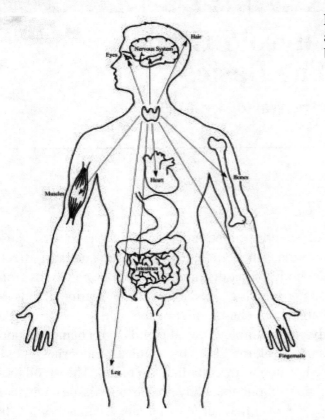

FIGURE 1: Thyroid hormone affects many organs of the body.

type. The heart is not the only organ affected. A variety of symptoms and manifestations of either hyperthyroidism or hypothyroidism will be expressed as a result of the effects of thyroid excess or deficiency in various tissues and organs (see figure 1). Some of these conditions will be discussed specifically below.

Where is the thyroid gland?

The thyroid gland is a butterfly shaped tissue located in the neck just below the Adam's apple and straddling the windpipe (trachea) (see figures 2a and 2b). The "butterfly" consists of left and right "wings" that are the two lobes of the gland and a connecting "body" of the butterfly that is known as the *isthmus*. In the early stages of development of the fetus, the cells that were to become the thyroid formed at the base of the tongue and then migrated down to their destined location. Occasionally a remnant or residual tract, called a *thyroglossal duct,* may remain in the migratory path. This tract of tissue can be the site of residual thyroid remnants that may form fluid-filled nodules (cysts) or solid cellular masses (tumors) that can be either benign or cancerous. Often, in cases where there is an overall stimulus for the thyroid gland to grow larger, the remnant of this thyroglossal tract that is attached to the top of the thyroid gland (typically the isthmus) can also enlarge and

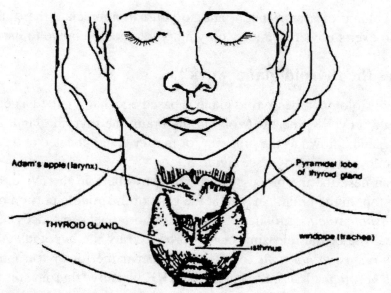

FIGURE 2A: Location and shape of the thyroid.

has been called a *pyramidal* lobe. Most people have only a right and left lobe of the gland. Some disorders of the thyroid will affect both lobes whereas others such as a solitary tumor may occur in either one lobe or the other. Rarely just one lobe of the thyroid develops (a "butterfly" with one wing), which is known as *hemiagenesis* of the thyroid.

Under normal circumstances, the size or weight of the thyroid gland will vary with the size of the individual person. Thus a 300-pound, 6-foot-6-inch football lineman will have a significantly larger thyroid gland than a 5-foot-tall, 95-pound ballerina. In average-sized women, the thyroid gland weighs 14 to 18 grams, and in most men, it weighs 16 to 20 grams. The latter represents about a half ounce or

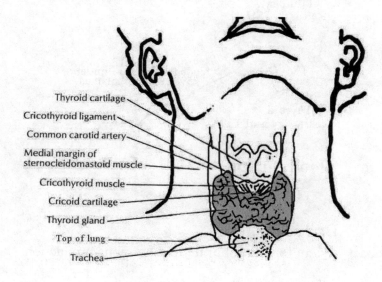

FIGURE 2B: Further anatomy around the thyroid gland.

about the volume of a tablespoon, and so you can appreciate that this relatively small gland exerts powerful effects on your whole body relative to its size.

How does the thyroid gland work?

The physiology of the thyroid gland is based on what is called a negative feedback system, a cyclic process involving the brain, the thyroid gland, and a small endocrine gland, known as the *pituitary*, or master gland, located at the base of the brain at the level of the nose (see figure 3.)

We can describe the process by starting anywhere in the cycle, but we will start at the top, in the brain. An area at the base of the middle portion of the brain, called the *hypothalamus*, produces a number of hormonal substances called *releasing factors*. One of the releasing factors produced by the hypothalamus is called *thyrotropin-releasing hormone*, or TRH. Another name for thyrotropin is *thyroid stimulating hormone* (TSH). So that means TRH is really "thyroid stimulating hormone-releasing hormone." The negative feedback system comes into play here because it is high levels of thyroid hormone circulating in the blood that signal the hypothalamus to turn off TRH. Similarly, low levels of thyroid hormone in the blood signal the hypothalamus to release more TRH.

The TRH released from the hypothalamus travels down to the pituitary gland, causing it to release the TSH that then enters the blood stream. Even though TSH

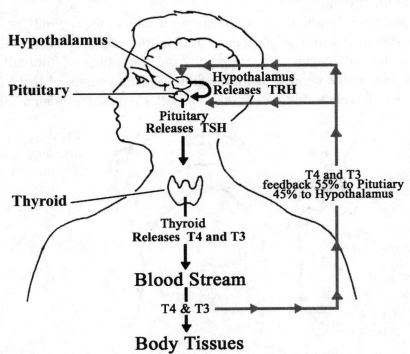

FIGURE 3: Negative feedback system for control of thyroid hormone production.

circulates throughout the entire body, its only known function is to attach to specific TSH receptor proteins on the surface of the thyroid cells.

Thyroid cells are normally arranged in units called follicles; the cells of these units are called follicular cells. These cells are formed into little circular units that look like rosettes. A jelly-like material within the rosettes is called *colloid*. The cells synthesize and release thyroid hormones into the colloid where it is stored until it is released into the blood. The rate of synthesis and release of thyroid hormones from the thyroid gland into the blood is controlled by TSH from the pituitary gland. Once a sufficient amount of thyroid hormone is established in the blood, the pituitary gland knows to reduce TSH production from the pituitary gland and TRH production from the hypothalamus.

This negative feedback system can be visualized if we imagine the blood flowing through the hypothalamus and that the blood is low in thyroid hormone levels due to deficient production by the thyroid gland or absence of the thyroid gland as would occur after thyroidectomy. As a result of sensing the low thyroid hormone levels, the hypothalamus will release TRH that passes down to the pituitary gland causing it to release TSH. Thus because the low thyroid hormone level triggered an increase in TSH, this is termed negative feedback. The TSH enters the blood, circulates to the thyroid gland and then stimulates the gland to trap more iodine out of the blood, make more thyroid hormone, and then release it into the blood. Eventually, in the healthy individual, thyroid hormone levels are restored to normal, and these now normal levels circulate back to the hypothalamus and pituitary where they will inhibit further production of TRH and TSH (again, negative feedback). All three levels (hypothalamus, pituitary, and thyroid) need to work properly to provide normal thyroid physiology.

What is the role of iodine in the thyroid?

A very important raw material that is used in the manufacture of thyroid hormones is *iodine*. This naturally occurring element is present in many of the foods we eat, seafoods in particular, and iodine can also exist in high concentrations in a number of drugs, preservatives, and X-ray contrast dyes. A common source of iodine in our diet in the United States is derived from salt. Iodine supplements have been added to salt since the mid 1920s, after the discovery that a lack of iodine or iodine deficiency could cause thyroid enlargement (*goiter*). Although iodine deficiency and iodine deficiency goiter and hypothyroidism are important world health problems, the program of adding iodine to salt has virtually abolished this deficiency in the United States. The amount of iodine in your diet can have important implications for the treatment of thyroid cancer after surgery. This will be discussed below in the section on low iodine diet.

Two thyroid hormones are produced in the thyroid gland: *thyroxine* (T4) and *triiodothyronine* (T3). These hormones are made by a complex mechanism that starts with the trapping of iodine out of the blood and into the thyroid gland under stimulation by TSH. The iodine is incorporated into the amino acid *tyrosine*, and these iodinated tyrosine molecules join together to form T4 and T3. The designations T4 and T3 reflect the number of iodine molecules that are present in each compound. Thus the "tri-iodo" prefix of T3 refers to its three iodine molecules, and the other name for thyroxine, *tetraiodothyronine*, refers to the four iodine molecules in T4.

What is the difference between thyroid hormone made by the thyroid gland and the thyroid hormone my doctor may give me?

Both T4 and T3 can be synthesized in pure form and are used in the treatment of underactive thyroid conditions and for thyroid cancer, as will be discussed below. T3 is approximately 10 times more potent metabolically than T4. Experimental data indicate that T4 circulating in the blood may serve primarily as a reservoir for the generation of T3. In fact, only 20 percent of the circulating T3 in the blood is actually derived from the thyroid gland itself. The remaining 80 percent comes from T4 circulating in blood and other tissues outside of the thyroid gland. This T3 is generated by a process that removes one iodine molecule from T4, thereby generating T3.

T3 rarely is used to treat hypothyroidism since the physiologic needs of the body are served by the normal generation of T3 from T4. There are circumstances, however, when an endocrinologist may prescribe a T3 medication for brief periods of time for patients preparing for radioactive iodine therapy, as will be discussed below. Once T4 and T3 are released by the thyroid gland into the blood, the hormones circulate almost entirely bound or tied to specific transport proteins (see chapter 2).

What does thyroid hormone do?

Once thyroid hormones enter the blood, they circulate to all the various tissues. While the thyroid hormone receptor proteins in each tissue of the body may be similar, the effects of thyroid hormone action will vary depending on the nature of the tissue. For example, in heart tissue thyroid hormone will increase the ability of the heart muscle to contract as well as increase the heart rate (the number of beats per minute). We believe that the T4 hormone may serve as a "pro-hormone" or reservoir for the production of the more active T3. Thus in tissues such as liver, kidney, and muscle, one iodine molecule is removed from T4, creating the more potent T3. T3 regulates the metabolic rates in virtually all of the tissues of the body; this includes the rates of metabolism of carbohydrate, protein, and fat; stimulation of growth and development; as well as our physical and mental development and function.

I notice how much better I feel when I take my thyroid hormone; would a little extra make me feel even better?

Because thyroid hormone causes the body to metabolize food faster, patients who have an excessive amount of thyroid hormone circulating in the blood (hyperthyroidism) may lose weight and may waste away. While abuse of thyroid hormone medication might, on the surface, appear to be a good way to gain energy and lose weight, it ultimately could be very destructive. This is because the body metabolizes not just fat but also protein, such as the protein in our muscles, and loss of muscle protein will lead to muscle wasting and weakness. Other adverse effects of excessive thyroid hormone include loss of calcium from bones that can lead to osteoporosis, heart rhythm disturbances, heart enlargement and heart failure.

How does my doctor determine exactly how much thyroid hormone I need to take?

Thyroid hormone therapy can be closely monitored to achieve normal or desirable levels by measuring the TSH and T4 circulating in the blood (see chapter 2). Based on these measurements, your doctor will adjust the dosage of thyroid hormone being administered. Once the appropriate dosage is reached, the danger or risk of either hyperthyroidism or hypothyroidism or any of the adverse effects or outcomes of these conditions is eliminated.

What is hypothyroidism? Will I get it?

Hypothyroidism happens when not enough thyroid hormone circulates in the blood. This deficiency results from any one of three mechanisms: disease of the hypothalamus with inadequate production of TRH, disease of the pituitary gland with inadequate production of TSH or primary thyroid disease within the thyroid gland itself. In the latter instance, the low thyroid hormone levels often will lead to extraordinarily elevated levels of TSH. The high TSH levels, per se, have no effect on you and simply represent the brain's response to the low thyroid hormone levels. Nevertheless and in spite of such high blood levels of TSH, there can be little response from the thyroid gland to the TSH when disease of the thyroid gland itself is present, and the patient remains hypothyroid. With hypothyroidism, laboratory measurements for T4 and TSH in blood will show elevated TSH and low T4 or free T4 (see chapter 2). You may have elevated TSH and low T4 if you have had your thyroid gland surgically removed (thyroidectomy) and are taking an insufficient amount of thyroxine replacement. Under certain circumstances temporary high TSH levels can be beneficial; however, and in fact endocrinologists often will intentionally allow patients to become hypothyroid to elevate their serum levels of TSH. They do this because patients with well-differentiated thyroid cancer often require treatment with radioactive iodine. The thyroid gland is most likely to take up iodine when stimulated by high levels of TSH. These high TSH levels will then facilitate the uptake of iodine (or in this case, radioiodine) to prepare the patient for radioiodine therapy. Patients preparing for therapy may become moderately to profoundly hypothyroid and symptomatic for as long as two to four weeks.

Must I always be hypothyroid to have diagnostic studies?

While thyroxine withdrawal to elevate serum TSH still is often necessary for optimal treatment of well-differentiated thyroid cancer, recent development of synthetic TSH (human recombinant TSH or *Thyrogen®*) has eliminated the need for many patients to become hypothyroid during their routine follow up and evaluation (see chapter 9). Thyrogen® was developed and is manufactured by the Genzyme Corporation and is essentially identical to the body's own TSH. Its availability has revolutionized the routine management of patients with well-differentiated thyroid cancer and greatly improved the comfort and well-being enjoyed by patients during these evaluations. It is administered by intramuscular injections, usually on two consecutive days, and results in elevations in serum TSH that are comparable to those achieved by withdrawal of thyroxine therapy. Hence the patient is allowed to continue taking synthetic thyroxine therapy, and the evaluation for residual disease is performed when possible using this synthetic TSH. Typical protocols for its use are described below (see chapter 13).

Patients allowed to become hypothyroid after thyroxine therapy is stopped can suffer from a variety of symptoms. These may include loss of menstrual periods or heavy menstrual flow, muscle weakness, accumulation of fluid or swelling (edema), weight gain, lethargy, intolerance to cold temperatures, reduced memory, decreased sex drive (libido), and constipation. Patients have been able to avoid all of these side effects by using Thyrogen® but should recognize that its use is not applicable or optimal in all clinical circumstances. However, more and more patients who otherwise would have had to stop thyroid hormone to become hypothyroid in order to increase their serum TSH are using Thyrogen®, and it is likely that use of this medication will be more broadly applied in the future.

Whether radioactive iodine therapy or ablation is performed after thyroxine withdrawal or after Thyrogen®, the immediate next step in the management of your well-differentiated thyroid cancer is to resume thyroxine therapy and bring the serum TSH back down to low levels. Thus after the radioactive iodine treatment, thyroid hormone therapy then can be initiated (or re-initiated) and normal metabolic function will be restored with elimination of all the above symptoms within days to weeks.

CHAPTER 2

Thyroid Hormone Measurements in Blood:

Thyroxine (T4), Triiodothyronine (T3), and TSH

Leonard Wartofsky, M.D.

What are all of the thyroid tests that my doctor wants to do and why are they needed?

Your doctor will use a variety of blood tests, biopsies, X-rays and nuclear scans during the course of your diagnostic evaluation, treatment, and further management. It may be useful for you to understand the principles behind these tests so that you can appreciate how your doctor is using them, when they are necessary and how they work.

In regard to blood tests for thyroid hormone, once T4 and T3 are released by the thyroid gland into the blood, the hormones circulate almost entirely bound or tied to specific transport proteins. Imagine a cartoon with miniature boats and passengers sailing through the blood. The boats represent the transport proteins and the passengers in the boats are T4 and T3. There are also some T4 and T3 swimmers who are not in the boats. Our modern laboratories can measure the T4 or T3 that is being transported in the "boats," just that fraction "swimming free" or both. Perhaps the most common laboratory assay measuring the level of circulating T4 or T3 is reported as total T4 or total T3. This designation reflects the entire amount of circulating T4 that is bound to the binding protein as well as those in a free or unbound form—in other words, all of the T4 or T3, both in the boats and swimming free in the blood.

A separate measurement done to assess the thyroid status of patients is the *"free T4"* measurement. More than 99 percent of circulating T4 or T3 is bound to its transport proteins (in the boats) and only a fraction of circulating T4 or T3 is not bound to its transport proteins and circulates (or swims) free. This free fraction of the total hormone is the most important because it is the concentration that is "seen" by the cells and tissues, i.e., the concentration that enters the cells and becomes bound to cellular receptors and then exerts the metabolic effects of thyroid hormone.

Your doctor may measure either total T4 or total T3 or free T4 or free T3 at various times and for varying purposes. Of all of these measurements of thyroid hormones, many endocrinologists believe the measurement of the free T4 concentration is the most useful. In addition to our ability to measure total T4, total T3, free T4 and free T3, perhaps the most critical measurement for assessing the thyroid status of an individual is the measurement of TSH itself. This is so even though TSH is not a thyroid hormone but a pituitary hormone, and the importance of its measurement is because the levels reflect whether the feedback system is functioning normally. Endocrinologists interpret a normal TSH level as indicating that the circulating thyroid hormone level is also normal because the pituitary gland is sensing or "seeing" that level as normal. Thus if the thyroid hormone level was slightly lower than optimal, TSH would be higher than normal as a means of trying to stimulate the thyroid gland to make and release more T4 and T3. Similarly, in someone who has been thyroidectomized and who relies on thyroid hormone medication, a high TSH level would indicate that the patient has not been taking enough thyroid hormone. Reliable assays for TSH are available in most commercial and hospital laboratories and can usually be performed within a day.

What is thyroglobulin and why is it important?

Within the colloid of the thyroid follicles is a large protein where the thyroid hormones T4 and T3 are kept inside the thyroid gland. This protein is called *thyroglobulin* and is produced only by thyroid cells. Thyroglobulin is not another thyroid hormone, and although it is not actively secreted by the thyroid gland, it does normally "leak" out of the thyroid into the bloodstream. We can measure the thyroglobulin levels in the blood, and it is arguably the most important measurement that is done to assess the status of any residual disease in a patient with well-differentiated thyroid cancer because it helps us determine whether there may be any residual tumor. Thyroglobulin is produced only by thyroid cells and should be low or undetectable in the blood after complete removal of the thyroid gland (thyroidectomy) and subsequent radioactive iodine destruction of any remaining thyroid cells. Its presence in the blood after effective therapy would indicate residual tumor, and therefore it may be thought of as a "tumor marker." Even though patients will be treated with thyroid hormone replacement, such as pure synthetic thyroxine (T4), after undergoing a thyroidectomy or radioiodine ablation, they still should not have any thyroglobulin in their blood because there is no thyroglobulin in the thyroxine tablets used for treatment. Therefore, any thyroglobulin present would indicate the patient still has thyroid cells, which would be making the thyroglobulin. Thyroglobulin is abbreviated as *Tg* and is not to be confused with the abbreviation for the binding protein for T4 and T3 that is *TBG* (thyroxine binding globulin). There will be further discussion below on the utility and clinical applications of thyroglobulin measurements in the management of patients with well-differentiated thyroid cancer.

What is the difference between thyroglobulin and anti-thyroglobulin antibodies?

In addition to the thyroglobulin result listed on your laboratory report, you may see a reference to another test result called *anti-thyroglobulin antibody*. This is not thyroglobulin per se but rather represents an antibody produced by the body's immune system. These antibodies are typically produced by white blood cells called lymphocytes, and they react with thyroglobulin. These anti-thyroglobulin antibodies may be present as a result of the patient's defense against a thyroid cancer. Unrelated to thyroid cancer, these antibodies are most typically common in patients with an autoimmune disease called *Hashimotos' thyroiditis* or *Hashimoto's disease*. In this disorder, the antibodies have the ability eventually to destroy thyroid cells (*cytotoxicity*) leading to a wasting away (atrophy) of the thyroid gland. Once a significant amount of normal thyroid cells are lost, the remaining thyroid tissue will under-function in that it will not produce enough thyroid hormone for the body. The hypothyroidism that will result will then require thyroxine replacement therapy to restore a normal thyroid state. Physicians managing patients with well-differentiated thyroid cancer rely on measurements of these anti-thyroid antibodies because, if they are present, they will interfere with the laboratory assay of thyroglobulin. Thus the thyroglobulin measurement will lose most of its value as an indicator of residual tumor or "tumor marker." While this problem of antibody interference is an area of active research and investigation, no scientist to date has developed a foolproof technique for accurately measuring thyroglobulin in the presence of anti-thyroglobulin antibodies. Fortunately, in many patients, the antibodies will disappear from the blood when the thyroid cancer is fully resolved and cured, thereby allowing meaningful future monitoring by measurements of thyroglobulin. Persistent antibody levels imply either the presence of residual cancer cells or underlying Hashimoto's disease.

CHAPTER 3

Thyroid Nodules

Leonard Wartofsky, M.D.

My interest in thyroid cancer all started with discovery of a thyroid "nodule." What is a thyroid nodule? Is it a goiter?

As described in chapter 1, "*goiter*" means enlargement of the thyroid gland from any cause. Goiters can be benign (non-cancerous) or due to malignancy (cancerous). Benign goiters can be classified as simple or toxic. Toxic refers typically to overproduction of thyroid hormone by the goiter leading to hyperthyroidism or *thyrotoxicosis*. Toxic goiters may be generally or diffusely enlarged, and this is referred to as *diffuse toxic goiter*. In most cases, diffuse toxic goiter is the same as *Graves' disease*, named after Dr. Robert Graves of Ireland who in the mid-19th century described patients with diffuse toxic goiter and thyrotoxicosis.

Goiters can also be nodular or harbor one or more small masses or tumors representing neoplastic (new growth), which are localized collections of thyroid cells. These are generally referred to as nodules, and these nodules may be benign or cancerous and may be toxic (over-functioning) or nontoxic. Later in this chapter, nodules will be described as warm, cold or hot in reference to their function and ability to trap and concentrate radioactive iodine within the nodules as demonstrated by a nuclear medicine scan. Typically, hot nodules are benign, but there is a significantly greater likelihood of cancer in a cold nodule. Nevertheless, 80 percent or more of cold nodules are also benign.

In population surveys, a single nodule of the thyroid gland may be detected in approximately 6 percent of women and $1^1/_2$ percent of men. The frequency of thyroid nodules increases with each passing decade of life and, in general, nodules are relatively rare in children. Your physician can detect thyroid nodules by physically examining your neck. With advancing age, it is very common to find multiple small nodules in the thyroid gland as may be incidentally found during neck surgery for non-thyroid purposes or by various X-ray or imaging techniques, such as ultrasound, computerized tomography (CT) or magnetic resonance imaging (MRI). Generally, a nodule must approach approximately 1 centimeter or $^1/_2$ inch in diameter in order to be detected by your physician on simple examination of the thyroid gland. Ultrasound, CT, and MRI are much more sensitive and will pick up tiny nodules of 1 to 2 millimeters. The clinical significance of such tiny nodules that are incidentally found during imaging of the neck region for other purposes remains controversial.

What causes thyroid nodules?

Iodine Deficiency: The exact cause of why certain people develop thyroid nodules is not known, but some factors have been identified. As described in Chapter 2, iodine is an important element for thyroid hormone production, and one such factor promoting nodule and goiter formation is lack of sufficient iodine (iodine deficiency). Insufficient iodine in the diet will lead to stimulation of the thyroid gland due to increases in circulating TSH (promoted by the negative feedback to the pituitary of reduced thyroid hormone production). Cold nodules of the thyroid occur some 2 to 3 times more commonly in geographic areas where the diet is low in iodine. Laboratory rats served a diet low in iodine, for example, experience increases in the levels of TSH in their blood, causing them to develop thyroid nodules, some of which may be cancerous.

High blood TSH levels lead to goiter or nodule formation because TSH is a growth stimulant (or mitogen) of the thyroid. This fact relates to the basis for the therapeutic use of thyroxine to lower TSH levels and reduce the stimulus for goiter or nodule formation. Thus, in physiological dosage, thyroxine therapy will restore normal thyroid function (euthyroidism). In a slightly excessive dose, thyroxine therapy will lower TSH even further and thereby eliminate possible stimulation of thyroid cells to grow. Your endocrinologist is following this reasoning when providing you with doses of thyroxine that suppress TSH in order to minimize growth or stimulation of any residual well-differentiated thyroid cancer cells.

This very same TSH suppression is the basis on which many physicians attempt to treat thyroid nodules with thyroxine therapy. The hope is to shrink the nodules or at least blunt their further growth. Unfortunately, this therapy works for some thyroid nodules but clearly not for all, and because shrinkage may be seen in only a small percentage of thyroid nodules, such therapy is often used on only a temporary or trial basis. On the other hand, clearly documented enlargement or growth of a thyroid nodule while a patient is taking sufficient thyroxine to suppress TSH levels is abnormal and may be a signal that the nodule is a cancer. TSH should be absent with suppressive dosage levels of thyroxine; thus any growth of a given nodule reflects autonomous behavior, which means growth that is independent of normal TSH regulation. This autonomous behavior is seen with thyroid cancers that will grow independent of TSH stimulation, although they often enlarge more rapidly in the presence of TSH stimulation. Enlargement of a nodule would be detected by either serial measurements or estimations of size by physical examination of the neck, or by imaging techniques such as ultrasound, CT scan or MRI.

Other causes of thyroid nodules include certain genetic or familial factors. Patients with a strong family history of thyroid nodular disease are more likely to have a benign cause for the nodules, which is called benign *multinodular goiter*.

Radiation and Thyroid Nodules: Another important cause for thyroid nodule formation and development of thyroid cancer is radiation exposure. Such exposure may be from either internal radiation absorbed into the body through the skin or by inhalation into the lung. The latter may be seen after accidental radiation exposures from nuclear fallout. The source of the radiation may also be external such as that given by radiation therapists or oncologists for treatment of other cancers occurring in the neck area. For example, patients with the disorder of Hodgkin's disease involving the neck area or patients with various head and neck cancers may be treated with external radiation, and the thyroid gland is within the field that is exposed in the process of the radiation therapy. The dosage of radiation in these cases could be so high as to permanently damage the thyroid gland and cause hypothyroidism. With lower doses of radiation, the thyroid cells could suffer genetic damage rather than total destruction, and this can lead to cell mutations, which then may lead to thyroid cancer. Indeed, there once was a vogue in this country and other parts of the world for low-dose radiation to the area of the head and neck for benign conditions such as enlargement of the thymus gland in the chest, recurrent tonsillitis or adenitis, and for acne. When such therapy is given without radiation shielding of the thyroid gland, a very high number of thyroid nodules and thyroid abnormalities will occur over the next 10 to 40 years.

Children are at greatest risk for radiation exposure of the thyroid as the adult thyroid gland is much less commonly damaged by radiation exposure. Among children receiving head-neck irradiation, 15 to 30 percent will develop thyroid nodules and one-third of these will be cancer. The most recent dramatic example of radiation-induced thyroid tumors occurred in the region of Belarus in the Soviet Union after the major nuclear accident at Chernobyl in 1986. The dramatic increase in cases of thyroid cancer in subsequent years in children exposed to fallout from this accident represented an increased incidence rate of more than 100 times, which occurred within 5 to 8 years after the accident.

Are all thyroid nodules cancer?

Most thyroid nodules are in fact benign (non-cancerous), and just the fact that you have a thyroid nodule should not create undue concern that it may be a cancer. Most nodules rather than being cancer (carcinomas) are actually tumorous collections of benign cells variously called adenomas or adenomatoid nodules. Whether nodules are "cold" or "hot" on thyroid nuclear scanning relates to their ability to trap and collect radioactive substances such as radioactive iodine or other radioactive elements used in nuclear medicine. These isotopes are either swallowed or injected intravenously, and their extraction from the blood and concentration within the nodules causes the areas corresponding to the nodules to show up as black "hot" spots on the scan image. Hot nodules are rarely cancer and most often represent benign follicular adenomas. In addition, such hot nodules may in fact be overproducing thyroid hormone and may cause hyperthyroidism. The larger the "hot" nodule the more likely it will be associated with hyperthyroidism. These nodules may produce either T4 or T3 or a combination of both.

Approximately 10 to 15 percent of patients with thyroid nodules that can be detected by physical examination will have cancerous nodules. Most commonly, these cancerous nodules will be a specific type of thyroid cancer derived from the thyroid gland itself; hence they are referred to as primary thyroid tumors. Less frequently, a nodule may represent spread of cancer from elsewhere in the body (metastatic or "secondary" cancer). Secondary tumors or metastases to the thyroid are not unusual, largely because of the rich blood supply to the thyroid gland that will carry cancer cells to the gland from cancers of other tissues in remote locations. Metastases to the thyroid can occur with cancers of the head and neck region because of their close proximity to the thyroid, but metastasis may also occur in patients with cancer of the esophagus, larynx, lung or breast, or with malignant melanoma.

How common is thyroid cancer?

The incidence of thyroid cancer in the United States seems to be increasing from approximately 11,000 new cases per year in 1990 to as many as 23,500 cases per year in 2004, as estimated by the American Cancer Society. The number of patients with thyroid cancer dying in 2004 in the United States is estimated to be 1,460. Thus with a relatively small percentage of the total new cases having a fatal outcome, it should be apparent that most patients will indeed survive and may have either a full cure of their disease or an extended life expectancy. In this regard, there is a statement that some healthcare providers are prone to make that goes something like: "If there is one cancer that you may get in life, it should be a thyroid cancer because it will rarely kill you." It can be falsely reassuring, dangerous and foolhardy to either make this statement or believe it. This is so in spite of the generally excellent prognosis with thyroid cancer. Clearly there is a population of thyroid cancer patients, albeit small, that will have a poor outcome with thyroid cancer even with the most optimal therapy. Therefore, it may not be possible to predict what course the tumor may take in a given patient until several years have elapsed. Years of follow-up (rather than months) are necessary because thyroid cancers are typically very slow growing. Because of the slow growth, a small tumor or tumor recurrence may not be obvious and require years of close monitoring to ensure its earliest possible detection and potential eradication. It might be said to patients on breaking the news to them that they have thyroid cancer that there is "good news and there is bad news," and both are the same. The fact that most thyroid cancer is slow growing is the good news in that the cancer will rarely kill as a result. The bad news is *also that it is slow growing* and therefore it is usually impossible to reassure a patient in any definitive way that the tumor is all gone at the time of surgery or at the time of initial radioiodine ablation. Rather, it may take years of close monitoring and surveillance to be sure no tumor remains. The monitoring for well-differentiated thyroid cancer is accomplished with periodic scans and serial measurements of the tumor marker, thyroglobulin, before determining there is no residual tumor. For medullary and anaplastic thyroid cancer, the treatments and follow-up are different. Having said that, there is good reason to be optimistic in the overwhelming majority of cases as long as this optimism is based on facts related to the different prognosis associated with different types of thyroid cancer and the stage at which the thyroid cancer was first discovered.

How does your doctor determine whether there is cancer within a thyroid nodule?

An endocrinologist confronted with a patient with a thyroid nodule first goes through a process designed to determine the likelihood of cancer. This process involves procedures such as fine needle aspiration (see chapter 6) for examination of the cells under a microscope (cytology) as well as isotope scans and other imaging tests. The results of these tests help us determine who is a candidate for surgery, i.e., those whose thyroid nodules have features suggestive of cancer. Because thyroid nodules are so common, it would not be medically or economically sound to consider operating on all patients with nodules. Indeed, the side effects or adverse outcomes of such surgeries might likely outweigh any benefit of finding an occasional thyroid cancer.

As mentioned, the overwhelming majority of such thyroid nodules are benign. However, certain elements in a patient's history and physical examination may suggest a greater likelihood that the nodule is cancerous. But even when such suggestive historical and physical findings are present, the overwhelming majority of these nodules are still benign. In the case of the patient's medical history, greater weight is placed on the risk of cancer in those patients who have been exposed to external radiation to the head and neck. The radiation risk does not apply to diagnostic X-rays such as dental X-rays or other occasional diagnostic X-rays of the head, neck or chest, whether by ordinary X-ray or computerized tomography (CT). Rather, the kind of radiation that will induce thyroid tumors includes radiation therapy for acne or hemangiomas of the skin or for large tonsils and adenoids that may be associated with frequent sore throats or upper respiratory infections in childhood. In the past two decades, physicians have been aware of the risks of radiation on the thyroid, and this awareness has led to the use of flexible lead shields or "aprons" over the neck to protect the thyroid from the radiation. Shields were not commonly in use between 1950 and 1975.

As mentioned above, internal radiation from the radiation fallout related to the nuclear plant accident in Chernobyl in April 1986 may also lead to the development of malignant tumors. As was seen after the Chernobyl accident, the greatest risk of thyroid tumor after radiation occurs in children and young adults up to approximately age 18. We believe this is true because of the relatively faster growth rates of thyroid cells in children. Cells are most vulnerable to radiation injury when they are actively growing and multiplying. Thus, before age 18, the growth activity of the thyroid with more cells undergoing cell division (mitosis) places the thyroid in a more critical or vulnerable phase for radiation damage. In older adults, tumors after radiation are quite rare.

Does genetics or family history play a role in thyroid cancer?

Also important in the evaluation of the patient with a thyroid nodule is the patient's family history. A family history of benign nodules or multi-nodular goiter suggests that the patient's nodule is also benign. Patients from a family with a history of rare forms of papillary carcinoma must be screened more carefully. Another type of thyroid cancer that quite commonly occurs in families is *medullary carcinoma (cancer) of the thyroid*. Medullary carcinoma occurs as part of a syndrome called *multiple endocrine neoplasia* (MEN), and such patients may have medullary carcinomas of the thyroid as well as a tumor of the adrenal that causes hypertension. These tumors are called *pheochromocytoma*. Thus a family history of either medullary carcinoma or pheochromocytoma would be of significant importance in a patient presenting with a thyroid nodule. If this family history were present, special blood tests would provide additional evidence supporting the diagnosis of these particular tumors. In the case of medullary cancer, the test performed is a measurement of another hormone produced by other cells ("C"-cells) within the thyroid gland called *calcitonin* or *thyrocalcitonin*. Should a patient with such a family history have both a thyroid nodule and high blood pressure (hypertension), an endocrinologist would likely want to measure both calcitonin and the hormones or products of pheochromocytomas, such as *metanephrines* in urine or *catecholamines* in blood. Further information on medullary thyroid cancer is available in chapter 24 entitled *Medullary Thyroid Cancer*.

What are the symptoms of a thyroid nodule?

Most thyroid nodules do not cause symptoms and are discovered almost accidentally. For example, the thyroid gland (and a thyroid nodule within it) will move upwards and downwards in the neck during swallowing. Thus it is not unusual for

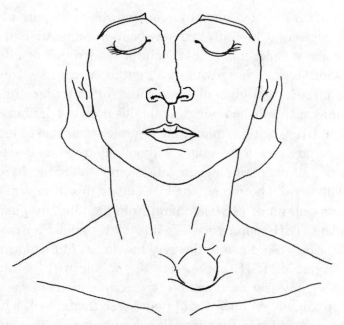

FIGURE 1: A nodule or bulge is seen in the lower aspect of the left neck region

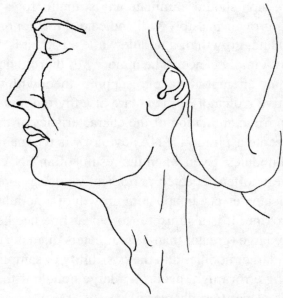

FIGURE 2: A nodule or bulge is seen from the side in the lower aspect of the left neck region

a spouse or family member to note fullness in the patient's neck due to the nodule at the dinner table while the patient is eating or drinking (see figures 1 and 2). Alternatively and very commonly, a primary care physician may detect a thyroid nodule during a routine physical examination of the neck.

Once a nodule is detected, the physician will likely inquire as to any associated symptoms. Signs or symptoms that may be more suggestive of cancer include rapid growth of the nodule, hoarseness, pain or tenderness, or difficulty or even painful swallowing. Extensive growth of a thyroid cancer may cause some interference with respiration and give a patient some difficulty breathing, particularly in certain positions such as when lying. Again this does not definitively imply cancer because some large, benign, multinodular goiters can cause similar degrees of obstruction due to pressure of the goiter without any invasion due to cancer.

Some but not all endocrinologists will attempt to shrink thyroid nodules by treating them with thyroid hormone. The idea behind this therapy is to suppress the thyroid stimulating hormone (TSH) coming from the pituitary gland because it is a growth stimulant. TSH suppression is achieved by giving a dosage of levothyroxine that will bring TSH down to the very low limits of the normal range. After achieving this degree of TSH suppression, the nodule will be followed by your physician by either physical examination or determinations of the nodule size on ultrasound. Approximately 40 percent of nodules so treated will have some reduction in size. The rest will stay the same size. Your endocrinologists may interpret any detectable growth in the nodule while on thyroxine as a sign of possible cancer since TSH suppression should eliminate any stimulus for a benign nodule to grow. In this setting, growth possibly will indicate the autonomous behavior of cancer. On the other hand, growth of a nodule while a patient is not taking thyroxine does not necessarily imply cancer. The majority of thyroid nodules will slowly grow with time when no attempt is made to suppress them with thyroxine therapy.

The most definitive indicator of the nature of a thyroid nodule is provided by fine needle aspiration for examination of the characteristics of the cells (cytologic examination). Fine needle aspiration (FNA) cytology is the mainstay of the initial evaluation of thyroid nodules. Even when the results of an FNA are interpreted as benign, the procedure is often repeated periodically during continued follow-up, such as when a physician detects an apparent growth of a nodule, particularly if it occurs while on thyroxine. It is also useful to repeat fine needle aspiration when nodules are extremely large (greater than 3 centimeters diameter) because we have greater concern about larger nodules and the possibility of sampling error. One can envision how sampling error might occur in a large nodule if the needle is inserted in just two or three places (see chapter 6).

In addition to the patient's medical history, there are some findings on physical examination of the neck that may be associated with possible cancer. The first relates to the nature of the nodule on palpation by the physician. The size of a nodule may vary from that comparable to a garden pea to one as large as a ping-pong ball. Most thyroid nodules will be firm in texture and feel to the physician like a small marble of the consistency of beefsteak. A cancerous thyroid nodule, on the other hand, will feel quite firm to very hard to the examining finger. This is so because such nodules may develop deposits of calcium within them (calcification). Typical of papillary carcinoma of the thyroid are microscopic calcium granules called *psammoma bodies*. Also, medullary carcinoma of the thyroid may have more dense calcium deposits due to calcification. Nevertheless, the presence of calcium in a nodule, while it may be suspicious, does not necessarily guarantee that the nodule is malignant. Benign nodules may outgrow their blood supply and through a process known as infarction (death of cells) may subsequently calcify. Again, the most important diagnostic procedure would be fine needle aspiration for cytology.

As the physician examines the thyroid nodule with his or her fingertips, the nodule should move freely up and down with swallowing. If it does not but rather remains attached to the surrounding tissue, the nodule may be cancerous since the fixation is due to local spread of the tumor cells into the surrounding tissues of the neck. Such fixation may cause discomfort during swallowing and hoarseness through involvement of the nerves to the vocal cords. The hoarseness does not mean that the tumor has invaded the vocal cords or larynx, just the nerves to the vocal cords. These nerves, called *recurrent laryngeal nerves*, pass under the thyroid gland on their way to innervate the vocal cords. Growth of a tumor toward the back of the neck (in the posterior direction) may impair the function of one of these laryngeal nerves and lead to poor function of the corresponding vocal cord that it innervates. As a result, one vocal cord will move sluggishly or not at all compared with the other cord, leading to failure of the two cords to meet and touch normally during speech. This is the cause of the hoarseness. Hoarseness with vocal cord paralysis, however, does not necessarily mean cancer because large, multi-nodular goiters also can cause this problem simply by putting external pressure on the laryngeal nerves.

What is the significance of lymph nodes?

Part of your physician's examination of the neck will be the careful assessment for enlarged lymph nodes outside the thyroid gland. The lymph nodes are collections of special white blood cells called lymphocytes, and the function of the lymph nodes is to filter tissue fluids called lymph. Lymph nodes are our first line of defense against foreign invasion by bacteria and other causes of infection. We have lymph nodes in all parts of the body, and they all drain specific tissues. The lymph fluid is "filtered" through the lymph nodes and then returned to the blood stream. A rich network of lymph nodes lying on both sides of the thyroid gland drains tissues in the head and neck. The most common cause of enlargement of these nodes would be infections of the scalp, face or throat. Other lymph nodes, for example, are located in relation to the elbow and the armpit and become enlarged with any sore or infection of the hand or arm. Lymph nodes are also a line of defense against cancer. This does not apply to all cancers, but many early cancers will invade the lymphatic system, and it is the presence of the tumor in the lymph nodes that will cause enlargement of these nodes and serve as a signal of disease to the physician. Cancer of the breast, for example, will typically spread to lymph nodes in the arm pit (axilla) if not caught early.

Since the lymph nodes in the neck (*cervical nodes*) drain the thyroid gland, these lymph nodes are the first place most types of cancer cells from the thyroid gland will show up. It is not unusual for cancer to be in the lymph nodes of the neck at the time of first diagnosis of thyroid cancer. This is often the case with papillary cancer and medullary thyroid cancer. A third type of thyroid cancer, follicular cancer, more typically invades capillaries and blood vessels and spreads by way of the blood rather than through the lymphatic system. Thus follicular thyroid cancer is more likely present as metastases to the lungs or bone rather than lymph nodes in the neck. However, because papillary thyroid cancer is the most common type of thyroid cancer, your endocrinologist will do a careful examination of the neck to determine if there is any enlargement of the lymph nodes (*lymphadenopathy*). When detected, such lymph nodes may also be candidates to undergo fine needle aspiration (FNA) for cytology to confirm whether they contain tumor.

Information about the presence of tumor in lymph nodes may help your endocrinologist decide the next step in managing your disease. Surgery may be required if FNA detects a significant number of enlarged lymph nodes or even a single lymph node positive for tumor. The FNA results, combined with imaging results by ultrasound or MRI, will alert the surgeon to the tumor in the lymph nodes, demonstrate the location of the lymph nodes and lead to a more extensive exploration of the neck and thyroidectomy to get rid of the involved lymph nodes. The neck is richly endowed with dozens and dozens of lymph nodes, and there is no longstanding harm done by removing those lymph nodes that are involved with tumor.

Many factors determine whether a 100 percent cure of thyroid cancer may be obtained, and these factors will be discussed at length throughout this book. In cases where the thyroid cancer has escaped from the thyroid and invaded lymph nodes, the thyroid cancer still potentially can be cured. Positive lymph nodes may alter the staging of the patient's cancer (see chapter 4) and imply a greater likelihood of recurrence of tumor after initial therapy. Therefore, the significance of the finding of enlarged lymph nodes is that they may represent a harbinger of cancer that demands the most thorough evaluation of both the thyroid gland and the lymph nodes such as by fine needle aspiration (FNA) for cytology.

What laboratory tests are done for thyroid nodule evaluation?

An endocrinologist may require a number of laboratory tests when evaluating a patient with a thyroid nodule, and several of these have been discussed in the prior chapter in specific clinical contexts. Common tests may include measurements in blood of thyroid hormone and of TSH to determine whether the nodule is not only functioning but *hyperfunctioning*. Hyperfunctioning nodules may produce an excessive amount of thyroid hormone leading to elevated serum levels of T4 and T3 and to a suppressed or low level of TSH. Such hyperfunctioning nodules are called "*hot*" and are almost always benign. Some studies indicate that hot nodules in children may harbor a cancer, but this would be extremely rare in an adult.

A thyroid scan using an isotope will demonstrate whether a nodule is hot or hyperfunctioning in that the nodule itself concentrates most of the administered isotope and shows up as an intense black spot on the scan (see figure 3). If the nodule is hyperfunctioning to where it completely suppresses TSH, the thyroid tissue outside the nodule will not pick up the isotope and will not be visualized. Fine needle aspiration for cytology, generally the most informative test or procedure in the evaluation of a thyroid nodule, may not be as effective for a "hot" or hyperfunctioning nodule. Nodules are extremely cellular, and the cytologic appearance under the microscope may not differ from a follicular cancer (carcinoma). Hence when the cytology has this appearance (sheets of follicular cells), the typical next step in the evaluation would be to perform a thyroid scan.

As mentioned above, the protein *thyroglobulin* is used routinely as a marker for well-differentiated thyroid cancer. As a diagnostic test, it is best used after total thyroidectomy and radioiodine ablation of any thyroid tissue because its presence

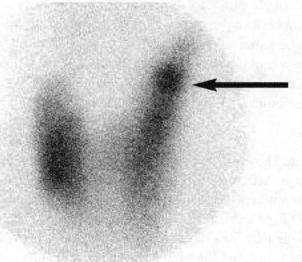

FIGURE 3: Hot or hyperfunctioning nodule (arrow).

would imply residual thyroid cancer. Thyroglobulin has very little utility in evaluating a thyroid nodule preoperatively.

Serum thyroglobulin may be elevated for many other reasons, including hyperfunction of the thyroid gland, Graves' disease (toxic diffuse goiter), thyroiditis (in that there is an inflammation of the thyroid that discharges thyroglobulin), multi-nodular toxic goiter and single hot nodules.

Thus prior to surgery with the thyroid gland in place and so many possible causes for a high serum thyroglobulin, it is unreliable to presume that an elevated thyroglobulin level means that a nodule is cancerous. Nevertheless, retrospective analysis of serum thyroglobulin in thyroid cancer patients before surgery may indicate slightly elevated serum levels of this protein. This finding implies that the tumor makes thyroglobulin and validates the subsequent utility of the thyroglobulin test as a tumor marker in such patients. Retrospective analysis of patients who had low or normal levels of serum thyroglobulin preoperatively may provide the opposite insight. That is, that the tumor may have lost its ability to produce thyroglobulin and therefore measurement of the protein is of little use subsequently as a tumor marker.

There is little utility to the measurement of *antithyroid antibodies* in the evaluation of patients with thyroid nodules. Laboratory tests may include measurements of antibodies called anti-thyroglobulin antibody or anti-thyroperoxidase (anti-TPO or anti-microsomal) antibodies. High levels in blood of one or both antibodies implies that the patient may have (in addition to the presenting thyroid nodule) coincident underlying autoimmune thyroid disease, most likely Hashimoto's thyroiditis. It is controversial whether thyroid cancer occurs with a greater frequency in the thyroid glands of patients with Hashimoto's thyroiditis. Coincidence of papillary thyroid cancer in a Hashimoto's thyroid gland is not unusual. One study indicated that a history of Hashimoto's disease in the background of a surgical specimen with thyroid cancer is a good indicator for ultimate cure of the thyroid cancer. As mentioned above, anti-thyroglobulin antibodies interfere with the laboratory assay of serum thyroglobulin. Hence, perhaps the only usefulness of the measurement of anti-thyroglobulin antibodies is to determine whether there will be difficulty monitoring thyroglobulin should the patient's thyroid nodule turn out to be cancer.

As explained in chapter 1, the thyroid produces only two thyroid hormones, thyroxine and triiodothyronine. The thyroid gland does produce one other hormone—although not by the thyroid follicular cells. Rather, so-called "C cells" scattered throughout the thyroid gland produce the hormone *calcitonin* or *thyrocalcitonin*. A malignant tumor composed of, or derived from, these C cells is called *medullary carcinoma* (see chapter 24). Medullary carcinoma or cancer may present as a single nodule although it commonly presents as several nodules that have spread to adjacent lymph nodes by the time of diagnosis. In such patients, calcitonin levels are elevated. Blood calcitonin measurements may be used as a marker for residual medullary carcinoma just as thyroglobulin is used as a tumor marker for papillary or follicular carcinoma of the thyroid. In a direct analogy to the use of thyroglobulin as a tumor marker, calcitonin is most useful after thyroidectomy and removal of the medullary cancer.

It is controversial whether endocrinologists should measure calcitonin when patients first present with a thyroid nodule. Most clinicians believe that it would not be cost effective to do so because medullary carcinoma is relatively rare and thyroid nodules are extremely common. On the other hand, medullary carcinoma of the thyroid can on occasion be an aggressive tumor and, like most cancers, offers the best prognosis when detected early and treated appropriately. Another protein that can be measured in the blood and that is useful as a tumor marker for medullary carcinoma of the thyroid is *carcinoembryonic antigen* or *CEA*.

What does the thyroid scan tell us about thyroid nodules?

A detailed description of the applications and utility of nuclear medicine scans in the diagnosis and management of patients with thyroid cancer is discussed in chapter 13. A short description of the principles underlying scanning may be helpful in this regard. In brief, the thyroid normally traps or collects iodine from the blood passing through it. This iodine is then protein bound and incorporated into the synthesis of the thyroid hormones, T4 and T3. The stable form of iodine is iodine-127 (^{127}I). Alterations in the atomic structure of iodine result in the formation of a variety of isotopes of iodine that are radioactive. These isotopes include iodine-123 (^{123}I), iodine-124 (^{124}I), iodine-125 (^{125}I), and iodine-131 (^{131}I). The physical characteristics of ^{131}I make it an ideal isotope for imaging the thyroid. The test is performed by the administration of a small "tracer" dose of ^{131}I followed by a scan 24 hours later. For the scan, the patient lies on a table while a special nuclear detector (gamma or scintillation camera) detects and collects the radiation emitted from the nodule or thyroid gland. The results are printed out on X-ray film or reviewed on a computer terminal.

Normal thyroid tissue will both trap the iodide and bind it to protein within the thyroid gland. A normal thyroid on thyroid scan is shown in figure 4. A normally functioning thyroid nodule will collect the iodine and show up as "warm" on the scan. Hot or hyperfunctioning nodules are described above (see figure 3). In the context of finding thyroid cancer, we are most concerned about "cold" or non-functioning nodules (see figure 5) since thyroid cancer is generally less functional than normal thyroid tissue and will show up as "cold" relative to the normal thyroid tissue outside of the cancerous nodule. In addition to cancer, a number of benign

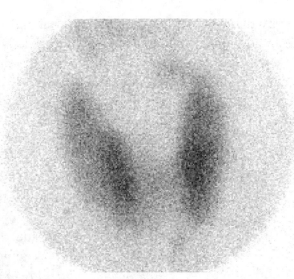

FIGURE 4: Normal thyroid gland on thyroid scan.

thyroid adenomas may also appear "cold" due to reduced trapping of the radioactive tracer material employed for the scan.

The thyroid scan is done in nuclear medicine or radiology departments of hospitals or radiology facilities, and the nuclear medicine physicians or nuclear radiologists interpret the images.

Two principal radioisotopes that are becoming more popular than ^{131}I are ^{123}I and [99m]technetium pertechnetate. [99m]technetium pertechnetate provides a lower radiation dose to the patient, is cheaper than ^{131}I and allows scanning to be done within an hour after the administered dose. [131]I requires a 24-hour delay and ^{123}I requires anywhere from four to 24 hours between the time of the administered isotope and performance of the scan. The scan will indicate how well a nodule is functioning and may also disclose other information to your physician. For example, although only one nodule may have been detected on physical examination, the scan may show multiple nodules.

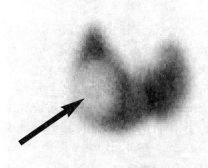

FIGURE 5: Thyroid gland with a "cold" (hypofunctioning) area in the right lobe (arrow).

Over the years, nuclear medicine physicians and nuclear radiologists have tried to improve on the sensitivity and specificity of different scanning agents to distinguish benign from cancerous thyroid nodules. For these purposes, isotopes such as [201]*thallium*, [75]*selenomethionine* and [67]*gallium* have been investigated. None has proved to be a reliable indicator for cancer (see chapter 16). In the case of medullary carcinoma of the thyroid, however, a radiolabeled material known as [131]I-*meta-iodobenzylguanidine (MIBG)* has been successfully used to locate tumor.

What does fine needle aspiration for cytology tell my doctor?

The fine needle aspiration (FNA) technique is described at length in chapter 6 entitled "Fine Needle Aspiration." Successful results with FNA cytology depend on two important factors. The first is the ability to obtain a good aspirate, which is a sample of cells to be examined under the microscope. The second is the skill and expertise of the cytopathologist interpreting the slides. When both of these criteria are met, the chance of missing or misdiagnosing a thyroid cancer (false negative) should be 1 percent or less (a missed diagnosis in one of 100 aspirates). Similarly, a mistaken impression that the cells may represent a thyroid cancer when they really do *not* (false positive) should occur less than 2 percent of the time. Based on the findings seen under the microscope, the thyroid cells are typically described by the cytopathologist as either clearly benign, suspicious for cancer, definitely cancer or inadequate for diagnosis. When the material is inadequate for diagnosis, the aspiration must be repeated.

Patients often ask whether needling these nodules may result in a spread of cancer should the nodule turn out to be malignant. This phenomenon, called "seeding" of the tumor along the needle track, has happened in cases involving other cancers and organs but not with thyroid cancer after FNA, possibly because such a fine caliber of needle is used. There is no other significant risk from having an FNA, although some patients may experience some bleeding, discomfort in the area for several days, and perhaps a bruise. In good hands, the FNA for cytology has been shown to significantly reduce the required frequency of surgical thyroidectomy by demonstrating that nodules are benign that might otherwise have been operated on. Finding malignant cells on FNA also confirms the necessity for thyroidectomy and will discourage temporizing or delaying the definitive therapy.

What is thyroid ultrasound or "echo"?

This technique is described at greater detail in Chapter 16, *Additional Diagnostic Imaging Studies*. In brief, *ultrasonography* involves the detection of sound waves passed through tissue or reflected back depending on the structure of the tissue. Ultrasonography is sometimes called *echography*, and the slang term for an ultrasound image is termed an "*echo*." When a tissue is solid, it creates echoes as the sound bounces off the solid or the cellular component. In the case of a thyroid nodule, echoes will be produced if the nodule is a solid cellular mass, benign or malignant. If the nodule is a fluid filled structure (*cyst*), it will have no echoes ("*anechoic*"). Echo-free true cysts are almost never malignant. Hence, the echo tells your endocrinologist whether a nodule is solid or cystic. When a cystic nodule undergoes FNA, a slightly larger bore needle may be used so that the fluid is drained off. The cytopathologist can confirm the benign nature of the cyst by examining the cells present within the cystic fluid.

Compared with physical examinations, ultrasound examinations of the thyroid are more specific and exact. A thyroid ultrasound, like a thyroid scan, often will detect multi-nodularity even though a physician may have found just a single nodule. Ultrasound may also detect the presence of tumor that has spread beyond the thyroid into lymph nodes. When we try to determine whether a thyroid nodule may be growing or shrinking during therapy, the most specific sizing of the nodule is done by ultrasound. For this technique, an ultrasound may be repeated six to 12 months after the initial evaluation, with the size of the nodule compared on the two studies. Ultrasound may be employed to guide fine needle aspiration. This is extremely useful when nodules are relatively small (less than 0.5 centimeters) or difficult to feel or locate during a physical exam. Nodules located toward the back of the thyroid gland, or "buried" within a large goiter, are particularly difficult to discover. During the followup of nodules proven to be benign on FNA cytology, ultrasound may be performed at three and six months and, if the size of the nodule does not change, repeated again in 12 to 18 months. As mentioned above, 40 percent of benign nodules may shrink on TSH suppression by thyroxine therapy. When this occurs, the intervals of follow up by ultrasound may be prolonged. Should the nodule fail to shrink with thyroxine therapy, a repeat FNA should be performed. When this is done, the original diagnosis tends to be confirmed in better than 95 percent of such nodules.

I have a history of radiation to the neck and was told that my thyroid had more than one nodule. What does that mean?

The thyroid glands in patients who have a history of exposure to radiation of the head and neck, and therefore a higher risk of thyroid cancer, tend to be multinodular. FNA in these cases may provide misleading results since there may be a mix of both benign and cancerous nodules. If only the benign nodules are needled, the results may give a patient false assurance that there is no cancer present. As a result, many endocrinologists will recommend thyroidectomy for the patient with a multi-nodular goiter who has a history of radiation to the head and neck. In general, whether the surgery should be a subtotal thyroidectomy or lobectomy (only one lobe with nodule removed) rather than a total thyroidectomy is discussed in chapter 7. Whether a single nodule or a multinodular gland is present, when the FNA definitively indicates cancer, we recommend total thyroidectomy. When the likelihood of cancer is significantly less but the indications for thyroidectomy remain, a subtotal thyroidectomy removing the lobe with the nodular tissue is an acceptable procedure. If the pathologic examination of the surgically removed lobe indicates thyroid cancer, then a second procedure (*completion thyroidectomy*) must be performed. A total or near total thyroidectomy is almost always recommended for patients with a history of irradiation to the thyroid because of the high incidence of disease on both sides of the thyroid gland. In such cases, the surgeon would look carefully for the presence of any lymph nodes that might be suspicious for involvement by tumor. This examination of the lymph nodes also would be performed in patients having a completion thyroidectomy after a first incomplete or subtotal surgery discloses thyroid surgery. Any large or suspicious looking nodes would be removed and examined by the pathologist for the presence of tumor. Once a thyroidectomy is done and malignancy confirmed, your physicians may periodically monitor and evaluate you for possible recurrence of tumor using high-sensitivity, high-resolution ultrasound or magnetic resonance imaging (MRI), in addition to physical examination and monitoring of serum thyroglobulin.

CHAPTER 4

Well-Differentiated Thyroid Cancer: Staging and Prognosis

Leonard Wartofsky, M.D.

What is meant by the "stage" of a tumor?

The "stage" of a disease, or in this case of cancer, refers to a phase in the course of the tumor when it has reached some defined level of extent. The extent of the tumor is a measure of its size and whether it has spread elsewhere. As thyroid cancers grow, they are first confined to the thyroid gland, may then extend in variable degrees to the region of the neck outside of the thyroid gland (for example, to the lymph nodes), and finally some types of thyroid cancer will spread to distant sites of the body. The process of "staging" was developed in order for physicians to more accurately describe the extent of disease in a given patient in objective and standardized terms. This then permits your physician to communicate accurately with other physicians about the degree of disease present and also to better select therapeutic approaches based on published literature on results of treatment in comparably staged patients.

Does stage affect prognosis?

Consulting the literature allows your physician to better predict the potential outcome of how you may fare with your tumor based on the results seen in hundreds or thousands of other patients at the same stage of disease (see figure 1). This prediction of outcome relates to "prognosis," which is a forecast of what is expected to come (based on the nature of disease present) and is usually given in terms related to life expectancy, or the likelihood of either full cure, remission, possible residual but non-life-threatening persistent disease, or, in the worst case scenario, of death. Tumors classified as Stage I or II are typically considered to be "low risk" tumors with excellent to good prognosis, whereas Stage III or IV tumors are often described as of "high risk," implying a higher risk of residual disease after initial treatment, or of recurrence. Fortunately, the overwhelming majority of patients will fall into Stages I and II and have an excellent prognoses with little risk for recurrence or death from their disease. In one large Mayo Clinic review of more than 1,400 patients, there was a remarkable 25-year survival of 97 percent in patients who had

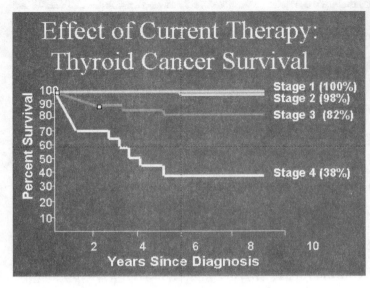

FIGURE 1: Effect of current therapy on thyroid cancer survival for papillary thyroid carcinoma. Cancer 1998; 83:1012-21. Copyright 1998 American Cancer Society. Reprinted by permission Wiley-Liss, a subsidiary of John Wiley & Sons, Inc., and the author, Steven I. Sherman, M.D.

complete surgical resection of their apparent disease. Thirty-year survival rates of 75-85 percent are not unusual for such patients, with low death rates. Stage II and III patients may have recurrences requiring additional therapy but may still have a relatively low risk for death. A worse prognosis is associated with extensive local invasion and even more so with distant metastases, especially those to bone.

How is staging done?

A number of clinical and pathologic characteristics have been evaluated as predictors of tumor behavior and ultimate patient prognosis. Some of the factors that may determine staging include the age of the patient, the original size of the cancer found at surgery, whether there was invasion into surrounding tissue, whether lymph nodes were involved with tumor and whether the nodes were on one or both sides of the neck, and if disease was found at sites distant from the thyroid gland, such as in the lungs or bones. Many types of staging systems have been developed over the past several decades, and different staging systems may be favored by various endocrinologists or more popular at certain specific medical centers. Moreover, some differences relate as well to staging systems used by clinical doctors versus those used by pathologists. One of the most popular staging systems is called the "TNM" system with the three letters referring to tumor size (T), involvement of lymph nodes (N), and the presence of distant metastases (M). When your doctor estimates, or "calculates," the stage of disease, he or she assigns a series of numerical scores to each of these characteristics reflecting the extent of disease present, ranging from 0 to 4, with 4 being the more severe or extensive degree of involvement (see Table 1). Thus a typical papillary cancer in a young patient might be described as Stage I (T1, N1, M0), meaning the tumor was less than two centimeters in size and that there was lymph node involvement but no distant metastases. Several of the grading or staging systems will include subcategories designated "A" or "B" so as to describe in abbreviated form, for example, whether the involved lymph nodes were on the side of the neck of the original cancer or on the opposite side of the neck (because this information may impact on prognosis).

Are all types of thyroid cancer staged similarly?

Because papillary thyroid cancer accounts for 65 to 80 percent of thyroid cancers, most of the discussion in this section will relate to this particular cancer and to follicular thyroid cancer, which accounts for almost another 15 percent of these tumors. Please see the chapters on medullary cancer (chapter 24) and anaplastic cancer (chapter 25) for more specific information about the prognosis of these particular tumors. Because anaplastic cancer always has a poor prognosis, it is automatically staged as Stage IV regardless of size of tumor, patient age or the presence of distant metastases. The current practice in staging anaplastic tumors is to break the category down into only Stage IV A (surgically removable), IV B (not surgically removable), or IV C (with distant metastases). Even when confining comments to the behavior of papillary cancer, the outcome may vary widely because some of these tumors may be very small (<1.0 cm), or so-called "microcarcinomas," and have an excellent outcome. In fact, these little tumors may be incidentally found in thyroid glands removed surgically for other reasons and as such show little evidence of invasion. On the other hand, other papillary thyroid cancers may grow rapidly, invade tissues aggressively, metastasize widely and ultimately cause death.

Does staging provide an accurate prediction of outcome?

Often it is the case that your physician may need to observe the course of your disease and the tumor's behavior over many months to many years before he or she may be able to give you a semblance of an accurate prognostication or prediction of the future. Therefore, because staging usually is done early in the course of the disease, i.e., shortly after thyroidectomy or the first administration of radioiodine, it may not accurately predict the outcome in a single given patient. This is so because the data on prognosis or outcome in published series of large numbers of patients reflect average data, and there can be outliers at either end, meaning some patients who do better than predicted and some who do worse. Those who have a worse outcome do so because their tumors turn out to be more aggressive with time than the averages anticipated for a given stage of tumor. Happily, the overwhelming majority of those tumors under 2.0 cm in diameter tend to behave in a more biologically benign manner, can be completely cured with definitive therapy, and thus have an excellent prognosis. As in all aspects of medicine, there are many things that we do not understand about the behavior of thyroid tumors, and new research continues to shed light on other characteristics that may affect prognosis. For example, as many as 20 to 30 percent of patients with thyroid cancer will have another underlying condition in their thyroid glands, a type of "autoimmune" (self-destructive) thyroiditis (inflammation) known as Hashimoto's disease. A recent study has indicated that such patients, those with thyroid cancer and underlying Hashimoto's disease, enjoy better success with therapy and hence a better prognosis than patients without Hashimoto's disease.

How does the initial clinical presentation affect staging?

As can be seen in Table 1, the size of the tumor found at surgery influences the "T" scores in the TNM system, but this is so only for patients over the age of 45. Because virtually all patients under age 45 fall into the category of "low risk" (Stages I or II), there are no young patients classified as having Stage III or Stage IV disease. In the majority of patients with thyroid cancer (about 70 percent), the tumor is confined to one lobe or one side of the thyroid gland, and in about 20 percent of patients the tumor is found in both lobes ("bilateral" disease). More rarely, some patients will have multiple tumors in several places throughout the thyroid gland ("multi-focal" disease), sometimes as many as 10 to 15 different little tumors. Some studies have suggested that multi-focal tumors may have a worse prognosis. This presentation may be related to "seeding" of the tumor throughout the gland, but sometimes such multiple tumors are the result of an environmental factor that causes cancer and affected the entire thyroid gland. An example of this would be seen in patients exposed to external or internal radiation such as the children in Belarus of the Soviet Union after the nuclear plant accident in April 1986 in Chernobyl.

Involvement of lymph nodes (the "N" in the TNM system) also affects staging. About 35 to 40 percent of patients presenting with thyroid cancer will already have some cancer in lymph nodes in the neck or upper mid chest ("mediastinum"). When a papillary cancer is more aggressive as evident by widespread involvement throughout the thyroid gland, the likelihood of lymph node metastases approaches 75 percent. In addition to staging of lymph node involvement based on the surgical findings, the extent of lymph node involvement can be determined by ultrasound or MRI examinations of the neck, or by CT scans of the chest and mediastinum. CT or MRI may be useful to determine if there are distant metastases as well, a finding that determines the "M" of the TNM Staging. Follicular thyroid cancer is the type that is most likely to spread to distant sites in lung or bone, and scans with radioactive iodine are generally more useful to detect metastases in bone than the radiopharmaceutical typically used for bone scans (such as [99m]technetium hydroxy methylene diphosphonate). However, combined scanning such as with the [99m]technetium-99m hydroxy methylene diphosphonate and [201]thallium may be useful to detect bone metastases. MRI is the most useful to image bone lesions, especially those of the lower spine and pelvis.

How does the initial clinical presentation affect prognosis?

The impact of some of the initial tumor characteristics on prognosis can be appreciated by considering the outcomes in a large series of patients with papillary thyroid cancer seen at the Mayo Clinic over a 40-year period. In reporting deaths by 20 years after diagnosis that were due to the cancer itself (so-called cancer-specific mortality), they observed that the rates of patients dying from their cancer increased with an increasing size of the tumor. There was a 20-year mortality of 0.8 percent for patients with tumors less than 2.0 cm in diameter, 6 percent for tumors 2.0 to 3.9 cm, 16 percent for tumors 4.0 to 6.9 cm, and 50 percent for tumors greater than 7 cm. When the tumor was confined to the thyroid, the death rate was 1.9 percent, whereas those patients whose tumor extended through the thyroid capsule into the surrounding tissues of the neck had a 20-year mortality of 28 percent. Outcomes were not as good in those patients with distant metastases at presentation. They experienced a 10-year mortality rate of 69 percent compared with 3 percent in patients with tumors confined to the neck.

Physicians at the Mayo Clinic and those at other centers have identified three varieties of initial clinical presentation, which can reflect a different prognostic category in regard to tumor recurrence. The three factors were (1) the presence of postoperative local metastatic lymph nodes, (2) local recurrence in the thyroid bed or adjacent tissue other than lymph nodes or (3) postoperative distant metastases. Rather than using the traditional TNM system of staging (see below), the Mayo group incorporates these factors into a different scoring system that is called MACIS. They feel that this scoring system can more reliably predict outcome based on data at initial presentation than the TNM system, which is limited to fewer characteristics.

What is the TNM Staging System?

The TNM (tumor-nodes-metastases) system of staging has been shown to be a useful method of staging in regard to correlation with observed outcomes based upon retrospective follow-up studies of the rates of cure, tumor recurrence and death in hundreds if not thousands of patients over many decades. The age of the patient is a very important prognostic factor influencing staging, and the designated age refers to the patient's age at the time of actual cancer diagnosis. More

		TABLE 1	
Tumor Size:	TX	Primary tumor cannot be assessed	
	T0	No evidence of primary tumor	
	T1	Tumor 2 cm or less in greatest dimension limited to thyroid	
	T2	Tumor larger than 2 cm but less than 4 cm in greatest dimension and limited to the thyroid	
	T3	Tumor larger than 4 cm in greatest dimension or tumor of any size extending to tissue around the thyroid	
	T4a	Tumor of any size extending beyond the thyroid capsule and invading local soft tissues	
	T4b	Tumor invading tissue on spine or wrapping around the carotid artery in the neck	
Nodes:	NX	Regional nodes cannot be assessed	
	N0	No metastases to regional nodes	
	N1	Metastases to regional nodes are present	
	N1A	Metastases to nodes around or in front of the windpipe and voice box (larynx)	
	N1B	Metastases to opposite side or both sides of neck or to upper chest (mediastinal) nodes	
Metastases:	MX	Presence of distant metastases cannot be assessed	
	M0	No distant metastases	
	M1	Distant metastases are present	

aggressive tumor behavior is likely after age 40 to 45, and the "cut-point" for staging has been set at age 45 (see below). In one large retrospective review of more than 15,000 cases of thyroid cancer, age was a stronger predictor of survival for patients with follicular carcinoma than for papillary carcinoma.

The TNM system is based on the following subgroups. Tumor size refers to the original single malignant nodule or the largest nodule in a gland with multifocal lesions. While not as important as age, the size of the original tumor is also important, with tumors less than 1.5 cm having the best prognosis and those which are larger than 4 cms having the worst prognosis. Regional lymph nodes are defined as bilateral neck (cervical) and upper mid chest (mediastinal) nodes.

What is the impact of age on TNM Staging?

Clinical Staging of Papillary Thyroid Cancer

The staging for papillary thyroid cancer is designated as Stage I, II, III or IV based on the TNM status and the age of the patient as follows:

	Age less than 45 years	Age of 45 years or older
Stage I	Any T, any N, M0	T1, N0, M0
Stage II	Any T, any N, M1	T2, N0, M0
Stage III	Not applicable	T3, N0, M0 or any T, N1, M0
Stage IV	Not applicable	Any T, any N, M1

The importance of age as a prognostic factor can be appreciated by noting that all patients less than 45 years old without distant metastases are classified as Stage I, and that there is no category of Stage III or IV for young persons who are not classified any higher than Stage II even with distant metastasis. The impact of age on prognosis can be seen by considering the outcomes in a large series of patients with papillary thyroid cancer seen at the Mayo Clinic over a 40-year period. In reporting deaths by 20 years after diagnosis that were due to the cancer itself (so-called cancer-specific mortality), they observed a death rate of 0.8 percent for patients less than 50 years of age, 7 percent for patients 50 to 59 years of age, 20 percent for patients 60 to 69 years of age, and 47 percent for patients aged 70 or more.

Clinical Staging of Medullary Thyroid Cancer

Stage I   C-cell Hyperplasia.

Stage II   Tumor less than 1 cm and negative lymph nodes.

Stage III   Tumors 1 cm or more or tumor of any size with positive nodes.

Stage IV   Tumors of any size with metastases outside the neck or with extra-thyroidal extension.

Examples of TNM Staging

PATIENT #1:	23 year old woman
SIZE OF TUMOR	1.0 cm papillary cancer
LYMPH NODES	3 of 5 biopsied nodes in side of neck positive for cancer
DISTANT METASTASES	No
WHAT IS THE TNM CLASSIFICATION?	T1, N1b, M0
WHAT IS THE STAGE?	Stage I
WHAT IS THE PROGNOSIS?	Excellent

While the presence of positive lymph nodes may imply potential for recurrence requiring additional radioiodine therapy, the possibility of a full cure is better than 95 percent.

PATIENT #2:	59 year old man
SIZE OF TUMOR	2.5 cm. papillary cancer
LYMPH NODES	3 of 5 biopsied nodes in side of neck positive for cancer
DISTANT METASTASES	Chest X-ray: 4-5 small densities suggestive of tumor, all of which are positive on post treatment radioiodine scan
WHAT IS THE TNM CLASSIFICATION?	T2, N1b, M1
WHAT IS THE STAGE?	Stage IV C
WHAT IS THE PROGNOSIS?	Poor

It is remarkable that the stage "jumps" from I to IV between Patient #1 and Patient #2 despite both having the same degree of lymph node involvement and Patient #2 having only a slightly larger tumor. This case illustrates the potentially profound effect of patient age and the presence of distant metastases in the lung on outcome.

PATIENT #3:	44 year old man
SIZE OF TUMOR	2.8 cm anaplastic cancer invading trachea and not readily resectable
LYMPH NODES	Extrathyroidal extension to cluster of lymph nodes on same side as tumor
DISTANT METASTASES	None detected
WHAT IS THE TNM CLASSIFICATION?	T4b, N1b, M0
WHAT IS THE STAGE?	Stage IV B
WHAT IS THE PROGNOSIS?	Very poor

Even though this patient is under age 45, any anaplastic cancer is considered to be Stage IV irrespective of patient age. The surgical non-resectability renders it a T4b. Although there are no apparent distant metastases, they may appear later in patients with this aggressive tumor, and the prognosis is poor in spite of the patient's age and the relatively small size of the tumor.

What is the impact of treatment on prognosis?

In regard to the initial management of a tumor by surgery, virtually all physicians who manage patients with thyroid cancer agree that a total or near total thyroidectomy is the procedure of choice, and that patients having a lesser procedure have a greater likelihood of tumor recurrence and a worse prognosis. For papillary and follicular thyroid cancer, the next step in management after surgery is often radioiodine ablation; however, the effect of ablation on prognosis or whether ablation is necessary in all patients is somewhat controversial. Early published series of patients indicated that ^{131}I ablation of thyroid remnants was followed by a significantly lower recurrence rate, but the conviction that such management is absolutely necessary in all patients and actually improves prognosis has been disputed by some experts. One of the early published series from the Mayo Clinic published a retrospective review of 1,500 papillary thyroid cancer patients in whom no difference in recurrence or cause-specific mortality was found among 946 patients treated with surgery alone and 220 patients treated with surgery plus radioiodine ablation. A equally well-controlled study from another medical center found that despite its patients having more advanced disease, those patients receiving post-operative radioiodine ablation for tumors greater than 1.5 cm and no distant metastases (Stages 2 and 3) had significantly lower rates of tumor recurrence (16 percent versus 38 percent) and cause-specific mortality (3 percent versus 9 percent) than patients not receiving radioiodine ablation. We believe that some of this controversy over the benefit of ablative therapy is due to differences in study design and the limitations of retrospective data and bias introduced by patient selection. This controversy notwithstanding, ablative therapy with radioiodine tends to be the standard of care in most centers, particularly in view of the fact that several analyses of large numbers of patients suggest that patients not treated with radioiodine ablation had a doubled risk of recurrence of their malignancy, although no difference in death rates. As discussed in chapters 24 and 25, radioiodine ablation is not indicated in medullary or anaplastic thyroid cancer.

Is the prognosis the same for all types of papillary thyroid cancer?

Most patients with thyroid cancer have a common variety of papillary thyroid cancer that is readily amenable to treatment, given a diagnosis at an early point in time, with tumor characteristics reflecting a low risk tumor, i.e., of Stage I or Stage II. However, there are some subtypes of papillary thyroid cancer that behave somewhat more aggressively and hence tend to have a poorer prognosis than the common form of papillary tumor. These subtypes are known by the pathologic terms used to describe the microscopic appearance of the cells and include tumors designated as the tall cell variant, the columnar variant and insular variant of papillary thyroid cancer. Not infrequently, pathologists will see many so-called follicular elements interspersed within the usual papillary cancer, and these tumors are designated as follicular variants of papillary thyroid cancer. However, in their biological and clinical course, these tumors tend to behave just like papillary cancers rather than like follicular thyroid cancers.

How does prognosis of follicular thyroid cancer differ from that of papillary thyroid cancer?

Staging for follicular thyroid cancer is done exactly the same as is done for papillary thyroid cancer. Stage I follicular tumors, like papillary tumors, tend to have an excellent prognosis. The key underlying difference between these two types of cancer is that the follicular cancers tend to be more invasive, invading blood vessels in the thyroid gland, entering the blood, and then being carried to distant parts of the body. Hence, follicular tumors are more likely to present with distant metastases, particularly in lungs and bones. Several studies have attempted to determine which features or characteristics of a follicular tumor might be associated with a poorer prognosis. It appears that these more "negative" features are similar to those for papillary tumors and include age greater than 45 years, tumor size greater than 4 cms, invasion of tumor into blood vessels or the capsule of the thyroid, extension of the cancer beyond the thyroid gland, and metastases to distant sites such as bones and the lungs. A retrospective analysis of 100 patients with follicular thyroid cancer from the Mayo Clinic over a 35-year period revealed that the overall cancer-related mortality was 29 percent at 20 years. A "multiplier" effect was seen with patients having several negative prognostic features doing more poorly than those with only one negative indicator. For example, patients with only one negative prognostic indicator had a 20-year mortality of 14 percent in contrast to a 92 percent likelihood of dying from thyroid cancer by 20 years with two or more negative risk predictors present.

Does staging and prognosis differ for well-differentiated (papillary and follicular) thyroid cancer in children compared with those for adults?

Well-differentiated thyroid cancer in children and adolescents is generally managed no differently than that in adults, with the same approaches including: near total thyroidectomy, radioiodine ablation, radioiodine therapy for recurrence and long-term monitoring with serum thyroglobulin measurements. Staging is done in a similar manner. For medullary and anaplastic cancer see chapters 5, 24 and 25. Because of the importance of age as a prognostic factor and the obvious fact that these patients are by definition young, the prognosis tends to be excellent in children even in the face of extensive local spread of disease. Indeed, in contrast to adults, the majority of children with thyroid cancer will already have local spread in the neck to lymph nodes at the time of initial diagnosis. Moreover, as many as 10–20 percent of children and adolescents will have distant metastases, such as tumor in the lung at diagnosis, compared with only 5 percent in adults. In spite of this apparently more aggressive appearance of these tumors in children, the prognosis for cure remains excellent with therapy, with less than 10 percent of children dying of their disease, a prognosis that is significantly better than mortality rates seen in adults. The excellent results with therapy have made some physicians question whether aggressive approaches to therapy with large-dose radioiodine are necessary in children as it may be in adults, given the long-term side effects that may ensue for these children. No definitive study answers this question as yet, but some physicians treating children with thyroid cancer will reserve aggressive radioiodine therapy only for those with disease spread to outside of the thyroid gland. Thus, as with adults, a reasonable approach often is to individualize therapy rather than adopt an arbitrary standard approach, and long-term follow-up and monitoring are essential given the slow-growing nature of thyroid cancer. Future research may help clarify which therapeutic approaches are both the safest and the most effective in both adults and children.

CHAPTER 5

Thyroid Cancer in the Child and Adolescent

Andrew J. Bauer, M.D., Maj, MC, USA

Gary L. Francis, M.D., Ph.D., Col, MC, USA

The opinions or assertions contained herein are the private views of the authors and are not to be construed as official or to reflect the opinions of the Uniformed Services University of the Health Sciences, the Department of the Army or the Department of Defense.

For the majority of our patients and families, the idea that your son or daughter would develop a thyroid nodule or thyroid cancer is something you probably never thought about. As you start down the road to diagnosis and treatment, questions and concerns will be a natural part of this journey. As is true with all new situations, the unknown can provide the greatest anxiety, and our goal is to keep this to a minimum with the understanding that it may not be possible to entirely eliminate it. There will likely be a list of new words that you haven't heard before. Keeping this in mind we refer you to the glossary at the end of this book for a list of explanations and definitions.

Overview

The most common reason that children are sent to our endocrinology clinic is because a primary health care provider has found an asymptomatic lump in the thyroid (a nodule) during routine physical exam for school or sports or during an evaluation of an unrelated acute illness. While you may know an adult friend or family member who has had a thyroid nodule, it turns out that they are found less frequently in children with only 1 or 2 out of 100 children affected. Nodules are more likely to occur in children with hyperthyroidism (Graves' disease), hypothyroidism (Hashimoto's thyroiditis or lymphocytic thyroiditis), and in survivors of childhood cancer (leukemia, lymphoma, brain tumors and others).

Over the past 10 to 15 years, the number of children with thyroid cancer has increased. This is likely due to a number of factors including changes in the environment, parents and health care providers being more aware of risk factors such as a family history of thyroid disease or radiation exposure from treatment of childhood cancer, and greater vigilance in the evaluation and earlier diagnosis of persistent lumps in the neck. There is convincing evidence that nodules found in children need a thorough evaluation because 30 to 50 percent of these thyroid nodules in children are found to be cancer. This is much different when compared with adults where only 10 to15 percent are found to be cancer.

Thyroid Nodules and Well–Differentiated Thyroid Cancer

In the evaluation of a thyroid nodule in a child, we often separate children into two groups: prepubertal (before the onset of puberty) and postpubertal (after puberty has begun). This separation is not absolute but does allow us to make several distinctions. For both groups of children, however, the children look perfectly healthy except for the finding of a lump or nodule in the thyroid and/or hard, persistent swollen lymph glands in the neck. This lack of any other signs or symptoms of a potentially medical problem is routine, but this does make it more difficult to accept that a thorough evaluation is needed and that thyroid cancer may be found and will need to be treated.

In general, prepubertal children with thyroid nodules have a greater chance of having a family or genetic risk factor (a history of thyroid disease or a medical syndrome associated with thyroid disease).

Teenagers are usually sent for evaluation after an asymptomatic nodule (lump) is found in the thyroid gland during a routine exam, such as a school sports physical. Thyroid disease of all forms, to include hypothyroidism (underactive), hyperthyroidism (overactive), thyroid nodules, and thyroid cancer, are more commonly found in adolescent girls than in adolescent boys. Compared with prepubertal children, it is more common to find thyroid nodules in this age group after the onset of puberty.

This is most likely because nodules are more commonly associated with autoimmune disease of the thyroid, particularly Hashimoto's thyroiditis (a common cause of hypothyroidism in young adult girls). While many nodules do not turn out to be cancer, overall a greater number of nodules are medically evaluated during this time.

Lastly, it is in the late teen years that survivors of childhood radiation therapy will begin to present with thyroid disease. The thyroid gland is particularly sensitive to radiation exposure, and the younger the patient at the time of the radiation therapy, the more quickly thyroid disease may develop. After radiation exposure, thyroid disease (hypothyroidism, nodules and/or cancer) may develop as soon as five years and as late as 30 years later. Examples of patients who may have received radiation therapy include Hodgkin's lymphoma and brain tumor survivors.

Why do children develop thyroid cancer?

We do not know why children develop thyroid cancer. We know that normal cells have a time-limited life expectancy whereas cancer cells are described as immortal—they keep on growing. One theory of cancer formation suggests that in order to become cancer, cells must be able to bypass certain key control biologic check points on growth, which then allow them to become immortal cells. Several specific abnormalities in DNA (mutations in specific genes that are associated with the development of cancer) and growth factors are believed to play a role in this process. The immune response (the system in our body that fights infections) and the fact that the child's thyroid gland is still growing even under normal conditions could also be important. As you can imagine, all of these factors are also important in the development of thyroid cancer in adults. In the final analysis, we currently do not have a unifying explanation as to what combination of the above factors makes childhood thyroid cancer behave differently than adult thyroid cancer.

Childhood cancer survivors

One subset of children at an increased risk of developing thyroid nodules and thyroid cancer are children who have been exposed to radiation. Before 1980, many children received radiation therapy for a variety of medical conditions to include ringworm of the scalp, facial acne, an enlarged thymus, and a whole host of other conditions. While these practices have been abandoned, what has been learned from this experience is that the younger the child at the time of exposure, then the greater the chance and the shorter the time for the child to develop thyroid cancer. In addition, small radiation doses appear to have a greater chance than larger doses of causing thyroid abnormalities such as cancer. This is so because larger doses usually kill all the cells whereas smaller doses cause damage to the nuclear genetic apparatus of the cell, which causes mutations through defective repair, which in turn increases the risk of developing thyroid nodules and/or cancer.

Today the children who may still receive radiation exposure to the thyroid are those who are being treated for other forms of childhood cancers such as brain tumors, leukemias, and lymphomas. Doses as small as 50 rads may cause enough damage to increase the risk of thyroid nodules and thyroid cancer, with the greatest risk occurring in patients who have received radiation doses of 200 to 2,000 cGy or rads to the head and neck prior to the age of 10 years.

In total, thyroid cancer may develop in as many as 10 percent of all tumor survivors after radiation treatments with an increasing risk related to the younger age the child was when they received radiation therapy. Most thyroid disease requires about 15 years to appear, but cases have been reported as late as 30 years after, or as short as five years later in younger children. What makes the child's thyroid gland more susceptible to radiation damage when compared to an adult's is not known.

Radiation exposure from the environment

One of our greatest concerns is the widespread increase in thyroid cancer among children exposed to environmental radiation. An extreme example of this is the Chernobyl nuclear accident in the Belarus region of Soviet Russia in April 1986. After the accident, childhood thyroid cancers began to appear around the region surrounding Chernobyl as early as five years after the accident. Because thyroid cancers usually develop slowly, the full impact of the accident may not be known for another 20 to 30 years

In the event of a nuclear accident, there are preventive measures that can be taken against radiation damage to the thyroid gland, which include the provision of stable iodine and non-radiation–contaminated water, milk, and food. The World Health Organization recommends stable iodine in doses of: 0.1 gm/day to adults, 0.05 gm/day to children over 3 years of age and 0.025 gm/day to children under 3 years of age. These doses should be given until food, water, and milk are free of contamination.

Other inherited thyroid cancer syndromes

As mentioned above, some forms of papillary thyroid cancer (PTC) may be inherited (passed from one generation to the next). In these families, inheritance follows a dominant pattern of transmission (one parent may pass on the risk of cancer independent of the other parent's genes). Although uncommon, these inherited causes should be considered in any family with cancer in multiple generations. Thyroid cancer may be one feature of a group of inherited tumor syndromes that have been named after the physicians who first described them and include Gardner's syndrome, Cowden's syndrome, and the Carney complex.

Are there differences in the presentation of thyroid nodules and thyroid cancer in adults and children?

As suggested above, the answer to this is *yes*. In fact, some of the differences in clinical findings between thyroid cancers in children versus thyroid cancers in adults may make it easier for you to understand the evaluation and treatment that we would recommend for your child or teen. As mentioned at the outset of this discussion, while the majority of thyroid nodules are not cancer, there is an increased risk that nodules in children, as compared to adults, are cancerous. Because of this, there is a greater need to more thoroughly and more quickly evaluate these when they are found. Unfortunately, there is no blood test or X-ray test that allows us to distinguish which nodule will be cancerous and which will not.

Unlike adults, more than half the children with thyroid cancer have swollen glands (enlarged lymph nodes in the neck that can be felt on exam). These lymph nodes are usually swollen because of small amounts of cancer that have spread to them, and while this finding predicts a worse outcome in adults, it does not predict a worse outcome in children. In fact, thyroid cancer should be considered in any child that presents with persistent enlargement of the neck lymph nodes.

In addition to lymph node involvement, almost 15 percent of children have cancer that has already spread to the lungs (pulmonary metastasis). In adults, this is associated with a significantly worse outcome. In children this does not appear to be the case. Many children will continue to have persistent disease; however, it often does not increase or worsen over 15 to 20 years, and in fact, over the same time period, some of these children's diseases may decrease to the point of being undetectable.

One of our greatest limitations in treating children with thyroid cancer is the relative lack of information concerning long-term outcome. Overall, we are fortunate that thyroid cancer in children is uncommon. However, because of the relative rarity compared to adults, we lack good data on a large collection of pediatric patients who have been followed over their lifetime. With these limitations in our knowledge in mind, the following is a discussion of our approach to the evaluation of thyroid nodules, and our treatment recommendations.

Evaluation

The tools used to assess thyroid nodules and the possibility that they might represent a thyroid cancer include: serum thyroid function tests (TSH and thyroid hormone level), thyroid ultrasound (US), radionuclide imaging (scan), and fine needle aspiration (FNA) for cytologic (cells) examination.

Thyroid function tests

Thyroid function tests (thyroid hormone and/or TSH levels) are not helpful for making a diagnosis of thyroid cancer, as most patients will have normal levels. However, high thyroid hormone levels (T4 or T3) and a low TSH level could indicate that the nodule is a benign hyperfunctioning nodule (adenoma), thereby tending to rule out thyroid cancer. In such cases, a thyroid scan would be done to show that the nodule is hyperfunctioning whereas thyroid cancers appear under-functioning ("cold") on scan. However, thyroid cancers can occur in children who have autoimmune thyroid disease (Hashimoto's thyroiditis or Graves' disease). In these patients, abnormal thyroid function tests reflect the underlying thyroid disease but do not exclude thyroid cancer. All nodules in the thyroid are suspicious, even in children with known autoimmune thyroid disease, and as we have already suggested, further evaluation of these nodules is required (see below).

Thyroid ultrasound

An ultrasound (echo or sonogram) uses sound waves to "take a picture" of the thyroid gland. This is a painless procedure in which your child will just need to lie still, have a warm jelly applied on the skin of their neck, and then have an ultrasound probe gently passed over the area. There is no radiation exposure. Ultrasound (US) is easy, painless and often provides useful information. US can detect lesions less than 1 cm in size (less than $1/2$ inch) and can find many other unsuspected nodules. Some physicians will use ultrasound to take a picture and to help with taking a biopsy (see below). For more information see chapter 16.

Radionuclide imaging

Radionuclide scans are generally unable to distinguish non-cancerous (benign) lesions from cancer. For this reason, some experts believe that radionuclide scans do not provide any benefit in the evaluation of thyroid nodules in children. However, these scans are very useful for the long-term follow up of patients with thyroid cancer, as they allow us to see if there is any new cancer growth. They are also useful to rule out hyperfunctioning nodules as described above.

Fine needle aspiration

Fine Needle Aspiration (FNA) is a form of minor biopsy in that only cells are removed and not tissue as in a true biopsy. With this technique, which is described in detail in chapter 6, a small needle is put into the nodule within the thyroid gland and a few cells are removed for evaluation under a microscopic. If an adequate number of cells can be collected, this allows us to determine if surgery to remove the thyroid is necessary (if the cells appear to be suspicious for cancer) or if the nodule can be followed without surgery. FNA has been used in children but can be performed only in a child who can hold still during the procedure. While the needle used and the puncture made is no more traumatic than drawing blood, in most patients there is some anxiety about having a needle inserted in the neck. A topical numbing or anesthetic cream can be placed on the area before the procedure, but even still, it is often harder to collect an adequate number of cells in younger children who cannot sit still. For this reason, some doctors recommend removal of all thyroid nodules in younger, prepubertal children without even attempting FNA.

Management of benign thyroid nodules in children

With the increasing use of FNA, benign (non-cancerous) nodules are being followed without surgery in children (most commonly in teenagers). In these cases, we often give thyroid hormone with the hope of possibly reducing the size of the nodule and decreasing the chance of other nodules forming. We use repeated, serial physical exams and ultrasound examinations to ensure that the nodule is not changing, as most benign nodules should not grow in size, even over long periods of time. Nodules that increase in size are worrisome and should either be re-evaluated with FNA or be surgically removed.

The best therapeutic approach to "hot" or hyperfunctioning thyroid nodules (nodules that produce an excess amount of thyroid hormone) has been debated, even in adults. Because several small, unsuspected cancers have been found associated with these nodules we recommend surgical removal of all "hot" nodules in children. If a decision is made not to remove the nodule, long-term follow-up is required as there is a risk that cancer could develop as a "hot" nodule.

Management of differentiated thyroid carcinoma

The types of thyroid cancers that are found in children are separated according to how they appear under the microscope into papillary (PTC) follicular (FTC), and medullary forms (medullary thyroid cancer is discussed later in this chapter). Both PTC and FTC are typically well differentiated (closer to normal cells in appearance) and appear to have a similar chance of cure or remission in children. As in adults, PTC is the most common form found in children.

Treatment overview

In general the initial approach to treating thyroid cancer is largely the same as described in great depth in several other chapters in this volume. The approach involves surgical removal of the thyroid, allowing the patient to become hypothyroid with a rise in serum TSH levels, and then treatment with an ablative dose of radioactive iodine. Thyroid cells absorb iodine, and if the iodine is radioactive any remaining cells will then be destroyed. This approach allows surgical removal of the bulk of tissue (thyroid nodule, surrounding thyroid gland tissue and any suspicious lymph nodes), followed by medical removal of any smaller amounts of thyroid tissue that may have been left behind by the surgeon. This post-surgical dose of iodine is called the "ablative" dose, as it ablates or destroys any remaining thyroid cells. Within the following week of the ablative iodine dose, a scan will be performed ("post-treatment scan") to see if any other areas absorbed the iodine that would indicate sites of residual tumor that could represent remaining, unsuspected disease (for instance in the lungs) that would need to be monitored in the future.

Surgical approach

Various experts debate the extent of initial thyroid and lymph node surgery that is necessary, as well as the use and dose of radioactive iodine, although it is not really very controversial. Those who argue in favor of more aggressive surgery (total or near-total thyroidectomy) cite improved disease-free survival and ease of finding recurrent disease. Those who argue in favor of less aggressive therapy (lobectomy or removal of only the segment of thyroid gland in which the cancer is found) cite the low mortality associated with thyroid cancer and reduced complication rates when less extensive surgery is used. In several studies of children and adolescents, treatment with total or near total thyroid removal, followed by radioactive iodine ablation, has led to remission in 70 percent of patients.

Many families ask why we recommend removal of the entire thyroid gland if we find a nodule on only one side. This recommendation is based on the fact that in both spontaneous and radiation-induced thyroid cancers of children, small (microscopic) areas of cancer are frequently found in more than one part of the thyroid (multi-focal tumor) despite finding only one nodule on physical examination of the neck or with ultrasound exam. For this reason, even though your child may have only one nodule on one side, we believe that removal of both lobes (both sides) decreases the risk of recurrence. In most cases, the patient will be taking lifelong thyroid hormone therapy irrespective of whether a subtotal or total thyroidectomy is performed.

Unfortunately, the risks of surgical complications are higher in young patients and highest when the surgery is not performed by a surgeon who specializes in thyroid surgery in children. It is difficult to balance these outcomes because the impact of recurrence on life span or quality of life is not well understood for young patients. Published survival data are favorable with the "long-term" risk of dying from thyroid cancer estimated at only 1 to 2 percent. Unfortunately, as mentioned above, this estimate may be falsely low because follow-up studies of childhood thyroid cancer beyond 10 years are rare. Even with extensive surgery, one in five children will have persistent or recurrent disease requiring additional therapy.

For adults, recurrent disease increases mortality, and in our opinion, this supports the use of somewhat more aggressive management in young patients. Total or near total thyroidectomy improves disease-free survival for young adults who have similar forms and extent of thyroid cancer as are found in children. In addition, removal of all lymph nodes in the central neck compartment also reduces the risk of recurrence.

Radioactive iodine

Studies of young adults (including some adolescents) have shown that recurrence can be further reduced by the use of radioactive iodine ablation after surgery. The optimal single and total doses have yet to be determined for children, but most experts suggest single doses for older children and adolescents of about 100 to 175 mCi, depending on the extent of disease at the time. For younger children, the dose of [131]Iodine is based on body weight. Some medical centers specializing in thyroid cancer use for each patient a sophisticated method of determining the maximal safe dose of radioactive iodine, called "dosimetry," but this is not done at all centers (see chapter 15).

Thyroid hormone suppression

Following surgery and radioactive iodine ablation, thyroid hormone is given to avoid hypothyroidism and to suppress thyroid stimulating hormone (TSH). For patients with persistent disease or metastasis, TSH levels should be reduced to as close to zero as can be achieved without causing clinical symptoms of hyperthyroidism (feeling warm, jittery, fidgety or nervous, having difficulty sleeping, a fast heart rate and an increased number of bowel movements per day, weight loss). A lower dose of thyroid hormone that would be associated with a slightly higher TSH levels is acceptable for lower-risk patients who appear to be free of disease for 5 to 10 years and have very low serum levels of the tumor marker, thyroglobulin (Tg).

Treatment outcomes

Although debate exists, the overall success of treatment of well-differentiated thyroid cancer is good. Many children with PTC enter into remission after the first treatment with surgery and radioactive iodine. However, some will require multiple doses of radioactive iodine but still achieve full cure.

Only about half of the children with distant metastasis such as in the lungs enter remission, and they require additional treatments with surgery, radioactive iodine or both. In addition, the risk of recurrence is higher if there was distant spread of cancer at the time of diagnosis, and the recurrence may occur sooner (within two years versus nine years). Depending on the location and size of recurrent disease, each recurrence is treated with surgery, radioactive iodine or both as warranted.

Persistent disease

For some children, thyroid cancer will persist despite the best treatment. This is more often seen in children with disease in the lungs. While no firm limit to the total dose of radioactive iodine has been set, doses exceeding 1000 mCi (1 curie) and approaching 3000 mCi (3 curies) have been used. Elimination of all disease is usually not achieved, but these large doses have reduced the amount of tumor in the body. If a decision is made to treat with more radioactive iodine (doses greater than a few hundred mCi), it may be best to have the therapy done at a medical center that can perform dosimetry (see chapter 15) to decide on the maximal, safe dose.

Recurrent disease

Despite favorable survival, recurrence is more common in children than adults. In young patients, the risk of recurrence is greatest during the first few years after initial treatment. One in five children will develop recurrent disease and require additional surgery, radioactive iodine treatments or both. For children, recurrent disease is more common when the age is less than 10 years old, in boys, with large tumors (greater than 2 cm in size), with multi-focal cancer, and with cancer that has spread to the lymph nodes of the neck or to the lungs.

Fortunately, the outcome in children with recurrent disease appears much better than in adults. In general, children with thyroid cancer are less likely to die from their disease than adults. This is very different from the outcome of any other solid tumor in children, for which spread of cancer into the lymph nodes, and especially to the lungs, has a higher mortality.

Surveillance for disease recurrence

In order to see if cancer has recurred, repeated [131]Iodine scans and measurements of blood Tg levels will be done at scheduled times over the next few years. Tg, or thyroglobulin, is a protein that is made exclusively by thyroid cells. Patients treated with total thyroidectomy and radioactive iodine ablation should have undetectable Tg levels while taking thyroid hormone with a very suppressed TSH.

Detection of thyroid tumor by measurement of Tg is most sensitive when the TSH is elevated, a state that may be achieved either after thyroxine withdrawal rendering patients hypothyroid or by administration of synthetic TSH (Thyrogen®). Thus patients will also have TSH-stimulated Tg levels and scans done at scheduled times. For these tests, thyroid hormone suppression will be stopped to purposefully let the TSH increase. Older children may be given synthetic TSH instead, called Thyrogen®. The TSH stimulation increases our ability to detect any smaller amount of thyroid cells that may still be present. Patients with Tg levels that remain under 2 ng/ml after stimulation are almost always free from disease, while those with stimulated Tg levels above 10 ng/mL most often have residual cancer.

Sometimes other tests will be needed. Suspicious lymph nodes can be evaluated with ultrasound (US) or magnetic resonance imaging (MRI). Suspected disease found by US or MRI may be subjected to fine needle aspiration for cytology and if found to be malignant could then be removed by surgery.

For children and adolescents, lifelong follow-up is required. Most recurrent disease occurs in the first seven years after treatment, but some patients will relapse after 20 to 30 years. The frequency and intensity of evaluation are debated, and there is no consensus on how often or for how many years children should have repeated radioactive iodine scans or be tested for Tg levels.

We recommend physical exams and Tg levels every 3 months, along with a yearly radioactive iodine scans for all patients until they are free from disease for at least two years. At that point, patients can be divided into those with low and high risk for recurrence based on clinical features. In general, patients older than 10 years of age with tumors less than 2 cm in size that have not spread beyond the thyroid have a lower risk of recurrence. All other patients are considered high risk.

After seven years, most patients will have a lower risk for recurrence. Lifelong surveillance, even for the lowest risk patients, is still needed. For low risk patients who remain free from disease, follow-up might include a thorough neck examination and yearly Tg levels while taking thyroid hormone. For younger patients, and those who originally had large tumors, TSH-stimulated Tg levels, with or without radioactive iodine scans, might still be done but not as often. Eventually all patients will need less frequent tests, but when to do so must be decided for each and every child.

Controversies in the treatment of thyroid cancer

Because every patient is different and each tumor may behave differently, generalizations are made in discussions such as in this chapter, but therapy and management always must be individualized. In this context, treatment in certain circumstances of some children and even adults is controversial. These include patients with high Tg levels but negative ^{131}I scans. This is a situation where we can detect by blood tests the presence of thyroid tissue, but the scan does not demonstrate it. The latter may occur because the remaining thyroid tissue has lost the ability to absorb iodine or the patient have very small cancers (less than 1 cm in size).

Patients with high Tg levels but negative scans can be imaged by other techniques such as CT, MRI and PET (see chapter 16). PET scans have been used in adults with good results. Unfortunately, normal lymph nodes or swollen or inflamed lymph nodes can also show up as positive on these scans, making it difficult to tell in children if this is cancer. Whether or not to treat with additional surgery or more radioactive iodine must be individualized especially as total doses of radioactive iodine approach 1000 mCi.

In regard to very small tumors (<1cm), there are data in adults to suggest that metastasis and recurrence can be seen just as in larger tumors, but there are few data to determine the impact of these small tumors on children. In each case the physician and family must weigh the risks of surgery against the risk of not performing surgery to remove the thyroid gland.

Prognosis

In general, children with thyroid cancer have a good prognosis. Many children (70 percent) will enter remission after the first treatment. For those children with persistent or recurrent disease, 3 out of 4 will eventually enter remission. Long-term follow-up for all children with thyroid cancer is required because there is always a risk of recurrence even as long as 20 to 30 years after treatment.

Medullary thyroid carcinoma in children

Background

Medullary Thyroid Cancer (MTC) is a unique form of thyroid cancer that requires a different approach than the more common types of thyroid cancer in its evaluation and treatment. MTC is often inherited as one part of a heritable disease abbreviated MEN or Multiple Endocrine Neoplasia (see below). Because this syndrome runs in families, other well–appearing family members, especially children, are often asked to be evaluated for possible MEN shortly after the first family member is diagnosed. MTC also differs from other forms of thyroid cancer in that removal of the thyroid gland prior to symptoms of the disease provides our best chance for cure. In the following section we will discuss these differences between MTC and other forms of thyroid cancer and hopefully shed light on the evaluation and treatment that may be suggested for you and your family.

What is MTC?

MTC is a form of thyroid cancer that develops from a distinct group of cells in the thyroid gland called chromaffin cells, or C-cells. The origin of C-cells is different from the origin of the cells that constitute other forms of thyroid cancer. C-cells develop from cells of the primitive nervous system of the embryo. Because of this, unlike other cells of the thyroid gland, these cells do not absorb or use iodine or make thyroid hormone. Unfortunately, this means that we cannot use radioactive iodine to treat MTC.

MTC develops because of an abnormality in one of the cell-growth pathways that causes the cell to constantly be in a growing phase. The specific abnormality is in a protein called a receptor on the surface of the C-cells, and it is called the RET-receptor. In the normal state this receptor is in the "off" or inactive position, and it requires a molecule to attach to it for it to turn on and be activated. The genetic abnormality in MTC is called an "activating mutation" because the receptor is turned on without any molecule attaching to it. The result is that the cells enter into a pattern of unregulated growth.

Individual genetic mutations are associated with specific clinical findings in the patient. The DNA coding instructions for how the receptor is built can be examined to determine if a patient has a RET mutation and if so, which mutation they have. This allows us to identify the specific risks any given patient or family may have for developing associated diseases. For example, specific RET mutations are associated with the different subtypes of clinical syndromes of MEN, which have been specifically subclassified and designated as either FMTC, MEN 2A or MEN 2B.

The same abnormality in the DNA can be inherited by anyone who has another person in his or her family with this disease. Knowing what DNA abnormality a particular person has allows us to make specific follow-up and treatment recommendation based on the clinical risk of potentially associated diseases. What is true for all family members found to have a RET-abnormality is that 100 percent will develop MTC. The time frame in which this may occur differs and is discussed in the "Treatment" section below.

Who gets MTC?

There are four different ways in which MTC can occur. It may occur as an isolated disease in a non-inherited form (only found in adults; called "sporadic" MTC), as an inherited form (called Familial Medullary Thyroid Cancer or FMTC), or it may be one part of an inherited tumor syndrome called Multiple Endocrine Neoplasia syndrome, more commonly abbreviated as MEN.

There are several forms of MEN, but MTC is associated only with types 2A and 2B. Knowing which form of MEN runs in a family is important, as the risk of MTC differs between the two both in the age at which MTC may develop and in how aggressive the type of MTC may behave. Fortunately there are differences in physical facial, tongue and other features between patients with MEN 2A and MEN 2B, and differences in DNA for which abnormalities can be tested.

How do patients come to medical attention?

The two most common reasons MTC patients are sent to a clinic are either from a referral of another health care provider who found a thyroid nodule that is ultimately found to contain MTC (more common in adults) or because another family member is known to have MTC and/or MEN (common for both children and adults).

What other tumors can MTC patients develop?

In Table 1 (below) is a summary of the differences among the inherited forms of MTC along with explanations of tumors that may be associated. This is also discussed in chapter 24.

TABLE 1

Tumor or Disease	MEN2A	MEN2B	FMTC
MTC	100%	100%	100%
Age when MTC presents	5 to 20 years	$1/2$ to 10 yrs	20 to 50 yrs
Pheochromocytoma	10–60%	50%	0%
Hyperparathyroidism	20–30%	0%	0%
Physical features*	0%	100%	0%

*Long face, soft nodules on the tongue or lips, loose joints and tall stature with long, thin fingers, arms and legs.

- **Pheochromocytoma** is a tumor of the adrenal gland that makes increased amounts of adrenaline-like hormones. Symptoms include headache, high blood pressure and spells where the face gets red and warm (flushing).

• *Hyperparathyroidism* is an abnormal growth of the parathyroid glands with increased production of the hormone made by the parathyroid glands. Symptoms include high serum calcium levels from an increased breakdown of bone that can lead to bone pain and osteoporosis.

MEN 2A

MEN 2A accounts for about 75 percent of all cases of MEN 2. Of all the DNA abnormalities found in MEN 2A, the most common abnormality is found at a specific location called codon 634. A *codon* is a small portion of DNA that provides information used to determine which one of 19 different building blocks is used to build a protein (in this case the RET receptor protein). The number, in this case #634, is an address defining the location in the DNA.

Knowing the specific location of the DNA abnormality allows us to predict if a person is at risk of other tumors and an estimate as to when the tumors most commonly develop. For example, almost half of the patients with MEN 2A and the #634 mutation develop a tumor of adrenal gland tissue called pheochromocytoma (see Table 1), and 20 to 30 percent also develop hyperparathyroidism (see Table 1). For patients with a 634 mutation, screening for these other tumors should begin immediately at the time of diagnosis and should continue every year throughout the patient's life. Many of these other tumors, for instance, pheochromocytoma, are found during the 3rd or 4th decade of life, but this does not always hold true, and children as young as 5 years of age have developed pheochromocytoma. The other mutations associated with MEN 2A have differing amounts of risk. Your physician will provide a specific screening recommendation schedule during the evaluation process.

MEN 2B

MEN 2B is less common than MEN 2A and is often diagnosed in a family without a previous history of MEN. This is called a new, or "novel," mutation. Two major differences in the MEN 2B syndrome have profound effects on the treatment. First, the form of MTC found in MEN 2B is the most aggressive MTC, and second, the MTC found in MEN 2B usually has its clinical presentation at a much younger age. Disease that has spread outside of the thyroid gland (to surrounding tissues, liver or bone) has been seen as early as 1 year of age. In addition, persistent or recurrent disease is also more likely in MEN 2B.

As mentioned, earlier specific physical features are found in MEN 2B and may alert doctors to the diagnosis. These include a long face, small soft nodules on the tongue or lips, "loose" or hyper-extensible joints and tall stature with long, thin fingers, arms and legs.

Evaluation

Nearly 100 percent of people found to have a RET mutations on DNA testing will eventually develop MTC. The goal of testing is to detect the RET mutation, thereby allowing the health care team to remove the thyroid gland before the cancer ever develops. This approach to diagnosis and treatment has dramatically improved the lives of our patients and their family members. Before the DNA test was available, the diagnosis of MTC was often delayed, resulting in the majority of patients having disease that had grown outside of the thyroid gland. Once this occurs, it is very difficult, if not impossible, to completely remove all of the cancer.

Over the years three common questions arise from patients with a family history of MEN 2. First, how should one test and treat children with a family history of MEN? Second, how should one test a child who has a family history of MTC but a negative lab test for the abnormal gene? Third, how should one test and treat children who have MTC but a negative family history?

The child with a family history of MEN

All children from a family with a history of MEN 2 should have blood tests for the RET mutation as soon as possible. The timing of surgery to remove the thyroid should be based on what DNA abnormality, or mutation, is found. RET mutations are divided into three classes. Class 3 has the most aggressive form of MTC and class 1 has the less aggressive form.

	TABLE 2	
	Mutation	**Recommended Age for Thyroid Removal**
Class 3	883, 922, 918 (MEN 2B)	within 1st few months of life
Class 2	611, 618, 620, 634 (MEN 2A)	before 5 years of age
Class 1	609, 768, 791, 804, 891 (FMTC)	before 10 years of age

Removal of the thyroid gland by the recommended age increases the chance of a surgical cure from the disease. The goal is to remove the thyroid gland before the cancer develops (called "prophylactic" or preventive removal of the thyroid gland). In other words, a successful surgery will result in removing a thyroid gland that appears normal. Because no cancer is found in the thyroid, one should not get the mistaken impression that the surgery was unnecessary. On the contrary, if the thyroid would not have been removed it would develop cancer (MTC) nearly 100 percent of the time.

Evaluation of the child from a family with a history of MEN but normal DNA testing

In rare families, the diseases associated with MEN (MTC, pheochromocytoma and/or hyperparathyroidism) may "run" in the family, but lab tests for the abnormal RET gene may not be found. This places children at unknown risk for MTC or the other endocrine tumors found in MEN2. In these cases, the method used for RET testing should be reviewed, as the lab may screen only for the most common abnormalities. A more complete test should be performed, but a research laboratory at a major medical center may need to be found in order to do the complete test.

For MEN 2B families this is uncommon as most abnormal RET genes are found at the same spot on the DNA (codon 918). In addition, patients with MEN 2B have unique physical features. Children with these physical features and a positive family history of MEN 2B should have their thyroid removed in the first few months of life, no matter what the blood test shows.

Evaluation of a child with MTC

Some children are found to have MTC when they are being evaluated for a thyroid nodule or enlarged lymph nodes in the neck. They have a much greater risk for local spread, metastases and persistent and recurrent disease. In these cases, a blood test for the RET abnormality should be sent and a more complete examination of the neck, chest and abdomen should be performed.

What other lab tests can be used to help follow success of treatment?

MTC can produce many hormones that can lead to symptoms both before the diagnosis of MTC is made and as an early sign that the MTC has grown back (recurred). These symptoms may include diarrhea, flushing, increased weight gain with purple-colored stretch marks and/or high blood pressure.

The cells that result in MTC also produce a hormone called *calcitonin*. If all of the MTC is removed, the calcitonin level in the blood should be undetectable. Some patients, however, have elevated levels of calcitonin without any evidence of detectable disease and still live long, productive lives. These patients, and indeed all patients with MTC, need close follow-up to include yearly (or more frequent) physical examinations, blood tests for calcitonin and carcinoembryonic antigen (CEA), and radiologic exams (ultrasound, MRI or other) for the rest of their lives.

What is the treatment and follow-up?

Surgery to remove the thyroid is the treatment of choice for MTC. Before surgery calcitonin should be measured to confirm the diagnosis and can be used later on to screen for the return of disease. If a child has a family history of MEN 2 and is over 5 years of age, screening for the other associated tumors (pheochromocytoma and hyperparathyroidism) should be done before removal of the thyroid gland is performed. Current recommended management guidelines support total removal of the thyroid gland by 4 to 5 years of age for all children with MEN 2A and total thyroid removal within the first few months of life for children with MEN 2B (see Table 2).

Blood calcitonin levels should be tested on a regular basis as soon as 4 to 6 months after surgery. It is best to wait a few months because blood calcitonin levels may fall more slowly in some cases and may raise false concern that all of the disease was not removed. After six months, the calcitonin level is a good test to detect any remaining disease. Only one in 20 patients with undetectable calcitonin levels will have their disease come back in the next five years. Even in patients with detectable calcitonin levels, many will lead long productive lives. The bottom line is that all patients are at risk of having the disease return and because of this will need life-long medical follow-up.

After thyroid surgery will I need to take any medications?

After removal of the thyroid gland, all patients will need replacement thyroid hormone. Thyroid hormone (thyroxine or levothyroxine) is available as a pill and is given on a once-a-day schedule. This is true even for infants. Blood testing will be done to measure if the correct dose is being given. When properly medicated, the TSH in patients who have MTC will be in the normal range. Taking the medication is extremely important as thyroid hormone is required for normal temperature control and energy levels, and for maintaining weight, bowel habits, heart rate and blood pressure, cholesterol metabolism, menstrual cycles and a long list of other key metabolic systems. In infants thyroid hormone is necessary for normal brain development. The need for this replacement will be life-long, and periodic monitoring to ensure appropriate dosage is mandatory.

What do we do about persistent or recurrent disease?

The risk of persistent or recurrent disease is high for children with cancer that has spread to the lymph nodes or to distant organs (most often the liver). CT scans, MRI or ultrasound should be done to assess enlarged lymph nodes and elevated or increasing levels of calcitonin or CEA.

Chemotherapy and radiation therapy have been tried in the past, and for some patients these treatments have stopped cancer growth, but only very rarely have patients been cured. In contrast to other forms of thyroid cancer, the cells that lead to MTC (C-cells) do not take up iodine, and neither radioiodine scans nor radioiodine treatment has any role in patients with MTC. Several new treatments show promise, but all of these are in the research phase and more time will be needed to see if these new treatments are really effective.

What should we do about our other children and family members?

The use of genetic tests for MEN 2 and FMTC has changed the approach to patients and their families. Prior to having other family members tested for the RET gene abnormality, the patient and the family should sit down and discuss what MTC and MEN are, what laboratory tests are necessary, and how the results are used to make decisions. We are very aware of the stress that this can have on your family and how difficult it may be to tell other family members who believe that they are healthy that they may be at risk of having MTC and/or MEN. Disbelief, guilt and anger are all normal reactions in these situations. Genetic counselors are available to help work through these stressful and difficult times.

Summary

Thyroid cancers are uncommon in children and adolescents but must be considered in children with thyroid nodules and persistent swollen glands, and in survivors of childhood cancers. Prior to surgery a biopsy can be done to speed the diagnosis. The current guideline is to remove all or almost all of the thyroid along with the lymph nodes in the neck. For non-MTC differentiated thyroid cancer, this is followed by radioactive iodine treatment and thyroid hormone suppression. With such treatment, the long-term prognosis is very good. However, patients must be monitored for recurrent disease on a lifelong basis.

For families with MTC, genetic testing allows early diagnosis and treatment. Performed early in life, removal of the thyroid offers nearly 100 percent "cure" and long-term survival. This approach has changed the lives of MEN2 families by allowing treatment and follow-up to be tailored to each form of the abnormal RET gene.

CHAPTER 6

Fine Needle Aspiration

Yolanda C. Oertel, M.D.

Your physician has just told you that you have a "lump" (or nodule) in your thyroid gland or you have felt a lump in your neck and have made an appointment to see your primary physician. If you are a woman from about 20 to 50 years old, you should understand that this is a common finding. Nevertheless, you may be concerned about the possibility of cancer. In fact, most nodules or "lumps" in the thyroid are **NOT** cancerous.

The challenge for the physician is to determine which nodules are benign and which nodules are cancerous. The following may provide useful information, but they will NOT determine whether the nodule is benign or malignant:

- How long the nodule has been present.
- Whether it is tender or not.
- Whether it feels soft, rubbery or firm to the touch.
- The blood tests of thyroid function.
- The response to thyroid hormone suppressive therapy.
- Ultrasound findings.
- Thyroid scans and uptake.

The only test prior to surgery that is proven to differentiate a benign from a malignant nodule is the fine needle aspiration (FNA). Hence your doctor will tell you that you need a fine needle aspiration of the nodule. What follows is some information about this procedure that will help you understand why and how it will be done.

Based on my experience as a pathologist who has been performing FNAs of palpable masses for 26 years (the last four years dedicated primarily to FNAs of thyroid nodules), I will try to answer the most frequently asked questions by patients. If you do not find an answer to your specific question, or if something is not clear, please do not hesitate to drop me a note (Yolanda C. Oertel, M.D., Director, Fine Needle Aspiration Service, Washington Cancer Institute (C-1219), Washington Hospital Center, 110 Irving Street, NW, Washington DC, 20010-2975). I will attempt to respond to all queries.

I. Before the FNA:

What is a fine needle aspiration?

It is a simple procedure, similar to drawing blood from your arm. The needle used is thinner than the one for drawing blood and is attached to a syringe in a syringe holder that allows the operator to apply suction easily. Cells from your thyroid lesion will be extracted through this thin needle. If there is fluid in the "lump," we will drain it. These cells will be smeared (spread) on glass slides, stained, and made ready to be examined under the microscope. After examining all the slides, the pathologist will make a cytologic diagnosis and issue a written report.

Do I really need an aspiration?

An FNA is the only non-surgical method of determining whether your thyroid nodule is benign or malignant.

"The tumor is large and has to be removed." In this instance, do I really need an aspiration (FNA)?

Yes, to avoid surprises for the surgeon. On rare occasions a patient may have a medullary carcinoma or anaplastic carcinoma of the thyroid. Knowing this in advance will help the surgeon plan accordingly. Additional tests will be needed to exclude the possibility of other tumors such as pheochromocytoma. This is important because pheochromocytomas occur with high frequency in patients with medullary thyroid cancer, and they need to be managed prior to undertaking thyroid surgery. In rare instances, cancer from other organs (breast, kidney, lung etc.) may have spread to the thyroid and may appear as if it had originated there.

Should I have an ultrasound prior to a FNA?

Most of the time it is not necessary. If your physician discovers a nodule and he or she (or the pathologist he or she works with) can perform an aspiration immediately, there is no need to wait for an ultrasound. You may have a diagnosis in 24 hours, and if the nodule is malignant, your appointment with a surgeon can be scheduled within a few days.

Do I need an FNA with ultrasound guidance?

This might be necessary if the nodule is not easily palpable (your physician can't feel it with his fingers), or is defined vaguely (your doctor is not quite sure he can detect it). For example, your lump was discovered by chance. You attended a "health fair" and had a scan of your neck to check your carotid arteries. The scan revealed that although your carotid arteries were fine, there was a nodule in your thyroid.

Is Fine Needle Aspiration (FNA) the same as a needle biopsy?

No, it is not. FNA is a much simpler procedure.

What about a needle biopsy?

With this procedure a core of tissue is removed from your thyroid gland by a "Tru-Cut" or "Vim-Silverman" needle with local anesthesia. The tissue then is processed in the pathology laboratory in the same manner as any other surgical biopsy.

Will I be given local anesthesia before the FNA?

We do not use or inject any local anesthetic. Similarly, no local anesthetic is used when drawing blood from your arm. Although the needle we use for FNA is thinner than that used for drawing blood, we apply an ice pack to numb the skin. Thus the needle prick is a minor discomfort.

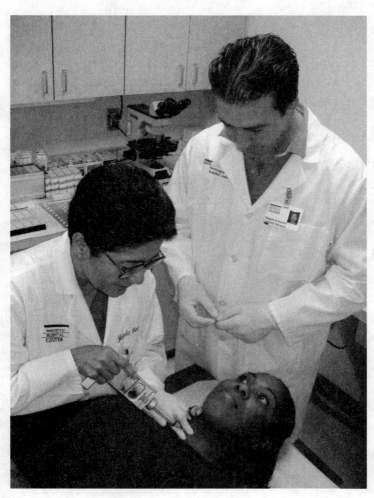

FIGURE 1: Procedure of fine needle aspiration

What does the procedure consist of?

The skin is cleaned with an alcohol swab (no iodine or betadyne is used), and then it is dried with a piece of gauze. Drying the skin avoids the "sting" that is felt when the skin is pierced if the alcohol has not evaporated from its surface. Then the needle is inserted (See figure 1).

How long will I spend in the doctor's office for an FNA?

The procedure usually takes about 20 minutes. Each "needle stick" requires only a few seconds. But be prepared to spend half an hour to 40 minutes in the doctor's office because you will need to fill in registration forms, insurance forms, etc. prior to being aspirated.

Should I fast before the FNA?

You do not need to skip a meal before the procedure. There are no restrictions on eating, either before or after the FNA.

Should I stop my medications before the FNA?

No, you do not need to stop any prescription medications. However, it is preferable to stop taking aspirin one or two days before and after the procedure. Please consult with your physician before stopping any medications.

I am on "blood-thinners." Should I stop taking them?

Please consult with the physician who prescribed the anticoagulants. He will advise you on the safety of discontinuing such medication. If this cannot be stopped for a couple of days prior to the FNA, make sure that the physician performing the FNA is aware of this medication so special precautions may be taken.

Can I wear a turtle-neck or a scarf?

When having a thyroid aspiration, you have to uncover your neck. It is easier for the doctor to perform the procedure if your clothing allows easy exposure of your neck. If you wear a turtleneck, it should have a zipper in back or front that will allow the collar to fold down. Better yet, wear a blouse without a collar, or one with buttons in front, or any clothing that will allow easy exposure of your neck. Also, avoid wearing jewelry around your neck.

How can I find out if the physician is skilled (or qualified) at performing FNAs?

Ask an endocrinologist or thyroidologist about this. To whom do they send their patients for FNAs? Or to whom would the doctor (or a member of the doctor's family) go if an aspiration was needed? Also, ask friends or acquaintances who have had the procedure whether they were satisfied with whomever performed it. Frequently, a "good aspirator" will be associated with a large medical institution.

How do I find out if the pathologist is experienced in diagnosing thyroid cancer?

If you have friends or coworkers who have had thyroid cancer, ask them. Go to the library and check publications such as "Who's Who." Ask the librarians, or if you are proficient at literature searches, find out the names of the pathologists who have published scientific articles on thyroid cancer and fine needle aspiration.

II. During the FNA:

How long will the needle be in my neck?

After inserting the needle and if the lesion is solid, the needle will be withdrawn in two or three seconds. If there is fluid in the lesion, it will take longer (maybe five to eight seconds).

Can I breathe while the doctor performs the procedure?

Yes, you can and should breathe while your doctor performs the procedure. However, you should NOT talk or swallow while the needle is in your neck.

How many "needle-sticks" are recommended to get a good sample?

There is considerable clinical judgment involved by the physician performing the FNA. In general, the size of the nodule or mass will determine the number of aspirates. An average of three needle-sticks should be done in nodules that are 1 to 2 cm in diameter. More aspirates are required for larger masses. If the lesion is cystic (contains fluid) and the first aspirate drains it completely and there is no residual mass palpable, then there is no need for a second needle-stick. If the lesion is firm and solid, then three or more aspirates are desirable to rule out a carcinoma.

III. After the FNA:

Will I need a bandage after the procedure?

No. Most of the time not even a Band-Aid is necessary.

May I drive after undergoing an FNA?

Yes, you may. An FNA is comparable to having blood drawn from your arm.

Will I need a painkiller after the FNA?

Most patients do not need any analgesics after the FNA. Some patients have a very low threshold for pain and take a Tylenol®. Aspirin should be avoided.

Will I be able to exercise or "workout" after the procedure?

Yes, you may exercise or workout after the FNA. You may swim, use a treadmill, etc., but try to avoid heavy weight lifting.

Should I plan on taking the day off from work after the FNA?

You may go back to work after the procedure. There are no restrictions.

What happens after the FNA is performed?

An endocrinologist, surgeon, internist or pathologist may have performed your aspiration. Regardless of who performed the aspiration, the sample obtained will be sent to a pathology laboratory. A laboratory technician will stain the slides, and a cytopathologist will examine them with a microscope and make a cytologic diagnosis. The cytopathologist then will issue a written report to communicate these findings to the physician who sent the slides or who referred you for FNA.

What is a pathology report?

A pathology (or cytopathology) report is a standardized written document that states what was found on the smears. In other words, it is a cytologic diagnosis — the results of your aspiration. Your treatment will depend upon it.

What are the possible cytologic results of the FNA?

Usually the results will fall into one of four categories: benign (70 to 75 percent of cases), malignant (4 to 7 percent), inconclusive (10 to 15 percent), and unsatisfactory (1 to 10 percent). We will explain the meaning of each of these.

What is a benign diagnosis?

This implies that your nodule or lump is not a malignant tumor. It could be due to inflammation (thyroiditis), accumulated secretion from your gland (colloid nodule), irregular growth of your gland (hyperplastic nodule) or a cyst (fluid-filled nodule).

What is a malignant diagnosis?

This implies that your nodule is cancerous. There are several types of thyroidal cancers. The most common and the easiest to treat successfully is papillary carcinoma.

What is an inconclusive diagnosis?

There is no certainty about the nature of your nodule; it could be either benign or malignant. Please make sure this is not confused with a benign diagnosis. This means that it is not possible to determine the nature of your lump. Either the FNA has to be repeated or the possibility of surgery should be discussed with your doctor.

What is an unsatisfactory diagnosis?

Whoever performed the FNA was not successful in obtaining enough cells from your thyroid to allow the pathologist to make a diagnosis. Most likely the doctor just obtained blood. The FNA has to be repeated (preferably by a more experienced aspirator). Please make sure that this is not confused with a benign diagnosis.

What happens next after my FNA is diagnosed as benign?

If your aspirate has been diagnosed as BENIGN, your physician will discuss with you whether you need to be given thyroid medication. Most of the time, if your thyroid function tests (your "blood-work") are normal, you will not require any medication. In other instances, you will need thyroid hormone "suppressive therapy," anti-thyroid drugs or radioactive iodine.

What happens next after my FNA is diagnosed as malignant?

If your aspirate has been diagnosed as MALIGNANT, you will need surgery. The extent of the operation should be discussed with your endocrinologist and surgeon.

What happens next after my FNA is diagnosed as inconclusive?

If your aspirate is INCONCLUSIVE, it may be the result of a scant or limited sample. It is wise to have it repeated by a more experienced physician who may obtain more abundant material. It may be due to lack of experience of the pathologist evaluating the smears. In this case sending the slides for a second opinion might solve the problem. It might occur because the thyroid mass is very cellular. Sometimes there is an overlap in the cytologic appearance of the benign and malignant follicular tumors. In such instances, your physician might consider it appropriate to give you thyroid hormone pills for six to eight months and then repeat the FNA. If the nodule or lesion is large or you cannot tolerate the uncertainty of not having a definite diagnosis, you might decide to undergo surgery.

What happens next after my FNA is diagnosed as unsatisfactory?

If your aspirate is diagnosed as UNSATISFACTORY or is said to be "non-diagnostic," you need another FNA.

What is a false negative diagnosis?

This occurs when the cytology report says that your nodule is benign and subsequent events prove that it was a cancer. This varies from one institution to another and has been reported to occur in 1 percent to 10 percent of FNAs with the frequency linked to the experience of the aspirator and cytopathologist. The drawback of a false negative diagnosis is the delay of treatment.

What is a false positive diagnosis?

This occurs when the cytology report says that your nodule is malignant, but after you undergo surgery, no cancer is found. This also varies with the experience from one institution to another and has been reported to occur in 1 percent to 5 percent of FNAs. The drawback of a false positive diagnosis is that the operation may not have been necessary. This is not the same as a "suspicious for malignancy" diagnosis, which may turn out to be benign with surgery, because the surgery was necessary to remove the entire nodule for definitive diagnosis.

Should I get a second opinion?

You always have the right to a second opinion. You should do this if you wish and if it will help you feel more comfortable. Remember that you must be willing to pay for it because it might not be covered by your medical insurance. If you have been diagnosed with cancer, a second opinion that confirms the diagnosis may make you feel more comfortable.

Why does an FNA have to be repeated?

The most frequent cause for a repeat FNA is a previous UNSATISFACTORY or "non-diagnostic" aspirate. There are other instances in which the FNA needs to be repeated:

- A nodule that enlarges while you are taking thyroid medication (which was prescribed to shrink the nodule)
- Follow-up of a previous inconclusive report
- The appearance of a new nodule
- Finding an enlarged lymph node adjacent to the thyroid gland
- One year follow up for persistent benign nodules.

When laboratory results do not clarify the case for the clinician or appear to be at odds with the clinical picture, they should be repeated.

Could I have cancer that is not detected on FNA?

Yes, because no technique is 100 percent accurate. If your lump is large and there is a small focus of cancer (next to it or in it), the cancer may not be detected.

What are the benefits of having an FNA?

If the nodule is benign, surgery can be avoided. If the nodule is malignant, surgery can be planned promptly and appropriately.

What are the risks, complications or side effects of FNA?

Complications may be immediate or delayed, and these are discussed below. All complications are rare and almost never serious.

What are the immediate complications of FNA?

1. The most commonly reported immediate complication is local bleeding. The patient might notice a bruise or swelling in the neck, with variable degrees of tenderness. This usually disappears in one or two weeks. It is extremely rare that this event may require any medical treatment. I am aware of only one case, aspirated by a surgeon, where severe hemorrhage occurred after a larger blood vessel was damaged and the patient required immediate surgery.

2. Vaso-vagal reaction (fainting). Some patients (particularly men) may faint during the procedure. These are the patients who often also faint when they have blood drawn.

What are the delayed complications of FNA?

Among the **delayed** complications are infection at the site of aspiration and damage to the recurrent laryngeal nerve in the neck.

1. Infection (suppurative thyroiditis) rarely has been reported. The patient may experience severe pain and swelling in the neck accompanied by fever and difficulty in swallowing. This requires prompt treatment with antibiotics prescribed by a physician.

2. The needle may hit the recurrent laryngeal nerve in which case there is immediate sharp pain or the nerve may be damaged either by bleeding or edema after the aspiration. This delayed injury will cause a temporary change in the voice and some hoarseness.

Can cancer cells spread (escape) as a result of the FNA?

Surgeons and patients frequently express their concern about "spread of the malignant cells along the needle tract." Needle aspiration has been in use at Memorial Sloan Kettering Medical Center in New York City for more than 80 years and at Karolinska Hospital in Stockholm for more than 50 years; they have yet to report a single case of such spread.

How much will it hurt after the FNA? Will my neck be sore?

The level of pain during and after the procedure is comparable to that experienced when blood is drawn from a vein in the arm. Usually it is less than that because the needle is thinner. Very few patients report using Tylenol" or an equivalent medication. Please try to avoid aspirin.

What are the recommended steps for someone whose results are reported as inconclusive?

The patient should discuss this interpretation with an endocrinologist. If the physician who ordered the FNA is an internist or family practitioner, I suggest that the patient consult an endocrinologist. If the FNA report is inconclusive because the nodule is cellular but not suspicious of malignancy, then the FNA should be repeated. Some endocrinologists believe that a trial of thyroid hormone therapy with subsequent repeat FNA in six to eight months might be appropriate. It might help to have the smears reviewed by another pathologist (second opinion) with a special interest or training in thyroid diseases who might be able to render a more definite diagnosis. If the diagnosis is "follicular neoplasm," then surgery is indicated.

What is the accuracy rate of FNA?

The rate of accurate results depends on the skill and experience of the physician obtaining the samples and interpreting the smears under the microscope. The results reported in the medical literature vary considerably and may be difficult to interpret accurately.

How long should it take for the results to come back?

Usually the pathologist will report results to the referring physician within 24 to 48 hours. Cases diagnosed as malignant are reported promptly (within 24 hours and by telephone). Then the referring physician has to decide how to convey the results to the patient. Some do it over the telephone, while others prefer to have the patient come to their offices to discuss results in person. Some patients have told me that their endocrinologist has advised them to "make an appointment to see them one week after the FNA." This seems very reasonable to me.

What about a second opinion?

It will vary depending on who requires it. It may be the pathologist, the endocrinologist, the surgeon or the patient. (1) The pathologist may not be absolutely certain of the interpretation or may "suspect cancer" but does not feel able to make a definite diagnosis. (2) The endocrinologist and/or the surgeon may receive a pathology report that does not appear to correspond to the clinical findings. (3) For any reason the patient is uncomfortable with the diagnosis, particularly if possible surgery is involved. Patients must be aware that doctors are not infallible and physicians are NOT God. No procedure or result is correct 100 percent of the time.

To a large extent, the patient may obtain a second opinion if the insurance or the patient is willing to pay for it.

IV. Miscellaneous

Who may perform FNAs?

Any physician who is interested in learning how to perform the procedure properly and who has adequate physical facilities (examining table, sink, counter space, slides, slide-holders, etc.).

Endocrinologists and internists have the advantage in that they can perform the FNA immediately after detecting the lump or nodule. Thus the workup may be more expeditious.

Surgeons should have the advantage of manual dexterity. However, the FNA technique is deceptively simple, and many surgeons are not proficient at it. Thyroids are particularly difficult to aspirate, in contrast to breast lesions. Also, surgeons do not have as many patients with thyroid lesions as the endocrinologists, so they lack practice.

Pathologists have the advantage that they can examine the smears immediately under the microscope and assess the adequacy of the specimen. Hence the rate of unsatisfactory specimens is much smaller. However, there are very few pathologists who are willing to perform this procedure. By training, pathologists are more involved with diagnostic issues rather than interacting with patients. Typically, we are the physicians "invisible to patients."

Radiologists have the advantage of being able to aspirate non-palpable lesions and deeply located masses in the chest and abdominal cavities (lungs, liver, etc). They use ultrasound, computerized tomography, and other imaging techniques to guide the needle to the nodule (that is not detectable by simple examination). However, they are not likely to have sufficiently large numbers of thyroid cases to become proficient at aspirating these nodules.

What makes someone skilled at performing FNAs?

The physician must be genuinely interested in mastering the technique and performing it often enough to gain expertise. As with any other procedure, "practice makes perfect." It is important to have manual dexterity and good "bedside manners" to make the patient feel comfortable. The ultimate measurement of the skill of the aspirator is the rate of unsatisfactory specimens. A 10 percent rate of unsatisfactory samples (which indicate technical failure) should disqualify the physician from continuing to perform aspirations.

How do you know that the cancer has already invaded the lymph nodes?

In 10 percent of patients with thyroid carcinoma the thyroid gland may be normal on palpation. There are no thyroid nodules palpable (or detected). Rather, the cancer may present as a lump in the side of the neck or as a metastasis to a lymph node in the neck. The aspirate of this lateral neck mass usually yields brownish fluid to the naked eye. Microscopic examination will reveal the malignant cells.

Why are some patients diagnosed incorrectly?

Because as hard as we try, physicians are not infallible. The errors can result from sampling problems (too few needle-sticks from a large lesion), unsatisfactory samples (due to poor technique), or errors of interpretation. The examination of smears is very demanding and tedious. The pathologist may not see the malignant cells, or there may be very few malignant cells (for example in cystic papillary carcinoma). In other cases, the technical preparation of the smears may be poor. In some cases, there is an overlap of cytologic patterns (cellular adenomatoid nodule, follicular neoplasm and follicular variant of papillary carcinoma).

I am not worried about the procedure, but I am worried about the results (having cancer). What should I do?

Please remember that most of the time the results are "benign." If the nodule is malignant, the likelihood of total cure may be excellent if diagnosed early. This should be discussed with your endocrinologist.

References:

Wartofsky L. The thyroid nodule. Pathogenesis, evaluation, and risk of malignancy. Wartofsky L. (ed.). Thyroid Cancer. A comprehensive guide to clinical management. Humana Press, New Jersey, 2000, pp1–7.

Oertel YC, Oertel JE: Thyroid Cytology and Histology. In: Meier CA (guest ed.). Thyroid Nodules and Thyroid Cancer. Baillière's Best Practice & Research. Clinical Endocrinology & Metabolism. Holly JMP (ed.-in-chief). Vol. 14, No 4, Harcourt Publishers Ltd., London, UK, 541–557, 2000.

CHAPTER 7

Surgery in Thyroid Cancer
Lisa Boyle, M.D.

Introduction

The overwhelming majority of patients with thyroid cancer will undergo surgery as the initial treatment for their disease. There are four primary goals for the surgical treatment of thyroid cancer. These goals are to:

- Remove the tumor in its entirety,
- Reduce the risks of the cancer recurring (or coming back),
- Facilitate additional treatments (for example, radioactive iodine), and
- Facilitate follow-up care.

Surgery to remove the thyroid (thyroidectomy) is a very effective treatment for eliminating thyroid cancer and serves to facilitate further treatments and follow-up care.

Structure & function

The thyroid is normally a very small gland that sits in the lower mid-portion of the neck and is attached to the underlying trachea (breathing tube). The thyroid is shaped like a butterfly and consists of two halves (or lobes)—one on the right side of the neck and one on the left. Thyroid tissue in the midline, called an *isthmus*, acts as a bridge connecting the two lobes (see figure 1). The thyroid gland is part of the endocrine system and functions in the body by making a hormone called thyroid hormone. Thyroid hormone is essential for the body to function normally. When all or most of the thyroid is removed, a substitute must be taken in the form of a pill to provide the body with the necessary amount of thyroid hormone. This is discussed in more detail in chapter 1.

Choice of operation

The most appropriate operations for patients with differentiated thyroid cancer (i.e. papillary and follicular carcinomas, which are discussed in more detail in

Lobes

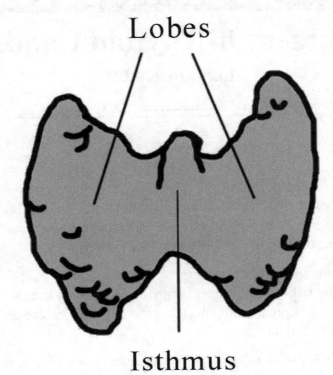

Isthmus

FIGURE 1: The thyroid has two lobes and a connecting isthmus.

chapter 4) remains, even today, a subject of some controversy. The reason for this is that to date there have been no scientific studies that have compared the various surgical treatment options in a way that would allow us to confidently say that one option is better than another. Each of the various surgical treatments has its advantages and disadvantages, and these should be carefully weighed in each patient prior to making a decision.

The following factors need to be taken into consideration when deciding what operative approach should be taken:

- **Size:** How large is the tumor? This can be determined on physical exam and by obtaining an ultrasound evaluation of the gland.
- **Extent of tumor:** Is the tumor confined to one lobe of the gland or side of the neck? Is there evidence of disease in the other lobe?
- **Is there any evidence that the tumor has spread beyond the thyroid to the surrounding lymph nodes of the neck?** Again, this can frequently be determined by physical exam or ultrasound evaluation.
- **Other risk factors:** Has the patient been exposed in the past to radiation to the thyroid area (See chapter 5)? This is known to predispose patients to a form of cancer that tends to affect the entire gland.

Surgical treatment options

The majority of patients with well-differentiated thyroid cancer can be treated successfully with one of two operations:

1. Unilateral lobectomy with isthmusectomy (or hemithyroidectomy)

This is considered to be the least invasive yet still effective operation for thyroid cancer. It involves removal of the lobe of the thyroid in which the tumor lies and the adjoining isthmus (see figure 2). For example, a tumor in the left lobe of the thyroid may be treated with a left lobectomy and isthmusectomy (or left hemithyroidectomy).

INDICATIONS: This operation is *sometimes* recommended if the following criteria are met:

- The tumor is very small or in a very early stage. For example:
  - papillary carcinoma, which is less than 1 to 1.5 cm in greatest diameter
  - follicular carcinoma, which has minimal invasion of the capsule by the tumor, as judged by the pathologists
- No evidence of disease in the lobe that is to be left behind,
- No evidence of tumor in the adjacent lymph nodes, and
- No history of radiation exposure.

What are the advantages of this operation?

This operation is associated with a slightly lower incidence of postoperative complications when compared to a total thyroidectomy. Specifically, the chance of

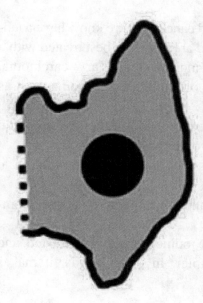

FIGURE 2: Unilateral lobectomy with isthmusectomy (or hemithyroidectomy)

low blood calcium (hypocalcemia) is essentially zero. This is discussed further below.

What are the disadvantages of this operation?

- There is a slightly higher chance of recurrence as time goes on, particularly in the remaining lobe,
- It may make the subsequent treatment with radioactive iodine more difficult,
- Because there is functioning thyroid tissue remaining, it makes the use of measurement of blood levels of thyroglobulin as a tumor marker in follow-up significantly less reliable if not virtually impossible. Thyroglobulin is a protein synthesized in the thyroid gland, and this is discussed in more detail in chapter 2.

2. Total (or near-total) thyroidectomy:

This operation involves removal of virtually all of the thyroid gland. In general, while the chances of long-term survival are very good for most patients, the majority of surgeons who deal with thyroid cancer patients believe that removal of the entire thyroid is the best option in all but a few select patients. While this operation does have a slightly higher risk of complications, these risks are minimal when performed by an experienced surgeon.

INDICATIONS: A total thyroidectomy is usually recommended in the following circumstances:

- The tumor is large. Although the definition of "large" varies, this generally refers to tumors greater than 1.5 to 2 cm.
- The tumor is ne of the several types of thyroid cancer that we know have a tendency to act in a more aggressive manner and are therefore best treated with a total thyroidectomy. Examples of these include medullary carcinoma, anaplastic carcinoma and specific variants of papillary carcinoma such as Tall Cell variant.
- If there is evidence that the cancer has spread outside of the thyroid gland to either the lymph nodes of the neck or to other parts of the body.

What are the advantages of this operation?

- The chance of recurrence is reduced since the thyroid gland has been completely removed,
- The subsequent administration of radioactive iodine therapy is facilitated, and
- This approach makes follow-up care simpler. In other words, it makes detection of recurrence much easier.

What are the disadvantages of this operation?

- Thyroid hormone replacement must be taken life long to support the body's need for thyroid hormone.
- The risk of complications from surgery including damage to the recurrent laryngeal nerve and hypocalcemia are slightly higher than with more limited procedures. This is also discussed further below.

Removal of lymph nodes at the time of thyroid surgery

Because some thyroid cancers will spread (metastasize) to the lymph nodes of the neck, your surgeon may remove the lymph nodes close to the thyroid gland at the time of thyroidectomy. In some cases there is evidence before surgery that the lymph nodes are involved with cancer; however, in many cases this is not obvious until the time of surgery. When surrounding lymph nodes are removed, the operation is called a *modified neck dissection*. After the operation, this area of the neck may be numb for a short period of time. Other than this numbness, there are no long-term effects of having these lymph nodes removed.

Risks of surgery

Thyroid surgery, like any surgery, is associated with risks, and the likelihood of these risks is low. In general, the risks of thyroid surgery include bleeding, infection, injury of the recurrent laryngeal nerve (RLN) and hypoparathyroidism (damage to the parathyroid glands resulting in low calcium levels).

BLEEDING: While bleeding from thyroid surgery can usually be controlled in the operative setting, there are times when bleeding occurs during the postoperative period. The development of a hematoma (a collection of blood) at the site of surgery can indicate ongoing bleeding. If this occurs, an immediate second operation is needed to find and control the source of bleeding. This complication is seen in less than 1 percent of patients undergoing thyroidectomy. It is important to let your doctor know if you have any unusual bleeding tendencies.

INFECTION: Infection is a very rare complication of thyroidectomy. However, this is usually easily treated with antibiotics.

INJURY TO THE RECURRENT LARYNGEAL NERVE (RLN): The most feared complication of thyroid surgery is damage to the recurrent laryngeal nerve (RLN), which can result in a change in the quality of the voice. The RLN runs directly behind the thyroid gland on its way to the vocal cords, which sit inside the larynx (voice box). The RLN gives the vocal cords their power to move and thus is responsible for our ability to speak. Injury to the RLN often is asymptomatic; however, 1 percent of patients who have had a thyroidectomy may experience vocal cord paralysis. This may result in hoarseness of the voice. These changes are usually of a temporary nature but may take up to 12 months to completely recover. In rare circumstances, these changes may be permanent. More subtle changes in the voice may also occur after surgery (for example, not being able to yell, talk loudly or reach high notes when singing), but these are also usually temporary in nature. A corrective procedure called thyroplasty may restore the voice in patients who experience vocal cord paralysis.

LOW CALCIUM LEVELS: A common problem after total (or complete) removal of the thyroid is a low calcium level in the blood. This complication is generally not seen when only one half of the thyroid is removed. This complication occurs because the glands that regulate calcium metabolism in the body are loosely attached to the back of the thyroid gland and need to be left behind as the thyroid is removed. We have four of these glands, which are called parathyroid glands (see figure 3). Two are on the right side and two on the left. They sometimes do not function efficiently in the postoperative period, and when they don't, the calcium level drops in the blood. While most patients have no symptoms from this, occasionally it can result in numbness and tingling around the lips and at the tips of the fingers and toes. Treatment usually involves taking calcium tablets by mouth.

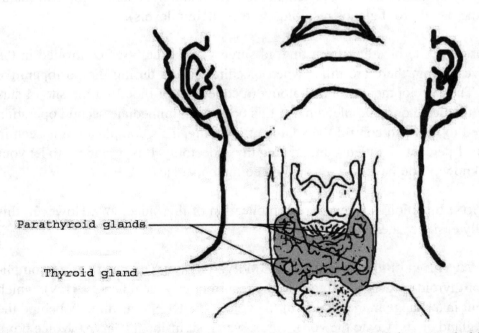

Parathyroid glands
Thyroid gland

FIGURE 3: Four parathyroid glands are typically present, and these are behind the thyroid gland as noted above.

Approximately 10 to 15 percent of patients will be required to take calcium for a brief period of time (2 to 4 weeks) after this operation. In a small number of cases (about 1 percent) this can actually be a permanent problem but is resolved by taking daily calcium tablets indefinitely.

Preoperative preparation

Because you will be having general anesthesia, there are a few simple tests that will be required prior to surgery. Your doctor will order the necessary tests based on your age and other medical problems that you might have. You will also be asked to refrain from eating or drinking anything after midnight the night prior to your surgery. Your doctor will advise you as to what you should do about taking any of your usual medications on the day of the operation.

Length of hospital stay

You will be admitted to the hospital the morning of the surgery. The operation generally lasts approximately two to three hours and is performed under general anesthesia (in other words, you are completely asleep). Most patients stay overnight in the hospital for observation and can be discharged the following morning. Your hospital stay will generally last no more than 1 to 2 days. There is relatively little pain from the surgery, though many people experience a sore throat for 24 hours. The sore throat is due primarily to the breathing (endotracheal) tube inserted by the anesthesiologist rather than to the surgery per se.

Will there be a scar?

Yes, there will be a scar on your neck, as this is the body's only mechanism for healing a wound, and a surgical incision is a wound. The ultimate cosmetic result depends on several factors, and the most important factor is an individual patient's healing characteristics. In general, however, this incision leaves a very acceptable result, and you can discuss this further with your surgeon. It usually takes between six months to a year for the scar to reach a mature stage.

CHAPTER 8

Low Iodine Diet

Kenneth D. Burman, M.D.

Low iodine diet

Adherence to a low iodine diet is generally regarded by thyroid cancer specialists to be extremely important to ensure that the diagnostic radioactive iodine scan is optimal and that radioiodine therapy will be maximally effective. Iodine is a chemical element found in a variety of foods and chemical agents, such as radiologic (X-ray) contrast dye. In its non-radioactive form, iodine has a molecular weight of 127. Physicians refer to this element as ^{127}I. Nature and humans have modified this substance into additional forms that are used for the diagnosis and treatment of clinical disease. Any form of iodine except ^{127}I is considered radioactive, which means it gives off radiation that can be measured or detected and used diagnostically or therapeutically. The medical use of radioactive iodine was discovered in the 1930s and was first used in humans in the 1940s. The most commonly used agent for treatment and follow-up scans in thyroid cancer patients is ^{131}I. It is also used in the treatment of patients with hyperthyroidism. Another form of the element, ^{123}I, can be used for thyroid scans, historically in patients without thyroid cancer and for determining thyroid uptake (a measure of thyroid function).

The thyroid gland handles all iodine molecules, including ^{131}I, ^{123}I, and "regular" non-radioactive ^{127}I, in the same way. That is, the thyroid gland is able to trap all forms of iodine and use them for thyroid hormone synthesis.

The thyroid gland cannot tell the difference between iodine molecules that will help it synthesize thyroid hormone (^{127}I) and those that will harm or destroy it (e.g., ^{131}I). The purpose of radioactive iodine therapy with ^{131}I is to be taken up by the thyroid gland and destroy it.

The major source of non-radioactive iodine for the thyroid gland is from the diet and the actual metabolic breakdown of the thyroid hormones. Under normal functioning conditions, the thyroid gland traps about 10 to 30 percent per day of the circulating iodine that is available to it. The normal thyroid gland contains approximately five to 10 milligrams (mg) of iodine, much of which is stored as the two thyroid hormones—thyroxine (T4) or triiodothyronine (T3).

Patients with thyroid cancer who are prepared for ^{131}I therapy will have had most or all of their thyroid gland removed surgically. Therefore, they will have a much lower percentage of iodine uptake, typically ranging from less than 1 to perhaps 10 percent, because most of the thyroid tissue has been removed, and there is very little left to take up the iodine. As will be explained below, ^{131}I scanning and treatment are most effective in a state of iodine deficiency, in other words, low circulating ^{127}I.

Any excess non-radioactive iodine available to the thyroid tissue will compete to get into the thyroid tissue, with both the radioactive and non-radioactive iodine on equal footing. But since the pool of non-radioactive iodine is enormous—and available to the thyroid gland at a ratio of about a million non-radioactive iodine molecules for every one radioactive iodine molecule—less radioactive iodine will be taken up by the thyroid gland. In fact, the radioactive iodine uptake frequently will be less than 1 percent.

In healthy people, the amount of non-radioactive iodine ingested daily in food, drink or medications equals the amount ultimately excreted in the urine. For example, if a person ingests 500 micrograms of iodine daily, he or she will discharge about 500 micrograms in the urine within the next 24 hours. Therefore, measuring urine iodine content can reasonably accurately reflect the average daily dietary consumption of iodine. A single random urine sample is adequate for this assessment in thyroid cancer patients because only an estimate is needed. The measurement is usually reported as micrograms per liter, and this value reflects daily intake because most patients excrete about a liter of urine daily. It is preferable to express the urine iodine excretion as mcg/g of creatinine. While clearly not performed at all medical centers, at the Washington Hospital Center we believe that every thyroid cancer patient being prepared for a radioactive scan or treatment should have a urine iodine measurement.

In the United States, people tend to ingest about 200 to 600 micrograms of iodine daily. Therefore, the urine measurement of iodine per person would be about 200 to 600 micrograms per day. The purpose of a low iodine diet is to decrease the amount of non-radioactive iodine available to be taken up by the thyroid gland. As a result, the thyroid gland will trap a greater proportion of the radioactive iodine, making the therapy more effective. It is only the amount of radioactive iodine that actually gets into the thyroid gland that determines effectiveness, not the amount taken orally. Adherence to a low iodine diet for about 2 to 4 weeks will decrease the urine iodine to less than 100 to 200 micrograms per day.

Because of the high iodine content in X-ray dyes, patients who have undergone tests such as a CT scan with contrast, cardiac angiogram or kidney intravenous pyelogram (IVP) will have been exposed to more than 100,000 micrograms of iodine, resulting in extremely high levels of iodine in the urine for the next two to three months. Over time, some of this iodine will be stored in the thyroid gland and gradually released into the circulation while the majority will be excreted in the urine. It takes an estimated six to eight weeks or longer for iodine levels in the urine to return to normal. In order to determine when a radioactive scan or treatment might be most optimally performed, the urine should be measured to determine exactly when this excess iodine load has been dissipated.

Let's consider a typical patient with thyroid cancer who is being prepared for a radioactive iodine scan or treatment. Before starting the low iodine diet, the patient would be ingesting and excreting about 200 to 600 micrograms of iodine daily. Adherence to the low iodine diet would decrease this person's iodine intake to less than 100 micrograms daily. In a few weeks the urine iodine would also drop to less than 100 micrograms per day or even lower than 50. This scenario assumes that the patient has not recently undergone a CT with contrast or other scan that would have exposed him or her to a large iodine load.

A normal person's thyroid gland will trap about 10 to 30 percent of the administered radioactive iodine dose. A patient who has had a thyroidectomy will have less thyroid tissue. As a result, his or her remaining thyroid tissue will have less ability to trap iodine, perhaps operating at just 1 to 10 percent of normal capacity. This thyroid tissue seeks out and traps any type of iodine, regardless of whether it is radioactive or non-radioactive. The important principle is that the thyroid tissue will trap radioactive and non-radioactive iodine with equal avidity. When a patient adheres to a low iodine diet, of perhaps 100 micrograms or less a day as compared with perhaps 500 micrograms under normal circumstances, the thyroid gland has less access to non-radioactive iodine and therefore will take up a higher percentage of the radioactive iodine. Thus the radioactive iodine has a greater chance of being effective.

A patient preparing for a radioactive scan or treatment should therefore avoid food and medicines that contain significant amounts of iodine. Among the types of food to avoid include iodized salt, sea salt, dairy products, seafood, others products from the sea, red dye #3, and processed, packaged or preserved canned foods. (See Table 1). It is critically important to read the labels of all foods to avoid those that contain iodized salt or other ingredients containing iodine. Even water may contain iodine as it is known to help kill bacteria and, therefore, distilled water is more desirable. Potassium iodate, a commonly used preservative in flour, pastry food or mixes, also should be avoided. Fresh fish and certain medications, particularly those that contain red food dyes, may contain large amounts of iodine, and kelp, seaweed, and cod liver oil should be avoided. In addition, some foods that are moderate in iodine (rather than low or high) should be eaten only in moderation.

TABLE 1
Food Items that Contain Significant Amounts of Iodine

Food Items	Avoid	Permitted
Drinks	Milk, hot chocolate, sodas with red dye #3	Coffee, tea, fruit juices, wine, beer, most sodas
Breads	Commercial products with iodate conditioners	Moderate amounts of plain cooked cereal and homemade bread products
Poultry and Red Meat	Canned and processed; read labels on fresh meats	Fresh, unsalted
Fruits	Canned or processed	Fresh fruits
Vegetables	Canned or preserved	Most fresh vegetables
Dairy products	All	None
Miscellaneous	Pickles, soy sauce, ketchup (read labels)	Non-preserved herbs and spices

This table has been adapted from information found on the ThyCa: Thyroid Cancer Survivors' Association Web site and the National Institutes of Health. The information is intended as a guide and is not meant to be all-inclusive. For more information and a free downloadable cookbook, visit the ThyCa Website at www.thyca.org.

For an authoritative resource used by physicians, please see other reference sources, such as "Principles and Practice of Endocrinology and Metabolism," Third Edition, edited by KL Becker, 2002, JB Lippincott Co. You may also obtain more information from the organization "The Light of Life Foundation." Their website is www.lightoflifefoundation.org, and a low iodine "cookbook" is available.

The Manischewitz Company, according to Deborah Ross, does not use iodized salt in its plant in Jersey City where all the matzo, crackers, meal products, and cake mixes are made. No iodized salt is used in the plant that makes its gefilte fish, canned soups, jarred soups, borscht, and shav. This is also true for Matzo Ball Mix, Matzo Ball, and Soup Mix plus Pilaf Mixes, potato based mixes plus a number of other items.

It is best to avoid foods whenever you are not sure of the iodine content. Even though this diet is relatively limited (and some would say bland and not exciting), it must be followed for only two to four weeks and will aid in the effectiveness of the radioactive iodine therapy. Many patients find it a rewarding challenge to adhere to this diet. It is possible to eat at a restaurant as long as you find out how a given meal is prepared, even to the point of asking to talk to the chef. Most restaurants are eager to please their customers and willing to prepare a dish with any requested modifications.

While adhering to a low iodine diet, patients should weigh themselves frequently and drink allowed fluids to prevent dehydration. Judgment should be used as to when the diagnostic scan or therapy is scheduled. Medical necessities must be met, but in general it is best to schedule the diagnostic scan or therapy at a time that does not coincide with vacations, business trips or family events such as a birthday or wedding. Many patients like to avoid scans during the holidays.

Patients are instructed to start the low iodine diet about two weeks before the diagnostic scan and continue it until after the radioactive iodine therapy. They may resume a normal diet after they are discharged from the hospital, usually the day after the radioactive iodine therapy.

Each of the issues just noted should be discussed with the health care team.

More about iodine

Iodine exists everywhere in the environment: in food, water, chemicals, and medications. Iodine is essential for life, and healthy adults are advised to take in at least 150 micrograms of iodine daily. Anyone deficient in iodine for several months may develop goiter or hypothyroidism. Newborns whose mothers were significantly deficient in iodine may display goiters and profound hypothyroidism including mental retardation. It is only during select circumstances such as preparation for ^{131}I therapy in a thyroid cancer patient that a low iodine diet during a short period of time is useful. Under most circumstances, no one should remain on this diet for more than a few weeks, but exceptions may be made for patients with persistent residual tumor that may require frequently repeated radioisotope scans and treatments.

Excess exogenous iodine, from food, water, chemicals, and medications, must be avoided to maximize the radioactive iodine effectiveness.

Radio contrast agents, which include intravenous radio contrast dyes used for CT and IVP scans, should be avoided for at least eight weeks and possibly longer before the scan or treatment (See Table 2). Angiographic dyes used for coronary or cardiac catheterization should also be avoided, although medical necessity may take precedence. Whenever there is a question relating to continued iodine excess in a patient, the most accurate method of determining whether to proceed with ^{131}I is to measure urine iodine to assure it is appropriate.

Dyes, contrast agents or radiopharmaceuticals used for Magnetic Resonance Imaging (MRI) or Positron Emission Tomography (PET) scans do not contain iodine and can be used during a low iodine diet. However, a PET scan does use radioactivity, and this in itself might interfere with a radioactive iodine scan. The radiation injected for a PET scan typically remains in the body for several hours and therefore should not be performed within 24 hours of a thyroid scan. Any questions should be discussed with your attending physician or nuclear medicine physician.

Amiodarone is a drug used for the treatment of some irregular heartbeats (arrhythmias). It has grown in popularity recently because of its proven effectiveness. However, this agent contains a significant amount of iodine, and it usually cannot be discontinued because of its beneficial cardiac effects. Amiodarone therapy will completely inhibit the ability to treat a patient with radioactive iodine. Even if it can be stopped, it takes months or years for the iodine to decrease sufficiently to allow radioactive iodine therapy. Patients requiring administration of a radio contrast agent or medication such as Amiodarone must weigh with their physicians the importance of continuing with their current therapies versus treating the thyroid cancer in a reasonable time frame.

TABLE 2
Iodine Content of Radio Contrast Dyes and Drugs or Medications

Agent	Use	Total iodine dose (mg)*
Ipodate, Telepaque	Hyperthyroidism	1650–6300
Diatrizoate, Iodamide	CAT scans, angiograms	540–4200
Metrizamide	Myelogram (study of the spinal cord)	450–4200
Amiodarone	Treat cardiac arrhythmias	75–300/daily
Potassium iodide	Cough medications	90–3900/daily
Iodide	Prenatal vitamins	15/tablet
Iodide	Kelp tablets	At least 15/tablet
Lugol' solution, SSKI	Treat hypothyroidism	378–760/daily
Povidone iodine (Betadine)	Skin antiseptic	Varies (about 10–100)

*(Note: There are 1000 ug (micrograms) in 1 mg (milligram.))

The data in this table are estimates adapted from Nuovo and Wartofsky, chapter 37, in "Principles and Practice of Endocrinology and Metabolism," Third Edition, edited by K.L. Becker, J.B. Lippincott Co, 2002.

CHAPTER 9

Withdrawal of Thyroid Hormones

Kenneth D. Burman, M.D.

Withdrawal of thyroid hormone in patients with well-differentiated thyroid cancer

As explained in chapters 1 and 2, blood TSH levels increase in hypothyroidism and a high TSH level is necessary to stimulate sufficient uptake of radioactive iodine to perform a scan or treatment in patients who have well-diferentiated thyroid cancer. Consequently, patients taking levothyroxine (T4) therapy must discontinue use of this medication before undergoing the isotope scan or treatment. There are several ways to accomplish this task. The first is simply to stop the levothyroxine and wait about five to six weeks before performing the scan or treatment. This period of time is necessary because of the half-life of T4, which is about seven days. This means that every seven days the level of serum T4 in the body decreases by half, so that after five to six half lives the serum T4 level would be less than 1 microgram per deci-liter (ug/dl) (normal total T4 is 4-8 ug/dl). Of course, the serum TSH should respond by increasing, and it is important to document that the TSH is elevated prior to administering radioiodine. We would prefer that the TSH be greater than an arbitrary level of 40 uU/ml and the serum total T4 should be less than 1 ug/dl or free T4 less than 0.1 ng/dl (normal free T4 is 0.8-1.8 ng/dl). Some clinicians prefer a slightly lower TSH level such as 25 or 30. Generally, it is necessary to document only that the TSH level is adequately elevated.

In rare circumstances, especially before the first scan or treatment and after the initial thyroidectomy has been performed, the TSH may not rise to greater than 40 uU/ml. One explanation for this observation is that the patient had inadvertently taken thyroid medication when he or she was supposed to have discontinued it. Other causes are that significant thyroid tissue remains after the initial surgery such that this tissue is making enough thyroid hormone to keep the blood levels of T4 and T3 normal. As a result, the TSH is suppressed and does not rise. In extremely unusual circumstances, a patient may have metastatic thyroid cancer that will synthesize and release enough thyroid hormone to prevent the TSH from rising.

For patients who have had a thyroidectomy, have had a previous ablation or treatment with ^{131}I, and have been on levothyroxine chronically, the physicians have two options for withdrawing levothyroxine. The first method is to stop levothyroxine and wait five to six weeks for TSH levels to rise before conducting the scan or treatment. The disadvantage of this approach is that as the serum T4 levels gradually decrease over the six-week period, the patient becomes increasingly hypothyroid with more symptoms becoming manifest. The alternative method for rendering patients hypothyroid in preparation for a ^{131}I therapy or whole body scan, and the one which most patients prefer, is to discontinue their levothyroxine (LT4) six weeks before the isotope administration and then substitute a shorter acting thyroid preparation with the brand name Cytomel® (T3), the active thyroid hormone. In practice, LT4 is stopped one day and T3 is started the next in a typical dose of 25 micrograms twice daily. The LT4 is stopped about six weeks prior to the scan, and the Cytomel® is taken for about four weeks. Cytomel® is then stopped for about two weeks prior to the scan. Because Cytomel® has a shorter half-life of only 24 to 30 hours, the patient can take this medication until about 10 days prior to the isotope administration. This regimen has the advantage of potentially keeping the patient "euthyroid" and thus feeling less hypothyroid for a longer time period. Cytomel® may keep patients feeling better especially during weeks three to five of thyroxine withdrawal. But after the T3 is discontinued, patients rapidly will manifest hypothyroid symptoms and the TSH will rise. In general, the hypothyroidism may appear several days after stopping Cytomel®.

Cytomel® itself has potential disadvantages such as causing a fast heart rate, nervousness, anxiety and, in rare circumstances, cardiac arrhythmias. These symptoms result because levels of serum T3 may actually increase above the normal range for part of the day. It is virtually impossible to maintain a constant blood level of T3 and TSH throughout the day because the T3 half-life is so rapid. This short half-life allows T3 to be used in the special circumstance of preparing a patient for ^{131}I, but this quality also becomes a disadvantage when using Cytomel® chronically. Cytomel®, in fact, should not be used for chronic treatment of hypothyroidism in thyroid cancer patients. In preparation for a radioiodine whole body scan, the typical dose of 25 micrograms of T3 twice a day is arbitrary, is occasionally excessive, and may need to be altered in selected patients, especially those with cardiac disease.

One specific schedule of activities in preparing a patient for a scan is as follows: If a patient just had an initial thyroidectomy, we would either start Cytomel® or keep the patient off all thyroid medications. If the patient is taking levothyroxine (LT4) chronically, we would switch to Cytomel®. Starting six weeks before the scan or treatment, the patient would stop LT4 and start on 25 micrograms of Cytomel® twice a day. Two weeks before the scan or treatment the patient would stop taking Cytomel® and start on a low iodine diet. Two or three days before the scan we would obtain lab studies to include a complete blood count (CBC), comprehensive metabolic profile (CMP), beta hCG (pregnancy test in all women with childbearing potential) and TSH. We would also test for serum thyroglobulin, as this withdrawal determination will be very useful in assessing the presence of residual disease (see chapter 10). Finally, we would obtain a random urine sample for iodine (see chapter 8). These tests must be completed and the results appropriate before we administer the isotope. In selected circumstances, when the TSH is not greater than 40 uU/ml, we will obtain a serum free T4 and total T3. Results of the urine iodine test may take several days to return depending on the laboratory used, so while we do not insist on the results returning before an isotope scan, we prefer having the results before the isotope treatment. The serum beta hCG (sensitive pregnancy test) must be negative prior to any isotope administration. Since the beta hCG is not a perfect test for detecting pregnancy, a patient of childbearing potential must fill out a questionnaire substantiating the fact that she is not pregnant. (The issues surrounding the administration of ^{131}I during very early pregnancy are beyond the scope of this chapter.) The purpose of the CBC and CMP are to make sure that the patient is not anemic and that the white blood cell count is appropriate, as previous ^{131}I therapy can cause bone marrow suppression. The CMP is helpful to ensure that the patient does not have low sodium (which can occur with hypothyroidism) or other problems with electrolytes or renal or liver disease.

The serum thyroglobulin level allows a more accurate assessment of the patient's residual thyroid tissue. If the serum thyroglobulin level is elevated, especially if it is unexpected, then we may consider obtaining additional radiologic tests, such as MRI or ultrasound of the neck and a chest CT without contrast (see chapter 16) in order to detect residual disease in the neck or metastatic deposits. This information may be useful in selected patients to allow a better assessment of whether ^{131}I therapy should be performed as planned or whether biopsy or surgery should be performed.

Once a patient has completed the scan or isotope treatment, he or she is restarted either on LT4 alone or a combination of LT4 and Cytomel® (T3). In most patients, particularly those under age 50, a full replacement dose of LT4 is started. In older or other selected patients, LT4 therapy is typically started at half of the regular dose for several days and then increased to the same dose that the patient was taking two months before the scan, and which caused an appropriately suppressed TSH. Great care is taken to individualize the process of restarting thyroid hormone because sudden elevations in blood levels of T4 and T3 may cause adverse effects in some patients. For example, an elderly patient with known cardiovascular disease should have his or her LT4 started very slowly to try to avoid cardiac arrhythmias or angina. This process is a balancing act between trying to restore the blood levels of T4 and T3 to a reasonable range to treat the symptoms of hypothyroidism while trying to avoid potential cardiac side effects.

Some clinicians will restore thyroid hormones by using a combination of T4 and T3. No single regimen is accepted, and physicians debate whether the combination of T4 and T3 restores normalcy faster than LT4 alone. If the physician and patient decide to try a combination T4 and T3, then a reasonable approach is to start half of the T4 dose that was previously shown to suppress TSH and 25 micrograms of Cytomel® twice a day. This combination is continued for 3 to 7 days, at which time the Cytomel® is stopped and the T4 dose is increased to the full dose.

There are two reasons for adding T3 for a short time when LT4 therapy is resumed. The first is to restore euthyroidism and reduce symptoms of hypothyroidism more quickly. The second reason relates to the concern that TSH may be stimulating growth of residual cancer cells, and therefore it might be beneficial to reduce the serum TSH as quickly as possible. T3 theoretically will do this more efficiently than will LT4 alone. However, neither approach is more medically correct than the other nor shown to be associated with a better outcome.

We typically restart thyroid hormone and institute a normal iodine diet immediately following a diagnostic scan, assuming the patient is not going to be treated with radioiodine, or one to two days after ^{131}I therapy.

Even after thyroid hormone therapy is restarted the patient will not immediately become free of symptoms of hypothyroidism. This is a gradual process as the thyroid hormone levels in the body's tissues are replenished. Some patients will feel much better within several days to a week, but it may require one to two months or more before they feel completely normal. Since the half-life of T4 is about seven days, it will take about four to six weeks for the serum thyroid hormone levels to rise and suppress TSH. That is why serum measurements of free T4 and TSH are measured six weeks after restarting LT4 therapy and only after this time period is the dose of LT4 modified in order to achieve the desired TSH value. Some patients need more than one dose adjustment over a period of several months.

Hypothyroidism

Weakness, lethargy, cold intolerance, paleness, dry skin, coarse hair, and constipation can occur with hypothyroidism (see Table 1). Other symptoms may include delayed reflexes (such as the knee jerk when the knee is hit with a reflex hammer), brittle nails, increased blood pressure, and a slow heart rate. Given that most patients with thyroid cancer will be hypothyroid for only about six weeks in preparation for an isotope scan or treatment, the manifestations of these symptoms will typically be minimal to moderate. Some patients will feel relatively well except for tiredness. Some patients will feel extremely fatigued. However, older patients have greater hypothyroid manifestations, and some patients will have a difficult time performing daily tasks. Thus, as a precaution, all patients who are hypothyroid should avoid making important decisions and driving or operating heavy machinery for one to two weeks before and after the scan or treatment. It is not true, despite the impressions that may be given in the lay media and press, that hypothyroidism is associated with significant weight gain. Indeed, in thyroid cancer patients undergoing withdrawal scans, only a few pounds of increased weight may occur, mainly due to water accumulation rather than fat. Once the patient is restored to normal thyroid levels, his or her weight should return to the level that it was prior to the withdrawal period.

TABLE 1
Manifestations of Hypothyroidism

Organ/Tissue	Sign/Symptoms
Skin/Hair	Dry, cold, pale, rough skin, brittle hair, hair loss.
Gastrointestinal	Decreased taste, constipation
Lungs	Shortness of breath
Blood	Anemia, increased bleeding tendency (slight)
Muscles/Nerves	Weakness, difficulty walking, difficulty concentrating, decreased attention span, muscle cramps.
Cardiac	Slow heart rate
Voice	Hoarness

Although we list here multiple possible signs or symptoms of hypothyroidism, in many patients few symptoms occur in the time required to prepare for a radioactive scan or treatment or during the weeks afterward restarting thyroid hormone. This list refers mainly to prolonged hypothyroidism, such as if a patient with thyroid cancer and a previous thyroidectomy did not take his or her medications for several months. This situation can be extremely dangerous and must be avoided, both to avoid unnecessarily prolonged hypothyroidism and undesirably prolonged possible stimulation of residual tumor cells by high TSH levels.

However, patients experience a wide spectrum of symptoms during their period of temporary hypothyroidism. A few patients feel the same as before. The great majority feel considerably slowed down, both physically and mentally. Some describe it as feeling mildly sedated. They can converse and do household chores, but their reaction times are slower. They are also more prone to errors when doing tasks involving attention to details. A few patients feel more severe symptoms from among those described above. The time of recovery from the symptoms of hypothyroidism also varies from weeks to months, and this at least in part depends on how long it takes to appropriately adjust the dose of thyroid hormone.

CHAPTER 10

Thyrogen®

Leonard Wartofsky, M.D.

As described in several of the chapters above, the routine management of a patient with thyroid cancer has included thyroidectomy followed by radioiodine ablation and thyroxine suppression of endogenous thyroid stimulating hormone (TSH). Longer-term follow up is designed to detect any residual or recurrent tumor and treat it before it grows further. The two important diagnostic mainstays to detect recurrence are performance of nuclear scans and measurement of the tumor marker, thyroglobulin (Tg), in blood. Both performance of a scan and optimal measurement of serum Tg require the patient to have a high serum TSH level. Prior to the year 2000, TSH elevation was achieved routinely by discontinuation of thyroxine therapy, rendering the patient hypothyroid in order to elevate serum TSH sufficiently to perform a whole body scan to detect residual or metastatic disease. When they are hypothyroid, patients will feel tired and sluggish, and have difficulty concentrating; dry skin and hair; declining memory; fluid retention with swelling (edema) of the legs, hands or face; constipation; menstrual irregularity; weight gain; and intolerance to low temperatures. The period of hypothyroidism might extend from three to six weeks or more, and the symptoms associated with this hypothyroidism are arguably the worst part of having a periodic evaluation. Use of Thyrogen® (a form of "synthetic" TSH) will allow a patient to avoid all of the above symptoms of hypothyroidism, for while Thyrogen® testing is occurring, the patient continues to take thyroxine replacement medication regularly. In addition to the symptomatic hypothyroidism after thyroxine withdrawal, some physicians have worried that the prolonged period of weeks of TSH elevation might have a stimulatory effect on the growth of any tumor that might be present.

Because the only source of serum Tg is from thyroid cells (there is none in thyroxine pills or thyroid hormone replacement therapy), measurement of serum Tg after thyroidectomy and remnant ablation serves as a potential marker for residual or recurrent tumor, and the magnitude of the serum Tg level reflects both the ability of the tumor to produce Tg as well as the volume or mass of tissue remaining. Detection of thyroid tumor by measurement of Tg is most sensitive when the TSH is elevated, a state that up until recently was achieved only after thyroxine withdrawal rendered patients hypothyroid. Thyroid cells producing Tg might be remaining in the neck near the original location of the thyroid gland prior to surgery, or they might be almost anywhere in the body, having spread (metastasized) via the bloodstream or lymphatic system. A rising Tg level in the blood provides your doctor with evidence of possible tumor somewhere, and the radioactive iodine whole body scan allows the site of the tumor cells to be localized and identified.

The recent availability of recombinant human TSH (rhTSH, Thyrogen®, thyrotropin alfa for injection) has radically altered routine follow-up evaluations for residual or recurrent disease of patients after their initial management by thyroidectomy and radioiodine ablation. Thyrogen® is TSH, which has been developed by the Genzyme Corporation and is virtually identical to TSH produced by the pituitary gland in your own body. So, just like the patient's own TSH derived from the pituitary while hypothyroid, Thyrogen® will stimulate any remaining thyroid cells to produce Tg and release it into the blood and to trap radioactive iodine out of the blood when it is given for a diagnostic scan or for a therapy.

Research has shown that administration of Thyrogen® improves sensitivity of thyroglobulin (Tg) testing to detect residual cancer cells and that iodine scans done after Thyrogen® stimulation are comparable to the diagnostic utility of iodine scans performed after thyroxine withdrawal. Consequently, the use of Thyrogen® has become a safe and effective alternative to thyroid hormone withdrawal in the detection of recurrent or residual thyroid cancer, and its use as an adjunct for diagnostic testing in patients with thyroid cancer is enabling physicians to limit the morbidity of hypothyroidism that has been traditionally associated with periodic monitoring. Indeed, based on the research, some experts in the field have suggested that there may be little need to do withdrawal of thyroxine any more, and that Thyrogen® scanning and Tg measurement would suffice in virtually all patients.

As this book goes to press, further studies and more extensive clinical experience are underway that are likely to fully delineate the role for this exciting new agent in the detection and treatment of thyroid cancer and other thyroid conditions. At the present time, however, there are several ways that your doctor might use Thyrogen®. First, because TSH stimulation is a more sensitive way to uncover Tg production from thyroid cells than simply measuring Tg while a patient is still taking their thyroxine, the option is then to either withdraw the thyroxine and make the patient hypothyroid with a high TSH or to administer synthetic TSH (Thyrogen®). Many patients who have had this done both ways prefer having the diagnostic studies done with Thyrogen® and thereby avoiding the effects of hypothyroidism.

The typical protocol for Thyrogen® testing is to monitor the serum Tg before and after Thyrogen® and perform a radioiodine scan after Thyrogen®. The radioactive iodine dosage used for the scan is typically 4 millicuries (mCi), which is a diagnostic dose that has been shown to provide a scan comparable to that achieved by withdrawal of thyroxine. After drawing the basal blood for Tg, Thyrogen® is administered by intramuscular injection on that day and again the following day. The 4 mCi dose of radioactive iodine is given on the next day, and the patient is scanned and a second blood drawn for Tg measurement is done 48 hours (2 days) later. The most common procedure is as follows:

Monday	Blood drawn for Tg
	Thyrogen® injection 0.9 milligrams
Tuesday	Thyrogen® injection 0.9 milligrams
Wednesday	4 mCi dose of radioactive iodine
Thursday	No procedures
Friday	Blood drawn for Tg
	Whole body scan

There are very few possible side effects from the administration of Thyrogen®. In the 48 hours or so after injection, a small percentage of patients have reported some transient lightheadedness, dizziness, headache, nausea, and very rarely vomiting. Some of the symptoms may be on a psycho-physiologic basis due to the stress of undergoing the studies. The Thyrogen® is injected by a needle into the muscle of your upper arm, thigh or buttock, and there can be a little pain, redness or itching at the site of the injection, but this is very temporary.

Something to be considered in electing to have Thyrogen® stimulation rather than undergo withdrawal is the cost of the Thyrogen®. It is rather expensive, and some insurance plans will resist paying for it unless the indications are clear. One such indication is when a patient may have an underlying other medical condition that makes superimposition of hypothyroidism after withdrawal more dangerous to their overall health. Another reason might be because there is concomitant pituitary disease from some cause totally unrelated to the history of thyroid cancer, but it is of such a nature that the pituitary will not produce sufficient TSH after thyroxine withdrawal to stimulate Tg production or radioiodine uptake for a scan or treatment. In such cases, administration of Thyrogen® is both indicated and a salvation for performing the required diagnostic studies. Most insurance plans, Medicare, and Medicaid generally cover the costs of Thyrogen®. However, it would be a good idea for you to check with your insurance carrier before undergoing the studies. The manufacturer of Thyrogen®, Genzyme Therapeutics, maintains a resource hotline (1-800-745-4447) that may be able to tell you whether your insurance provider will cover your costs. If you discover that the cost is not covered, you should inform your endocrinologist who may be able to help you appeal this decision.

Most well-differentiated thyroid cancers can be cured if the management is consistent with recommended approaches of total thyroidectomy and radioiodine ablation as indicated, and close periodic monitoring for recurrent or residual disease by scanning and measurement of thyroglobulin. With the availability of Thyrogen®, we now are able to detect disease with greater sensitivity and at an earlier time, because evaluation has been made relatively simple compared with the past when patients may have been reluctant to undergo thyroxine withdrawal.

Essentially all of the discussion of the use of Thyrogen® above has been in the context of diagnosis, that is, looking for tumor. Studies are currently underway to examine the efficacy of Thyrogen® for therapy as well. Such use would include Thyrogen® administration prior to radioiodine treatment for either or both the initial ablation and for subsequent therapies for persistent disease. If the data being collected now support efficacy of Thyrogen® for therapy purposes that is comparable to that seen after thyroxine withdrawal, patients with thyroid cancer may never again have to undergo the misery of having to be hypothyroid.

CHAPTER 11

The Role of Various Physicians, Specialists, and Second Opinions

Kenneth D. Burman, M.D.

The role of the primary care physician

The primary care physician, who can be the family practitioner, internist or obstetrician/gynecologist, plays a critical role in managing the patient with thyroid cancer. Initially the primary care physician will examine the neck closely to detect a thyroid nodule, goiter or cervical lymphadenopathy. A careful history will focus on signs or symptoms related to possible thyroid masses or thyroid dysfunction. If the primary care physician is familiar with modern methods of diagnosing thyroid cancer and the case is uncomplicated, then the primary care physician can perform initial evaluation of a patient with one or more thyroid nodules. He or she can work closely with an experienced thyroid cytologist, nuclear medicine physician and nuclear radiologist. If the primary care physician is less familiar with the modern methods of evaluating a thyroid nodule or thyroid cancer, then the primary care physician will usually refer the patient to an endocrinologist.

Once the diagnosis of thyroid cancer is made and after the patient's surgery, the endocrinologist will typically arrange the radioiodine scans and other procedures. The endocrinologist will work closely with the primary care physician to help arrange these tests as well as to plan the routine thyroid tests and, for patients with well-differentiated thyroid cancer, the measurement of thyroglobulin levels. After the first year of follow-up, the primary care physician will usually assume more responsibility for care, and the endocrinologist may see the patient two to three times a year and arrange the follow-up radiologic tests. Over time, as it becomes clear that there is little likelihood of any residual cancer, the primary care physician will see the patient more frequently, and the endocrinologist will become less involved. These guidelines may be altered depending on the patient's overall condition and the arrangement between the primary care physician and the endocrinologist.

The role of the endocrinologist

The endocrinologist will typically take primary responsibility for care during the first one to two years after the diagnosis of thyroid cancer. The endocrinologist will determine the timing of both the isotope studies and the periodic physical examinations and radiologic studies. In patients for whom the evidence of any disease subsides, the primary care physician will assume more responsibility for care. The cooperative arrangement between the primary care physician and the endocrinologist will vary based on their relationship and the clinical context. Nonetheless, close cooperation among the entire health care team is very important.

The role of the nuclear medicine physician or nuclear radiologist

Typically the nuclear medicine physician or nuclear radiologist will be a supporting member of the team of physicians performing and interpreting the nuclear medicine scans and X-rays as well as performing the radioiodine therapies in patients with well-differentiated thyroid cancer. However, the level of participation of the nuclear medicine physician or nuclear radiologist may also vary and is dependent upon the relationship of the physicians, the clinical context and the qualifications of the physicians. Some nuclear medicine physicians or nuclear radiologists will evaluate, manage and treat patients with thyroid cancer, and some endocrinologists will perform the radioiodine therapies. This may depend in part on the geography or locale in which the patient resides and the availability of specialists in more rural areas as opposed to major cities with larger hospitals and more specialists.

When to get a second opinion.

Whenever a patient desires a second opinion, he or she should get one. Patients and their families should feel comfortable visiting other doctors regardless of the original physician's experience or medical background. Patients with complex cases may find it particularly reassuring to get a second opinion. The more knowledge and discussion that occurs regarding an individual case the more likely an optimal treatment plan will be devised and an informed decision made.

However, decisions can be difficult, and more than one course of diagnosis or treatment may be appropriate. Although it is possible that a second opinion may lead to more confusion on the patient's part, it is more likely that the added discussion will be beneficial. Relevant issues will be discussed in more detail, which should give the patient even more information to use in deciding on a course of treatment that makes him or her most comfortable. Most of the time, the second opinion will agree with that of the first opinion, which is directly helpful for the patient and health care team.

In addition to discussing these issues with their physician, it is important in this process that the patient consult books such as this one and reputable on-line information and discuss the issues with knowledgeable people he or she respects. Further sources of information are noted in appendixes C and D. Participating in thyroid cancer patient support groups such as ThyCa may also be helpful.

Who should perform the second opinion? Generally, getting the second opinion from someone recommended by friends or primary care physicians is appropriate. Consulting an endocrinologist at a large medical center is another good option. Physicians who specialize in thyroid-related diseases can be identified by contacting national or local endocrine societies such as the American Thyroid Association, the Endocrine Society or the American Association of Clinical Endocrinologists (see appendix C).

To ensure that a consulting physician will provide you with the most informed opinion, it is very important that all relevant medical information be transmitted, including correspondences, radiologic reports and biopsy reports. In many cases, the actual biopsy slides and radiologic films will be requested so that these materials also can be reviewed and the interpretations confirmed.

CHAPTER 12

Radiation, Carcinogens, Chernobyl, Genes, and Thyroid Cancer

James John Figge, M.D.

In most cases, the origin of thyroid cancer is unknown. However, radiation is one of the few well-established causes of thyroid cancer, and radioactive iodine, which accumulates in the thyroid gland, is now recognized as a thyroid carcinogen (cancer-causing agent). This relates to accidental or unintentional exposures to radioactive iodine and should not be confused with the diagnostic and therapeutic uses of radioiodine described elsewhere in this book. The first section of this chapter reviews the wealth of information on this topic, culminating in a discussion of a catastrophic event that resulted in a surge of thyroid cancer diagnoses, the Chernobyl nuclear reactor accident. Recent discoveries have pinpointed two human genes, *ret* and p53, that are involved in radiation-induced thyroid cancer. The second section of the chapter focuses on these cancer-related genes and includes a summary of the effects of radiation on human genetic material, or chromosomes.

Radiation and thyroid cancer: evidence for cause and effect

Abundant evidence links radiation exposure to the subsequent development of thyroid cancer. The evidence is now strong enough to implicate thyroid irradiation as a direct cause of thyroid cancer. The risk of developing thyroid cancer is especially high among children younger than 10 at the moment of radiation exposure. Thyroid cancer risk is moderately increased in individuals ages 10 through 19 who are exposed to radiation. The time lag (known as the latency period) between the moment of radiation exposure and the subsequent appearance of a thyroid malignancy can be as short as four years but more commonly extends for 10 to 15 years. An individual exposed to radiation as a child likely will remain at increased risk for the development of thyroid cancer throughout his or her lifetime.

The link between radiation exposure and thyroid cancer, first suspected in the 1940s, was demonstrated in studies of thyroid cancer cases that were detected in the 1940s and 1950s. Many of these cancers arose in individuals who had received radiation treatments as children for a variety of benign problems. Beginning in about 1920, doctors routinely used radiation to treat children for acne, swollen tonsils or adenoids, enlarged thymus glands, fungal infections of the skin and other conditions. Often X-rays, or the more potent gamma radiation, were employed. The thyroid gland was often directly in the path of the radiation, resulting in significant levels of exposure to the thyroid tissue. No one at the time linked this procedure with a future risk of cancer. But as many as 25 to 30 years later, cancers of the thyroid appeared in these exposed individuals, and by 1960 the relationship between radiation exposure and thyroid cancer was widely appreciated, and this medical practice in children was abandoned.

Further evidence linking radiation and thyroid cancer originated from the study of nearly 80,000 atomic bomb survivors from the Japanese cities of Hiroshima and Nagasaki. After tracking the survivors for 40 years, researchers found that radiation-exposed children younger than 10 were significantly more likely to develop thyroid cancer than unexposed children. A strong relationship was found to exist between the radiation doses received by the thyroid gland and the subsequent likelihood of developing thyroid cancer. In children and adolescents younger than 15, the relationship between the dose and the development of cancer is linear, which means that as the dose increases so does the risk of cancer. We now know that even low-dose radiation exposure confers risk. Adults exposed to the atomic bomb radiation, however, experienced no increased thyroid cancer risk, possibly because thyroid cells grow more actively in young people and are more vulnerable to damage or mutation.

Between 1950 and 1960, above-ground nuclear weapons testing in Nevada released radioactive iodine (^{131}I) throughout the continental United States. The highest deposits occurred immediately downwind of the test site. In the eastern part of the country, rain washed most ^{131}I deposits from the atmosphere onto the ground, while in the west, dry particles settled onto the ground. It is now recognized that radioactive iodine is a thyroid carcinogen. The National Cancer Institute in 1997 published an extensive analysis of the radiation doses to the thyroid people received as a result of these weapons tests, and as a consequence, the Institute of Medicine estimated that a considerable excess of thyroid cancer had occurred.

The Chernobyl nuclear reactor accident on April 26, 1986, was the worst technological disaster in the history of nuclear power generation. Two explosions occurred in the fourth reactor of the Chernobyl nuclear power station in the Ukraine, releasing massive amounts of radioactive materials into the atmosphere. Operator error has been identified as the immediate cause of the accident, but the reactor design, which lacked a reinforced concrete containment vessel, has been implicated in the serious consequences of the accident. More than 80 types of radioactive substances were released. Several of these were volatile, meaning that they were taken up into the atmosphere and distributed over large geographic

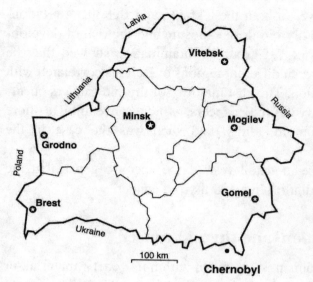

FIGURE 1: Map of Belarus. The Gomel region of Belarus, just to the north of the Chernobyl reactor site, was heavily contaminated by ^{131}I. The highest incidence of thyroid cancer in children was documented in the Gomel region following the Chernobyl accident.

regions. As in the Nevada tests, ^{131}I was the most important of the volatile radioactive substances released at Chernobyl. A large plume of radioactive iodine drifted over the northern part of the Ukraine and the southern part of Belarus (see figure 1), both now independent of the former Soviet Union. Just north of the reactor site, the Gomel region of Belarus received the highest level of ground contamination from ^{131}I. The prevailing winds moved contaminated air masses to the west and then the northwest, resulting in the detection of radiation in Sweden on April 27, 1986. By April 29, the wind had shifted east and a large cloud of radioactivity entered the southwestern corner of Russia. Rainstorms during April 28 to 30 washed some of the radioactive agents out of the atmosphere and onto the ground in Belarus and Russia.

Most residents of the contaminated regions of Ukraine, Belarus, and Russia lived in rural agricultural settlements. Deposits of radioactive iodine on pasturelands and gardens introduced ^{131}I into milk from cows grazing on the land and other parts of the food supply. Some children who ingested contaminated dairy products and vegetables and inhaled ^{131}I from the air ended up with substantial radiation doses to the thyroid tissue.

Four years after the Chernobyl accident, an increase in pediatric thyroid cancer cases was noted in northern Ukraine and in southern Belarus, particularly in the Gomel region. Between 1986 and 1994, 333 cases of pediatric thyroid cancer were diagnosed in Belarus. By comparison, only seven cases of pediatric thyroid cancer had been diagnosed in Belarus in the nine years prior to the Chernobyl accident. The largest number of cases occurred in children who were younger than 4 at the moment of the accident. Five- to 9-year-olds were at the next highest risk level, and 10- to 19-year-olds were at moderate risk, in agreement with the observations from other exposures, as discussed above. In both the Ukraine and Belarus, a relationship was documented between ^{131}I thyroid dose exposure and the risk of developing thyroid cancer. Measurements of ^{131}I ground contamination showed that the incidence of pediatric thyroid cancer in different regions of Belarus correlated with the level of ^{131}I ground contamination. The vast majority of thyroid cancers occurring post-Chernobyl were papillary thyroid cancers, which can exhibit a more aggressive course in children than in adults, and such was the case in the Chernobyl-related cancers.

The next section will explore in detail two of the specific genes that are involved in the development of radiation-induced thyroid cancer.

Chromosomes, genes, radiation, and thyroid cancer

The blueprint for a living organism is contained within its genetic material, or chromosomes. In each human cell, there are 46 chromosomes, consisting of a set of 23 pairs. One member of each pair is maternal in origin and the other is paternal. The chromosomes contain DNA, which is the chemical substance that actually carries the genetic blueprint for the organism. DNA is a long chain built from four components, known as A, G, C, and T (similar to a four-character alphabet). The exact combinations of A, G, C, and T within the linear DNA sequence comprise a functional program for the cell, similar to a computer program. The DNA is, in essence, a program to direct the normal functioning of a cell. As long as the DNA is intact, the cell will function normally. If the DNA becomes damaged (mutated), the program for the cell may become deranged, and the cell may exhibit abnormal properties. We now know that cancer is a disease of the DNA. Any physical agent (such as radiation) or chemical substance (such as a chemical carcinogen) that can alter or mutate the DNA can potentially cause cancer.

The DNA within a chromosome is organized into functional units called genes. Genes contain specific sequences of codes (composed of combinations of A, G, C, and T) to direct the production of proteins, which are one of the major building blocks of cells. In humans, approximately 30,000 genes are distributed among the 23 pairs of chromosomes. Genes can be regulated (turned on or off) so that only selected proteins are produced in specific cell types. For example, the genes within a thyroid cell are regulated so that the proteins critical for thyroid hormone synthesis are produced. Genes encoding proteins that are not needed in the thyroid cells are generally turned off.

As an organism develops, cells need to grow and divide. In an adult organism, many cells, including thyroid cells, grow more slowly. Several types of genes regulate this process. Some genes encode proteins that can stimulate cell growth and cell division. Other genes code for proteins that slow the pace of cell growth and division. Still other genes encode proteins that regulate the death of cells. These various proteins are components of complex regulatory circuits that control the pace of cell growth, cell division and cell death. During the process of cell division, the cell must produce an exact copy of its DNA to pass on to each of two "daughter" cells. Rarely, an error can occur in the process of DNA replication. As a safeguard to ensure the integrity of the DNA, proteins encoded by certain genes in cells repair defective DNA. These genes are known as DNA-repair genes. It is now understood that cancer results from deleterious alterations (mutations) in genes that control cell growth and division, cell death and DNA repair.

Radiation can damage DNA and, as a consequence, induce abnormalities in genes. A radiation-induced alteration or mutation in genes that control cell growth and division, cell death or DNA repair could generate a cancer cell. Two genes appear to have been "targeted" by radiation-induced alterations following the Chernobyl accident. One of these, the *ret* gene, resides on chromosome number 10. The *ret* gene encodes a protein that is activated by a specific growth factor and is able to stimulate the growth and division of certain cell types. This gene is normally silent in thyroid cells, so that *ret* protein is not found in these cells. However, it appears that radiation can damage chromosome number 10 in the vicinity of the *ret* gene, resulting in a rearrangement of the chromosome (see figure 2). This radiation-induced chromosomal rearrangement can lead to an unusual situation where part of the *ret* gene DNA becomes directly linked to the DNA of an unrelated gene on chromosome 10. This rearrangement creates a mixed, or "hybrid," gene that contains a portion of the original *ret* gene as well as a segment of the unrelated gene. The hybrid gene can sometimes be expressed in thyroid cells, so that an abnormal form of *ret* protein will be produced in these cells. The abnormal *ret* protein is often biologically active even in the absence of the specific growth factor. Therefore, the abnormal *ret* protein will stimulate thyroid cells to continuously undergo growth and cell division in an unregulated fashion. Each new thyroid cell will retain a copy of the abnormal *ret* gene, thereby perpetuating the process of abnormal cell growth and division. This unregulated process contributes to the formation of radiation-induced papillary thyroid carcinomas. Indeed, following the Chernobyl accident, many papillary thyroid carcinomas arising in children were found to have chromosome 10 rearrangements, featuring an abnormal hybrid *ret* gene. Several specific types of abnormal hybrid *ret* genes have been identified in post-Chernobyl thyroid cancers; the most common forms are called *ret*/PTC1 and *ret*/PTC3.

The integrity of DNA is critical to the maintenance of normal cellular function in the living organism. As noted above, DNA-repair genes are present in cells and produce proteins that can repair damaged DNA. One critical gene, p53, encodes a protein that helps coordinate the DNA repair process. When damaged

Intrachromosomal Rearrangement

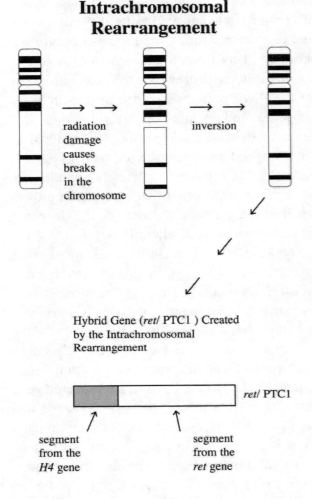

radiation damage causes breaks in the chromosome

inversion

Hybrid Gene (*ret*/ PTC1) Created by the Intrachromosomal Rearrangement

ret/ PTC1

segment from the *H4* gene

segment from the *ret* gene

FIGURE 2: The upper half of the illustration demonstrates radiation-induced rearrangement of chromosome number 10 in the vicinity of the *ret* gene. As a result of the chromosome 10 rearrangement, a segment of the *ret* gene becomes directly linked to a segment of an unrelated gene known as H4 as noted in the lower half of the illustration. This results in the creation of a hybrid gene known as *ret*/PTC1, which directs the expression of *ret*/PTC1 protein in thyroid cells. The *ret*/PTC1 protein is biologically active (it does not need to be activated by a growth factor) and stimulates unregulated thyroid cell growth and division.

DNA is detected within a cell, the p53 protein functions to prevent the replication of DNA until the damage can be repaired. This effectively stops damaged DNA from being passed on to daughter cells. In this regard, the p53 gene has been called the "guardian of the genome"—the genome being the complete genetic information contained in each cell. The p53 gene, however, is not foolproof, and in fact cancer researchers have found that the p53 gene itself is mutated in about 50 percent of human cancers. The mutated p53 gene produces a defective p53 protein, which no longer "guards" the genome. As a consequence, defective DNA is replicated and passed along to daughter cells. Since the process to coordinate the repair of DNA is broken, additional mutations can occur and will be passed along when the cells divide. This process eventually results in an accumulation of genetic defects, a phenomenon called genomic instability. Other critical genes that control the growth of cells can be damaged in this process. Mutations of the p53 gene, therefore, are extremely bad for cells and may lead to the development of cancer.

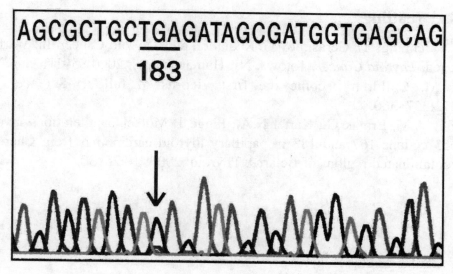

FIGURE 3: Output from an automated DNA sequencing machine showing a mutation (arrow) in the p53 gene originating from a post-Chernobyl papillary thyroid cancer. Reprinted with permission from Pisarchik AV, Ermak G, Kartel NA, Figge J. Thyroid. 2000; 10:25-30 and Mary Ann Liebert, Inc. Combinations of A's, G's, C's, and T's, taken three at a time, code for specific chemical components called amino acids, which are the building blocks of proteins. Position 183 of the p53 protein is normally coded in the p53 gene as "TCA." However, in this thyroid cancer specimen, the p53 gene has been mutated (most likely by radiation) and contains the code sequence "TGA" for position 183. This particular code, "TGA," is read by the cell as a "stop" signal and results in the premature termination of the p53 protein. As a consequence, the p53 protein in affected thyroid cells will be nonfunctional.

Specific mutations have been identified in the DNA sequence of the p53 gene in some post-Chernobyl papillary thyroid cancers. Researchers believe radiation was a direct cause of these mutations (see figure 3). DNA sequence data, derived from an automated DNA sequencing machine using DNA extracted from the thyroid cancer of a Chernobyl victim, demonstrate that there is a specific mutation at one point in the p53 gene from the thyroid cancer tissue, which is denoted by the arrow in figure 3. This mutation was not found in DNA from normal tissue originating from the same patient, illustrating that the mutation is specific to the cancer cells. In this case, the mutation will result in the production of a defective, shortened p53 protein that cannot function to protect the genome.

It is likely that other genes, in addition to *ret* and p53, can be damaged by radiation and may participate in the formation of thyroid cancer. Future research will be required to identify all of the genes involved in this process and to further understand the functions of the relevant genes in the cell.

Further reading

Figge J., Jennings T., Gerasimov G. Radiation and Thyroid Cancer. In: Wartofsky L, ed. *Thyroid Cancer*. Totowa, NJ: Humana Press; 2000:85–116.

Balter M. Children become the first victims of fallout. Science. 1996; 272:357–360.

Pisarchik A.V., Ermak G., Kartel N.A., Figge J. Molecular alterations involving p53 codons 167 and 183 in papillary thyroid carcinomas from Chernobyl-contaminated regions of Belarus. Thyroid. 2000; 10:25–30.

CHAPTER 13

Radioiodine Whole Body Scanning:
Overview and the Different Types of Scans
for Well-differentiated Thyroid Cancer

Douglas Van Nostrand, M.D.

Introduction

Radioiodine whole body scanning for well-differentiated (papillary and follicular) thyroid cancer is a valuable diagnostic imaging tool, which your physician may use to help evaluate, manage, and monitor these types of thyroid cancer. It has been in use for many decades and is a relatively simple procedure that offers minimal radiation exposure. However, radioiodine whole body scanning can be very confusing. The scans can be performed many different, yet appropriate, ways, and the terminology not only varies from one imaging facility to another but also within the same imaging facility. This section presents an overview of some of the different ways in which radioiodine whole body scans are performed and the terms frequently used. Although it is not our intent to make you an expert in radioiodine whole body scanning, it is our hope that this section will make whole body scanning a little less confusing.

Types of scans

To more easily understand radioiodine whole body scans and to better understand why your physician has chosen one type over another, keep in mind the following three factors:

A. The point in time during your medical care at which the scan is performed,

B. The type of "thyroid stimulation" before the scan, and

C. The type of radioiodine used.

A. The point in time during your medical care at which the scan is performed.

Scans are typically performed at four time points during your medical care.

Time Point 1: Pre-ablation scan, also known as the first scan, diagnostic scan or post-operative scan:

This first scan typically is performed four to six weeks after your initial thyroid surgery, hence the term "post-operative" scan. It also is performed before your first radioiodine treatment to destroy (ablate) any remaining thyroid tissue, and hence the term "pre-ablation."

The purpose of this scan is to determine how much normal thyroid tissue remains after your surgery. Almost all surgeons will leave some thyroid tissue in your neck to minimize the risk of damage to your recurrent laryngeal nerve and to leave some parathyroid gland tissue for regulation of your blood levels of calcium. Side effects of injury of the recurrent laryngeal nerve and removal of too much parathyroid gland tissue are discussed in more detail in chapters 7 and 18. This scan also can provide evidence of possible spread of your thyroid cancer, and all of this information along with other clinical information will help your physician determine the best treatment plan for you.

Of note, some imaging facilities have eliminated these scans. These facilities typically will use the same dose of radioiodine for all initial ablations (treatments) regardless of what the results have been on an initial pre-ablation scan. However, most imaging facilities continue to perform these scans because the results may change the treatment plan. There is no conclusive scientific data indicating whether one approach is better than the other. Your physician will advise you regarding the plan that he or she thinks is best for you.

Time Point 2: Surveillance scan:

A surveillance scan may be performed at routine intervals as part of monitoring your thyroid cancer. These scans may be performed as soon as six months or possibly as long as two years after your initial ablation or treatment, although most are performed after one year. The availability of the blood test to determine the level of the thyroid cancer tumor marker, thyroglobulin (see chapter 3), has led some physicians to stop performing surveillance scans routinely. Rather, they may request a surveillance scan only if an increase in serum thyroglobulin is detected.

The procedure for this scan is identical to the first, post-operative, pre-ablation scan. Your physician will determine if and when you need a surveillance scan.

Time Point 3: When metastasis is suspected:

A scan may also be performed when there are other indications that your thyroid cancer may have spread. Signs of metastasis may include a new mass on your physical exam, a rise in your thyroglobulin blood level or changes detected on other imaging exams such as CT or ultrasound. The protocol for this scan varies from one imaging facility to another. For instance, it may be performed exactly the same way as your first, post-operative, pre-ablation scan, or it may be a more complex procedure that includes dosimetry. For a further discussion of scans performed with dosimetry, please see chapter 15.

Time Point 4: Post-therapy scan:

This scan is typically performed seven to 14 days after your radioiodine ablation or treatment. Ablation and treatment are discussed further in chapter 17. The procedure for a post-therapy scan is identical to that of the first, post-operative, pre-ablation scan except that you do not receive any additional radioiodine. The camera will obtain images based upon the dose of radioiodine you received earlier for your ablation or treatment. This is a very important scan. It is well-known that imaging performed after the larger dosages of radioiodine used for ablation or treatment can better detect small areas of normal thyroid tissue and spread of thyroid cancer (metastasis). Thus, the post-therapy scan takes advantage of the higher dose of radioiodine used for your ablation or therapy and could demonstrate thyroid tissue that may not have been detected on the first, post-operative, pre-ablation scan, which was performed with a much lower dose of the isotope.

B. The type of "thyroid stimulation" before the scan.

A radioiodine scan may visualize either normal or cancerous thyroid tissue provided that the tissue first takes up the radioiodine, which you swallowed by mouth. To do this, the thyroid tissue must be stimulated, which can be accomplished by either "withdrawal" of thyroid hormone (see chapter 9) or "Thyrogen®" (see chapter 10).

By withdrawing (not taking) thyroid hormone medication, the pituitary gland in your head will sense over several weeks that you no longer have enough thyroid hormone circulating in your blood. In response, the gland produces a hormone, which stimulates any thyroid tissue present in your body. This hormone is called thyroid stimulating hormone, or TSH (see chapter 2). As the amount of thyroid hormone in your blood decreases, or withdraws, the TSH level increases and stimulates any remaining thyroid tissue to produce thyroid hormone by taking up more of the radioiodine. A key ingredient in this thyroid hormone is iodine, and therefore the thyroid tissue will extract any iodine circulating in the blood including all

Withdrawal of Thyroid Hormone

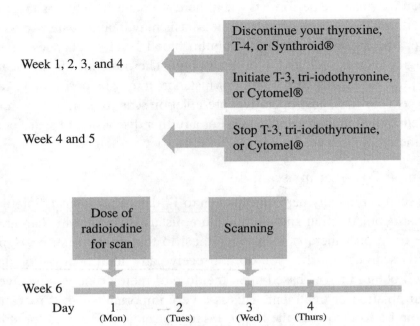

FIGURE 1

Thyrogen® Injections
Pre-ablation post-operative schedule

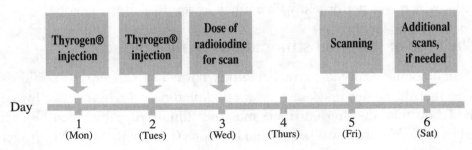

FIGURE 2

radioactive forms of iodine. One typical protocol for withdrawal of your thyroid hormone is shown in figure 1.

Until recently withdrawal of your thyroid hormone has been the only way to stimulate thyroid tissue to take up the radioiodine. However, there is now an alternative way to stimulate your thyroid tissue, which involves two or more injections of the hormone Thyrogen®. Thyrogen® stimulates your thyroid tissue in a manner similar to your own TSH. More information about Thyrogen® is available in chapter 10. One protocol frequently used for preparation with Thyrogen® is shown in figure 2.

Your physician will decide whether to prepare you by withdrawal or Thyrogen® depending on whether you receive a surveillance, first-post operative (pre-ablation), post-therapy or post-therapy with dosimetry scan.

i. Surveillance scans:

The Food and Drug Administration (FDA) has approved Thyrogen® injections as preparation for surveillance scans and as an acceptable alternative to thyroid hormone withdrawal. Eliminating the need to stop your thyroid hormone avoids the unpleasant side effects of hypothyroidism. Your physician will discuss this topic with you to determine whether you will have thyroid stimulation with withdrawal or Thyrogen®.

ii. First post-operative pre-ablation scans:

Although preparation with Thyrogen® injections has been predominantly used for surveillance scans, several institutions now use Thyrogen® injections for preparation for first-time (post-operative, pre-ablation) scans. Initial data for this approach is very promising, but it is still unclear whether preparation with Thyrogen® for these scans is equal to or better or worse than preparation with withdrawal of thyroid hormone. Your physician will advise you of any new information and the best approach for you. However, the data available as this book is being prepared appear to be very favorable for the utility of Thyrogen® for the preparation for these scans.

The use of Thyrogen® may be less important in patients having their first post-operative pre-ablation scan, as the major benefit of using Thyrogen® injections is to avoid the unpleasant symptoms of hypothyroidism. These symptoms are usually less frequent and less severe in patients having their first post-operative pre-ablation scan because some thyroid tissue usually remains after the initial surgery. This residual thyroid tissue usually can produce at least a small amount of thyroid hormone and in some patients considerably more thyroid hormone such that the patient experiences significantly less or sometimes no symptoms of hypothyroidism. On the other hand, patients who are scheduled to have a surveillance scan typically have had at least one ablation or treatment. Consequently, these patients will have little to no thyroid tissue remaining that can produce even a small amount of thyroid hormone, and they typically experience more significant symptoms of hypothyroidism during the withdrawal period. Thus these patients benefit more from Thyrogen® injections.

iii. Post-therapy scans:

Neither Thyrogen® nor withdrawal as a preparation is necessary for post-therapy scans. You will have restarted your thyroid replacement hormone shortly after your radioiodine therapy and continue this without interruption.

iv. Whole body scans with dosimetry:

For patients undergoing dosimetry, Thyrogen® preparation has also been used. Little information was available at the printing of this book to indicate whether the preparation with Thyrogen® is equal to or better or worse than withdrawal when done in conjunction with dosimetry. Your physician will advise you about your options, any new information, and the best approach for you.

C. The type of radioiodine used.

Many different types of iodine elements can be made by man or exist in nature, and each different element of iodine is designated by a number such as 123, 124, and 131. Likewise, each type of iodine element has different physical characteristics such as its method of decay and its half-life. Based upon these different physical characteristics, each element of iodine has advantages and disadvantages, and these determine when a particular element of iodine may be used by a nuclear medicine physician or nuclear radiologist and for what goal. A full discussion regarding how the elements of iodine are assigned their number, the physical characteristics of the various elements of iodine, and the advantages and disadvantages of each are discussed in detail in the section entitled *"I'm Sorry I Asked,"* which concludes this chapter.

Nevertheless, as a result of the advantages and disadvantages and based upon the goals of your physician, various elements of radioiodine will be used. For example, for the first post-operative pre-ablation scan, your physician may choose ^{123}I, ^{131}I, or not perform a scan at all. Because of the concern about stunning, which is discussed further in the section entitled *"I'm Sorry I Asked About Stunning,"* the radiopharmaceutical of choice in many facilities is ^{123}I. For surveillance scans performed after withdrawal of your thyroid hormone, your physician may choose again either ^{123}I or ^{131}I. As above, the radiopharmaceutical of choice in more and more facilities is ^{123}I. Further studies are under way to confirm that ^{123}I is an acceptable replacement for ^{131}I for withdrawal surveillance scans. For surveillance scans performed with the preparation of Thyrogen®, ^{131}I has been used more frequently because the original research that evaluated Thyrogen® used ^{131}I. However, additional research is under way comparing ^{123}I and ^{131}I after preparation with Thyrogen®. For dosimetry, ^{131}I is used. Dosimetry requires imaging as well as blood samples, and both have to be repeated for five to seven days after the dosing of the ^{131}I. Because of the characteristics and dosage of ^{123}I, it is presently not used for dosimetry. ^{124}I holds promise for imaging and dosimetry but is limited because of the cost and availability. In the end, your physicians will select the type of iodine, preparation and scan that is best suited for your situation.

Putting it all together

By knowing **(1) the time point during your medical care that the scan is performed, (2) the type of "thyroid stimulation" before the scan and (3) the**

type of radioiodine used, you will have a better understanding of the radioiodine whole body scan that your physician is performing. These scans are also presented in outline format in Table 1. Based on combinations of the above, some of the names used to refer to various whole body radioiodine scans by different facilities are listed in Table 2. Three examples of radioiodine scans are shown in figures 1, 2, and 3 below.

TABLE 1
Scans by Time Point, Thyroid Stimulation, and Type of Radioiodine

Post-Operative Scan (First-time Scan) (Pre-Ablation Scan)
   ^{123}I or ^{131}I
      Withdrawal
      Thyrogen®

Surveillance Scan
   ^{123}I or ^{131}I
      Withdrawal
      Thyrogen®

Dosimetry and Scan
   ^{123}I or ^{131}I
      Withdrawal
      Thyrogen®

Post-Therapy Scan

TABLE 2
Examples of Numerous Names Used for Radioiodine While Body Scans

• ^{123}I post-operative withdrawal scan	• ^{131}I first-time withdrawal scan
• ^{123}I post-operative Thyrogen® scan	• ^{131}I first-time Thyrogen® scan
• ^{123}I pre-ablation withdrawal scan	• ^{123}I surveillance withdrawal scan
• ^{123}I pre-ablation Thyrogen® scan	• ^{123}I surveillance Thyrogen® scan
• ^{123}I first-time withdrawal scan	• ^{131}I surveillance withdrawal scan
• ^{123}I first-time Thyrogen® scan	• ^{131}I surveillance Thyrogen® scan
• ^{131}I post-operative withdrawal scan	• ^{131}I withdrawal scan and dosimetry
• ^{131}I post-operative Thyrogen® scan	• ^{131}I Thyrogen® scan and dosimetry
• ^{131}I pre-ablation withdrawal scan	• Post-therapy scan
• ^{131}I pre-ablation Thyrogen® scan	

"I'm Sorry I Asked About Atoms"

An atom is made up of a center (the nucleus) and electrons, which circle around the nucleus as satellites orbit the earth. The atom is labeled with a letter such as I for iodine, and this is a chemical element. The nucleus is made up of

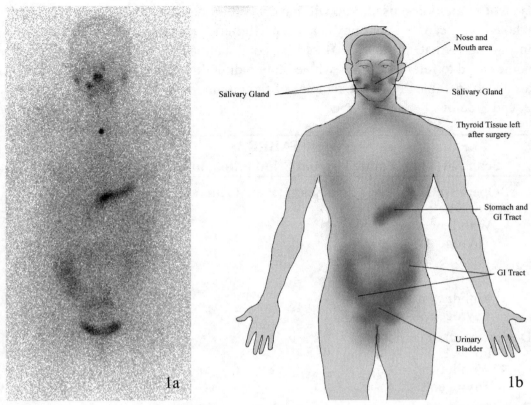

FIGURE 1A: Radioiodine whole body scan performed approximately one month after initial surgery with ^{123}I scan. A small area of activity is present in the thyroid bed region. In order to minimize complications, surgeons typically leave behind some thyroid tissue. This tissue will be ablated with the first dose of radioiodine. Normal activity is seen in the mouth, nose, and urinary bladder. See figure 1b for identification of some of the structures in the scan.

FIGURE 1B: Identification of some of the structures in figure 1a.

protons and neutrons. The total number of protons and neutrons equals the mass number, which is labeled as "A." The total number of protons equals the atomic number, which is labeled as "Z." These labels are usually placed above and below the letter or letters used to designate the chemical element as noted here:

$$^{A}_{Z}I$$

Often this label is shortened to simply ^{131}I. Thus, the "I" represents the chemical element of iodine, and the "131" indicates the total number of protons and neutrons in the atom of which 53 are protons and 78 are neutrons.

Although a chemical element such as iodine must always have the same numbers of protons, the number of neutrons may vary. In other words, the atomic

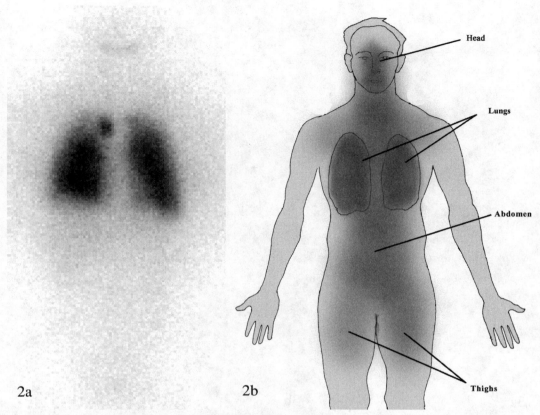

2a   2b

FIGURE 2A: This ^{131}I whole body scan was performed after withdrawal of the patient's thyroid hormone and demonstrates radioactivity throughout both lungs. This is due to spread of the cancer to both lungs and can be treated with radioiodine. Because of the significant radioiodine in the lungs, most of the rest of the body is not seen. See figure 2b for identification of some of the structures in the scan.

FIGURE 2B: Identification of some of the structures in figure 2a.

number (Z) must always be the same, but the mass number (A) may change, as there are more or less neutrons in the nucleus. When there is a different number of neutrons, these different atoms of the same element are called isotopes. [131]I, ^{123}I, [124]I, and [127]I are all isotopes of the same chemical element iodine and are different because of a different number neutrons in the nucleus. While all have 53 protons, ^{131}I has 78 neutrons, ^{123}I has 70 neutrons, [124]I has 71 neutrons, and [127]I has 74 neutrons. The number of neutrons affects the isotope's physical characteristics, which include the half-life and decay (see below) but has no effect on its chemical behavior. For thyroid carcinoma two isotopes, ^{131}I and ^{123}I, are used clinically, and one isotope, [124]I, is used in research studies.

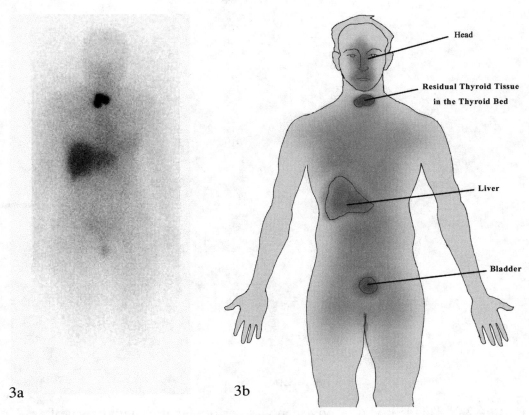

3a   3b

FIGURE 3A: This is a post-therapy ^{131}I whole body scan, which was performed approximately 14 days after ablation with [131]I. A large area of activity is present in the thyroid bed region, which represents good uptake of the ablation dose in normal residual thyroid tissue. As noted above, the surgeon typically leaves behind some thyroid tissue in order to minimize complications. Normal activity is seen in the liver. See figure 3b for identification of some of the structures in the scan.

FIGURE 3B: Identification of some of the structures in figure 3a.

"I'm Sorry I Asked about Half-life and Decay"

Half-life: An important characteristic of an element of radioiodine is its half-life. In nature, some elements such as the different types of radioiodine can change spontaneously into a different element. The time it takes for half of the atoms to change to the other element is called the half-life, and this time is precise. The half-life could be seconds, minutes, hours or days, but it is the same for all atoms of a given type. For example, if you had 100 atoms of ^{131}I, it would take 8.06 days for half of them to turn into the element Xenon. For ^{123}I, it would take 13.3 hours for half of the atoms to change to tellurium. For [124]I, it would take 4.2 days for half of the atoms to change to tellurium. The half-life is important because the longer the half-life, the longer the radioiodine exists. This in turn may be useful because images may be obtained later after the dosing of your radioiodine, and later images may increase your physician's ability to image smaller areas of thyroid tissue.

Decay: Another important characteristic of different elements of radioiodine is how radioiodine releases its energy when it is changing from one element to another. This release of energy is frequently called decay, but this is misleading. Although decay suggests deterioration, nothing is being destroyed. The element is only changing to another form with the release of energy.

Many different methods of releasing energy (decay) exist. One method is releasing a wave. These waves are similar to light but cannot be seen by the human eye and can pass through tissue. These "waves of energy" are called *gamma waves* and can be seen only by special cameras called *gamma cameras.* Just as there are different types of light, there are different types of gamma waves. The gamma camera used by the nuclear medicine physician or nuclear radiologist not only has the ability to see the gamma waves but also can identify the types of gamma waves.

Another way of releasing energy is the release of a particle, which is similar to the current that flows to and through a light bulb. The particle could be negatively or positively charged. Negatively charged particles are called electrons or beta particles. Positively charged particles are called positrons. With this method, the energy is released by the element "throwing off" an electron or positron.

TABLE 3			
	^{131}I	^{123}I	^{124}I
Negative particle (also known as beta particle, or electron)	Yes	No	No
Gamma wave	Yes	Yes	Yes
Positive particle (also known as positron)	No	No	Yes

Although there are other methods of release of energy, a more detailed discussion is outside the scope of this book and not essential for understanding ^{123}I, ^{124}I, and ^{131}I. The methods of release of energy for ^{123}I, ^{124}I, and ^{131}I are listed in Table 3. When ^{123}I changes, it releases gamma waves. When ^{131}I changes, it releases several types of gamma waves as well as a beta particle, which is a negatively charged electron particle. When ^{124}I releases energy, it releases a positron. This positron collides with an electron, and both the positron and electron disintegrate. This disintegration results in two gamma waves of the same energy being sent out in two opposite directions. A special positron camera, or PET (positron emission tomography) camera, can see these specific types of gamma waves and is discussed further in chapter 16.

"I'm Sorry I Asked About Stunning"

As noted above ^{131}I releases a particle and a wave. The advantage of the particle is that it can be used to treat cancer, and thus ^{131}I is used for ablation of normal thyroid tissue and treatment of metastatic thyroid cancer. The advantage of the wave is that ^{131}I can also be used to image your normal thyroid tissue as well as possible thyroid cancer. As a result ^{131}I has been used for many years for whole body scanning. However, when ^{131}I is used to obtain images of your whole body, the particle becomes a potential disadvantage. Although the amount of ^{131}I used for imaging is low, the particle may still partially injure the thyroid cells. This phenomenon is called "stunning" and comes from the expression used when somebody hits his or her head in an injury and is "stunned." Injury to your thyroid tissue in and of itself is not a problem because usually your physician plans to treat and hopefully kill these cells. However, if those particles from the dose of ^{131}I for your scan injure the cells slightly, then these injured cells, or "stunned" cells, may not take up as much of the treatment dose of iodine given shortly thereafter. This in turn may reduce the overall effectiveness of the treatment dose of ^{131}I and is a potential disadvantage for ^{131}I for imaging.

Unlike ^{131}I, ^{123}I has no particle and thus no stunning at the doses administered for scanning. As result, ^{123}I has become the radiopharmaceutical of choice for many facilities for the initial post-operative radioiodine whole body scan. In some facilities it has become the radiopharmaceutical of choice also for surveillance scans. The radiopharmaceutical, ^{123}I, has been an important addition for radioiodine whole body scans.

TABLE 4*
[131]I

Advantages	Disadvantages
Least expensive	Potential stunning (discussed in text)
Readily available	Requirement of possible radiation safety precautions for family and friends
Can be used for imaging	
Allows longer delay between dosing and imaging	
Can be used for treatment of thyroid cancer	
Can be used for dosimetry (see chapter 15)	

*Advantages and disadvantages at the time of publication.

"I'm Sorry I Asked about Advantages and Disadvantages of ^{123}I, ^{131}I, and ^{124}I"

Some of the advantages and disadvantages of ^{123}I, ^{131}I, and ^{124}I are summarized in Tables 4, 5, and 6, respectively. The content of these tables may change over time as a result of a change in the cost of these isotopes or new information derived from further research.

TABLE 5*	
^{123}I	
Advantages	**Disadvantages**
No stunning	At least presently, it cannot be used for dosimetry
Good image quality	
Although the availability was previously limited, it is now widely available.	
Although the price was initially expensive, the price is now more reasonable and is reimbursed by Medicare.	
Significantly less or no radiation precautions for family or friends (see chapter 14).	

*Advantages and disadvantages at the time of publication.

TABLE 6*	
^{124}I	
Advantages	**Disadvantages**
Superior image quality	Very expensive
Potential ability to detect smaller areas of thyroid tissue	Limited availability
Allows intermediate delay between dosing and imaging	Primarily used for research
Can be used not only for bone marrow dosimetry but also lesional dosimetry	Not reimbursed by insurance companies
Tomographic images	

*Advantages and disadvantages at the time of publication.

CHAPTER 14

Radioiodine Whole Body Scanning:
Preparation, What to Expect and
Radiation Safety Precautions for
Well-Differentiated Thyroid Cancer

Douglas Van Nostrand, M.D.

This chapter is divided into the following sections regarding radioiodine whole body scanning:

    I. Preparation for radioiodine whole body scans,
    II. What you may expect when you go for a whole body scan, and
    III. General radiation safety guidelines.

I. Preparation for radioiodine whole body scans

Summary Checklist:
    ☑ **Withdrawal of thyroid hormone or Thyrogen® injections**
    ☑ **Diet**
    ☑ **Laboratory Tests**

A. Withdrawal of thyroid hormone or Thyrogen® injections

In preparation for your radioiodine scan or ablation (treatment), your thyroid tissue must be stimulated to take up the radioiodine that will be administered to you. For an in-depth discussion about how your thyroid works, withdrawal of thyroid hormone, and Thyrogen®, please see chapters 1, 9, and 10, respectively. To stimulate your thyroid tissue to take up radioiodine, there are two options: withdrawal of your thyroid hormone and injections of Thyrogen®.

If the preparation is by withdrawal of your thyroid hormone, your endocrinologist, nuclear medicine physician or nuclear radiologist will give you instructions regarding the schedule for stopping your thyroid hormone medication. This schedule may vary among physicians; however, the differences generally are not significant (see chapter 9). A typical protocol is as follows. Your physician will discontinue the thyroid hormone you are taking and at the same time initiate

Cytomel® (or T3), a shorter acting thyroid hormone preparation. This allows time for the longer acting thyroid hormone to clear your body. When the long-acting preparation has cleared, then the Cytomel® is stopped, which clears rapidly. This helps reduce the length of time that you are hypothyroid. The dose of Cytomel® is typically 25 micrograms two to three times each day. Your physician will determine the dose and the frequency based on such factors as the amount of thyroid hormone you are presently taking, any previous experience you have taking Cytomel®, your weight, and other health conditions. The Cytomel® typically is taken for two to four weeks and then discontinued. The whole body scan is then performed anytime between 10 days to two weeks after discontinuing the Cytomel®. Any ablation or treatment would be performed within a week after the scan. Some institutions may not routinely perform a scan before the first ablation. This is discussed further in the chapter 15. Once you are off your thyroid hormone and your Cytomel®, you will most likely become hypothyroid (See chapter 9).

For patients receiving Thyrogen® injections, there are also several protocols, which will be determined by your physician. You may receive either two or three injections of Thyrogen® followed by your scan. One common protocol is an injection of Thyrogen® on Monday and then again on Tuesday. On Wednesday, the dose of radioiodine for the scan is given, and on Friday the whole body images are obtained.

B. Diet

Your physician may also instruct you to follow a low iodine diet. Thyroid tissue needs iodine to make thyroid hormone. Thyroid tissue "starved" of iodine will be stimulated to take up as much radioiodine as possible. A more detailed discussion of a low iodine diet along with specific examples of low iodine foods are noted in chapter 8. Patients generally adhere to the diet for two or more weeks before their scan.

C. Laboratory tests

Your physician will order various blood tests prior to your whole body scan. These tests may include a complete blood count, thyroid tests, kidney function tests, liver function tests, and thyroglobulin blood levels. Women of childbearing age may also be required to have a pregnancy test.

II: What you may expect when you go for a whole body scan

You will be asked to swallow either a capsule or a small amount of liquid that contains iodine. The iodine is identical to the iodine added to foods such as many breads and table salt except that this iodine is radioactive (see glossary). The iodine

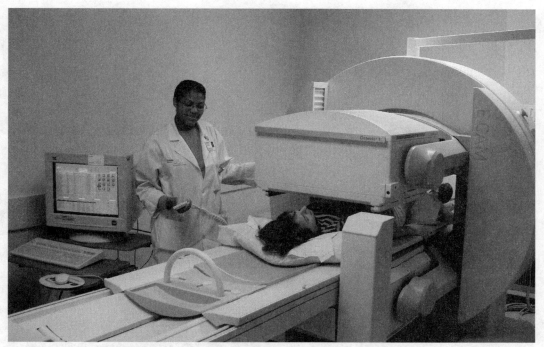

FIGURE 1: The camera has two imaging surfaces—one above and one below your body. The camera will sweep across your body to obtain your images. Different facilities may use different types of cameras.

is then absorbed through your stomach and intestines into your blood. Because thyroid tissue needs iodine to make thyroid hormone, the thyroid tissue will "pull" the iodine out of the blood, where it then accumulates in your thyroid tissue cells. Because the iodine is radioactive, the iodine will send out energy, which can be imaged with the special gamma camera.

Approximately 24 to 72 hours after you receive the radioactive iodine, you will return to your medical facility to be imaged by the camera. You will typically lie on a table on your back, and the camera will sweep over your entire body (see figure 1). Some cameras will sweep the front and back of your body concurrently while others will do one side at a time. Other cameras will image your whole body one section at a time. Depending on the type of camera, the time for scanning your entire whole body can be as short as 30 minutes or as long as two hours. But do not assume that the camera that obtains the images faster is better. Slower imaging in some cases may result in better quality images. Your nuclear medicine physician or nuclear radiologist will determine what is the best imaging time for the camera that is being used to image you.

After completing your whole body scan, a nuclear medicine physician or nuclear radiologist will review your images. Additional views may be requested as

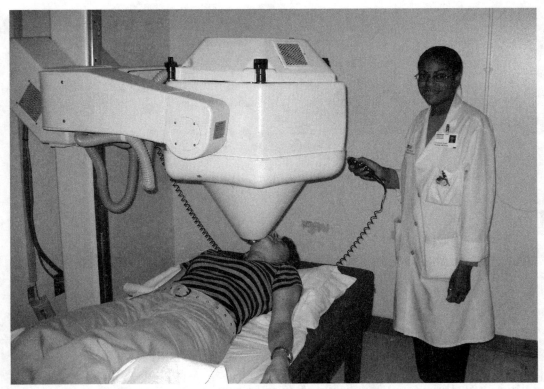

FIGURE 2: This camera has a funnel shape attachment and is called a pinhole collimator or pinhole camera. It is used to obtain high quality images of selected areas of your body.

routine or to clarify an area. Do not assume that because you are getting extra views that there is something worrisome. This can be part of the clinic's standard routine or an attempt by your nuclear medicine physician or nuclear radiologist to get the very best images possible. Obtaining extra views on a different camera is also not necessarily indicative of a problem with your scan. Some clinics automatically take additional views with a different camera, which is called a pinhole camera, to maximize the visualization of an area (see figure 2).

After completion of your images, you will be released. A nuclear medicine physician or nuclear radiologist performing the images for a referring endocrinologist or other physician will probably not review the results with you. Rather, the report will be forwarded to your referring physician. If your nuclear medicine physician or nuclear radiologist is performing the images as part of his or her clinical management of your care for possible treatment or ablation, then the nuclear medicine physician or nuclear radiologist may review the results of the scan with you as well as go over the plan, schedule, and other aspects of your possible radioiodine ablation or treatment.

III. General radiation safety guidelines and recommendations after receiving doses for radioiodine whole body scans

Except for woman who are pregnant or lactating, there are no special safety guidelines for patients who receive ^{123}I for their scans. The radiation dose is very small. However, if you are concerned about any radiation dose to any family member, then you may consider reducing close contact for the first 12 hours. This will make a very small radiation dose exposure even smaller.

For patients who receive ^{131}I radioiodine, many different guidelines are available, and this may vary among facilities because of different amounts of radioactivity administered and different preferences regarding reasonable actions to take to minimize radiation exposure to others. Regardless of the indications, it is important to appreciate that the overall radiation exposure to others is <u>very small</u> following diagnostic doses of ^{131}I radioiodine.

An example of a radiation safety guideline with recommendations for patients who have received diagnostic doses of ^{131}I radioiodine is included below. We are not proposing that this is the only or best guideline, and as always, you should follow the instructions from your facility. The guidelines and recommendations may also be different depending upon the dose of ^{131}I radioiodine.

GENERAL SAFETY GUIDELINES AND RECOMMENDATIONS AFTER DIAGNOSTIC DOSE OF ^{131}I RADIOIODINE

After a dose of ^{131}I for scan, you will be slightly radioactive. Although the radiation exposure you receive is beneficial to you, the radioactivity remaining within you will expose other individuals. Although this exposure is minimal, it provides no benefit to them. To reduce the radiation exposure to others, please follow the general safety guidelines noted below.

I. DURING THE FIRST ONE TO THREE DAYS AFTER THE DOSE FOR SCANNING, PRACTICE THE FOLLOWING THREE BASIC PRINCIPLES:

Principles 1 and 2: Time & Distance

The radiation exposure given by you to your family, friends, and caregivers depends on how long you stay close to them and how close you are to them. A few feet can make a big difference. So, minimize *prolonged close* contact with any individual (more than one hour at less than 3 feet).

For example:
• Do not sleep in the same bed as your spouse or significant other.

- Do not sit next to someone in a movie theater or other enclosed close space for more than one hour.
- Do not take a trip requiring more than one hour of travel time during which you would be sitting next to someone such as in an airplane, train or car.

Principle 3: Hygiene

Radioiodine comes out in your saliva, urine, and perspiration. Proper hygiene decreases the likelihood that anyone else will be exposed to any of your body fluids. Good toilet hygiene and thorough hand washing are essential to reduce the possibility of exposure to others.

For example:
- Avoid kissing and sexual intercourse.
- Wash your eating utensils and clothes separately.
- Avoid contamination with urine (e.g., wash your hands well and flush the toilet twice after each use).
- Bathe or shower frequently.
- Use ONLY YOUR OWN towels and washcloths, and these should not be shared with others.
- Do not prepare food for others. If you must prepare food for others, then use disposable gloves.
- Special note: Contact your physician if you vomit within the first four hours after you receive your diagnostic dose of ^{131}I radioiodine.

II. WITH REGARD TO EXPOSURE TO CHILDREN LESS THAN TWO YEARS OF AGE AND PREGNANT WOMEN:

Practice all of the above basic principles of time, distance, and hygiene for at least FIVE DAYS. In addition, children should sleep in a separate room during this time.

III. NURSING MOTHERS *MUST* STOP BREAST-FEEDING THEIR BABIES BEFORE RECEIVING ^{131}I, AS THE IODINE IS SECRETED IN BREAST MILK AND WILL DAMAGE THE INFANT'S THYROID GLAND.

Any additional questions regarding restrictions for work or personal lifestyle should be directed to your nuclear medicine physician or nuclear radiologist.

Again, this is only one example. The instructions given to you at your facility may vary, and you should follow those instructions.

CHAPTER 15

Dosimetry

Frank Atkins, Ph.D.

The word "dosimetry" has its roots in the Greek "meter," which means to measure. In this case the measurement that we are interested in performing is the determination of "dose." There are also many different ways in which the word "dose" is used. For example, your endocrinologist has prescribed for you a certain "dose" or "dosage" of thyroid hormone to be taken every day. However, in the case of dosimetry we are interested in measuring a very different quantity, namely the radiation dose (see glossary). To make matters even more confusing, the term dosimetry has even been used in several different ways within the medical community, but for our purposes this refers to the radiation dose that would be delivered to your organ(s) following the administration of radioactive iodine ^{131}I. In order to have a better understanding of this section, please make sure that you are familiar with the following terms, which are further discussed in the glossary: activity, exposure, half-life, ionizing radiation, rad, radiation beta particles, radioactivity, and radioiodine.

Overview of Dosimetry

When your physician recommends radioiodine therapy as a treatment for your well-differentiated thyroid cancer, he or she must first decide on the appropriate quantity or dosage to use. In most cases the choice is simple. A standard (also referred to as "empiric") dosage is used, which is based on a general consensus of the medical and scientific communities, decades of experience, and long term follow-ups of the results of these treatments. With an empiric standard dose, however, the choice of the dosage has little to do with the individual patient. For example, there are no established factors or adjustments that would be made in a consistent and universal manner to the **standard dosage** that are based on your height, weight, age or sex. Furthermore, how your body processes iodine, that is, how quickly or slowly is it removed by your kidneys and how much is circulating in your blood at any point in time following the administration, does not enter into the dosage selection. Each of these factors can influence not only the success of the treatment but also the severity of some of the potential side effects, most notably a short–term and possibly permanent suppression of your bone marrow (see chapter 18 which discusses side-effects in more detail). Since bone marrow is very sensitive to the effects of radiation, then a "standard" (empiric) dosage acceptable for everyone must be set at a somewhat lower value in order to minimize the chance of unintentionally giving too much radiation to some patient's bone marrow. Alternatively, a treatment dosage can be derived based on how your body handles radioiodine, which is called dosimetry.

Dosimetry involves a mathematical analysis of a series of measurements to determine how much radioiodine is present in your body, your blood, and possibly your thyroid cancer itself, at a number of time points. These measurements are performed following the administration of a relatively small amount of ^{131}I over the course of four to seven days. From this information it is then possible to estimate how much of a radiation dose would be delivered to your bone marrow from the therapeutic dosage of radioiodine. Your physician would then be able to make a more informed decision on what adjustments (if any) should be made to the standard (empiric) dosage for your treatment. This does not directly address the question of what effect the radioiodine treatment might have on your thyroid cancer. In order to do this we need to know how much radiation, that is dose, would your thyroid tumor (frequently referred to as a lesion) receive. Such a determination is also referred to as a dosimetry. This is a more difficult and complicated procedure and in many cases not possible to perform. A discussion of this can be found at the end of this chapter. Table 1 below provides a summary of the different approaches used to determine a treatment dosage of radioiodine.

TABLE 1
Similarities and differences between dosimetry and empiric approaches

	Empiric	Bone Marrow Dosimetry	Lesion Dosimetry
Blood Samples	No	Yes	No
Additional Clinic Visits	None	3–5	3–5
Additional Time for Data Collection	0	4 hrs	6 hrs
Additional Time off Thyroid Hormones	0	7–10 days	7–10 days
Radiation Dose to Thyroid Cancer*	75–100%	50–400%	50–500%
Side Effects	Low	May be reduced or elevated	May be reduced or elevated

*Relative to an empiric dose of 200mCi

Background (medical use of radioiodine)

Radioiodine has a long and significant history in the diagnosis and treatment of thyroid disease and cancer. Hertz, Roberts and Evans, using ^{128}I, performed the first studies that demonstrated the uptake of radioactive iodine in thyroid tissue in 1938. Unfortunately only very small amounts of ^{128}I could be produced, and its short half-life of only 25 minutes limited its usefulness. However, in the same year Livingood and Seaborg discovered radioactive ^{131}I. The longer half-life of this radioiodine led to the development of many important diagnostic and therapeutic procedures in which ^{131}I was a key component. In 1921 Lawrence invented the cyclotron, and in 1938 the first cyclotron dedicated to medical applications was installed at MIT under the direction of Evans. This device was then able to supply a mixture of ^{130}I (half-life 12 hrs) and ^{131}I to a number of investigators. One of these was Samuel M. Seidlin, M.D., chief of endocrinology at Montefiore Hospital in New York City. At considerable expense (adjusting for inflation, equivalent to about $15,000 today) of research funds he persuaded Evans to produce enough radioiodine to be used for a patient experiment. This was done with the approval of the hospital's chief of medicine and the collaboration of L.D. Marinelli, Ph.D., a medical physicist, at the facility that is now called the Memorial Sloan-Kettering Cancer Center. The patient had a thyroidectomy in 1928 and was then demonstrating thyroid metastases in the lungs, ribs, skull, and other bones. In 1943 this patient received the first medical treatment of thyroid cancer with an injection of radioiodine. Today we have available much more technically advanced imaging systems, but at that time Dr. Seidlin used a hand-held Geiger counter to determine the locations in the body where the radioiodine concentrated. He found that all of these locations corresponded to the known sites of metastases plus two additional ones, which they had not known about. Despite the advanced nature of this patient's disease, the patient did surprisingly well following this treatment, and thus another weapon was added to the medical arsenal in the fight against well-differentiated thyroid cancer. To understand how this benefit is achieved, we need to know a little about the effects of radiation on living things.

Sensitivity of man/woman to radiation (biological effects)

Radiation is something that none of us can avoid. Our atmosphere is constantly being bombarded with radiation from the sun and universe. There are also naturally occurring radioactive materials found in the Earth's crust and interior. Radioactivity is in the air that we breathe and the food that we eat and drink. All living beings are even radioactive, because they all contain small amounts of potassium-40 (^{40}K) and carbon-12 (^{12}C) in their bodies, both of which are radioactive. It has been estimated that something of the order of 60,000 radioactive disintegrations are occurring every second within our bodies from ^{40}K and ^{12}C alone.

When we administer a radionuclide either orally or intravenously for treatment purposes, the ideal situation would be if all of this radioactivity accumulated very rapidly in the tumor(s) to be treated and nowhere else within your body. Unfortunately, methods have not yet been developed to achieve this objective, nor is it ever likely. Instead we must rely on a preferential accumulation of the radioactivity in the tumor(s) compared to all of the other tissues and organs. This is the case for iodine, whether radioactive or not, for normal thyroid cells and to a lesser extent thyroid cancer cells. For example, if ^{131}I was given orally to the average adult with a normally functioning thyroid, then after 24 hours the distribution of the radioiodine might be approximately:

- 20 percent localized in the thyroid gland
- 50 percent localized in the remainder of the body including circulating in the blood
- 30 percent excreted from the body, mostly in the urine.

As a result, the radiation will affect not only the targeted tumor cells but also some of the patient's normal cells as well.

The various cells that make up the different organs and tissues in the human body also respond differently to radiation. All human cells possess the capacity to repair the damage from radiation to some extent. However, this ability varies considerably from one type of cell to another. In general, those cells that are more active in dividing and producing other cells are more sensitive to the effects of radiation. In addition, how quickly the radiation is delivered will also have an effect on

Sensitivity of Cells to Radiation

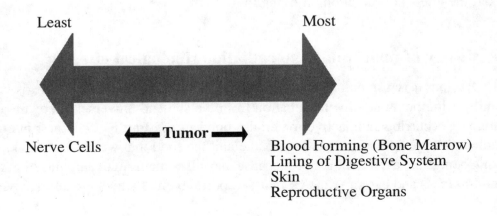

the cell's ultimate fate. If the exposure is over a short time (seconds to minutes) the cell's repair mechanisms may not be able to compensate for the damage to the same extent it would if the dose was given over a much longer time interval.

In all cases the biological effect of ionizing radiation (see glossary) begins with the ionizing process itself. Occasionally, the electron that is dislodged from an atom (ionization) by the radiation was responsible for bonding several atoms together into a larger, more complex structure called a molecule. As a consequence, the molecule falls apart. If this molecule just happened to belong to a critical component of the cell, namely the genetic material or DNA, which contains the information and instructions that allow the cell to perform its functions and to divide when necessary, then the effects can be significant. Each time a radioactive transformation occurs within the body the radiation released can result in thousands of these ionizing events. For each of these ionizing events there are different consequences:

- Cells are undamaged (nothing critical was hit)
- Cells are damaged but successfully repair the damage and operate normally
- Cells are damaged but cannot fully repair the damage and operate abnormally
- Cells die

Determination of treatment dose

Individuals are unique in many respects, and this includes the way in which their body handles iodine. Rather than treat everyone with the same quantity of ^{131}I, many facilities now try to customize the dose given to the patient. One approach that was adopted in the early 1960s was by Benua and Leeper at Memorial Sloan-Kettering Cancer Institute, and the goal was to administer the maximum amount of ^{131}I that could be "safely" administered to the patient. As previously discussed, different organs are more sensitive to radiation than others, and the most sensitive organ for ^{131}I, which is called the critical organ, is the bone marrow. Based on the experience of these early investigators, it was observed that none of the patients suffered any serious complications or side effects when the radiation dose to their blood (bone marrow) was less than 200 rads. The question is then, "How do we determine this radiation dose for the patient?"

When we talk about radioactivity what we mean is that eventually all of the atoms of that substance will transform into a different form through a process referred to as decay. In the case of ^{131}I, it decays into a gas, which is named xenon and is no longer radioactive. During this process of decay, the nucleus of the ^{131}I releases energy. It is this energy which gives rise to the radiation dose. However, this energy is released in several different forms. One of these forms is called beta radiation. These are particles that are identical to those involved in the generation of electricity. These beta particles travel very short distances (typically less than one quarter of an inch) before they have deposited all of their energy. Another form is called gamma radiation. This radiation can travel much larger distances through your body (several inches to several feet) without losing any of its energy. Occasionally a gamma ray will interact at some point within your body and transfer some and possibly all of its energy to the tissue at that location. Since energy is released each time an ^{131}I atom decays, we need to know how many of these decays occur while the ^{131}I remains within you. In addition, we need to know the distribution of the ^{131}I within you: (1) how much is in the blood and (2) how much is spread throughout your body. This is in fact the essence of what we mean by thyroid cancer dosimetry. Since each patient handles radioiodine differently, some will have a large fraction of the ^{131}I circulating in the blood, while others will have much less. Some will eliminate the ^{131}I from the body through the kidneys very rapidly, while others much more slowly. If the ^{131}I is removed from the body before it has had a chance to decay, then those atoms will not contribute to any radiation dose to you. It is only those atoms of ^{131}I that decay while still inside you that contribute to the radiation dose to your blood and hopefully the thyroid cancer being treated.

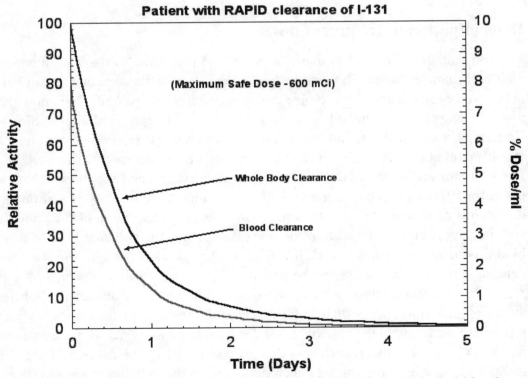

GRAPH 1: The curves represent the clearance from the whole body and blood as noted. This patient has faster clearance than the patient denoted in Graph 2 below. Hence the patient in this graph has a higher permissible dose of radioiodine for treatment.

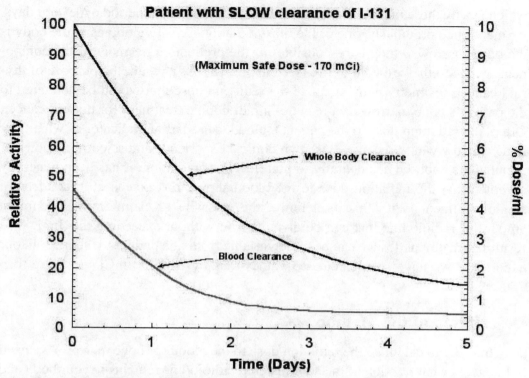

GRAPH 2: The curves represent the clearance from the whole body and blood as noted. This patient has slower clearance than the patient denoted in Graph 1 above. Hence the patient has a lower permissible dose of radioiodine for treatment.

Therefore, the faster you clear or remove the radioiodine then the more that can be given to you initially. This is illustrated in the curves above. This patient has a very rapid clearance of the radioactivity from both the blood and the body and hence a permissible treatment dose would be 600 mCi (see Graph 1). However, for another patient with a much slower clearance (see Graph 2) a permissible treatment dose is only 170 mCi. For this patient the maximum permissible dose is less than what many medical facilities might routinely use, namely 200 mCi, and in this case the 200 mCi may have resulted in a significant effect on the bone marrow in this patient.

The dosimetry procedure

Each time an atom of ^{131}I undergoes a decay, some energy is released and a small dose of radiation is delivered to the tissue surrounding that atom. Since the radioactivity decays occur over several days to a week or so, we must add all of these individual, very small doses together in order to determine the "total radiation dose." The biological effect is determined largely by this cumulative dose, which is why these measurements must be performed over a period of several days. As mentioned previously, one of the most radiation–sensitive organs in the body is the bone marrow, which is responsible for the production of many of the components of blood that are vital to life (see chapter 18). As a result, the purpose of thyroid cancer dosimetry is to calculate the radiation dose that would be delivered to the patient's bone marrow as a result of a radioiodine treatment for thyroid cancer. Often, the radiation dose to the patient's blood is used as an indicator of what their bone marrow would receive. Based on clinical experience and scientific studies of populations exposed accidentally to high levels of radiation, it has been generally accepted that the radiation dose to the blood should not exceed 200 rads from a single treatment. With this as a limit, it is possible to estimate the maximum amount of radioiodine that can be given to you without exceeding this limit. The resulting treatment dosage can be quite variable from one patient to the next. In our experience we have seen calculated values ranging from 50 mCi's to more than 700 mCi's.

Description of the Method

In order to calculate the radiation dose to the blood (or bone marrow) we need to know (1) what fraction of the administered radioiodine remains in your body and (2) how much of this is in your blood. There are several different ways to determine the activity in your body. One approach uses a small radiation detector, usually called a probe, which is positioned some distance away from the patient. This is typically about 10 feet but may be more. This device will detect radiation originating from anywhere within your body. Often readings will be obtained with you both facing towards the probe and away. Since the probe is usually small, each measurement may require five to 10 minutes to complete. Alternatively, this information could be obtained using the same imaging system that was used to generate an image of the radioiodine within your body (see chapter 13). Since the purpose is only to determine the amount of radioiodine in your body and not where it might have accumulated, the time required for this measurement is considerably less than that required for imaging purposes and is usually only about five to 10 minutes. Since many imaging camera systems today use two camera heads, the counts from both sides of your body are obtained during the same sweep across your body from head to foot. A third possibility is to have you collect all of your urine during each 24-hour period. Since almost all of the radioiodine is eliminated from the body by means of the kidneys, then the difference between what was administered and what is contained in the urine represents the amount of radioiodine that remains within you. However, urine collection is very inconvenient and poses unnecessary risks to other family members. Furthermore, it is not as reliable as the other two methods. Consequently, most facilities performing dosimetry no longer require urine collection. To determine the radioactivity in the blood, a small (3-5 ml) sample of blood is obtained. From this vial a small, but accurately measured, volume can be counted in a radiation-measuring device to determine the amount of radioiodine present in each milliliter of blood.

Time points

In order to determine the total radiation dose to your bone marrow, we need to know how much of the administered radioiodine remains in your body and blood at several time points over a period of four or more days following the administration of the ^{131}I. Generally one or two measurements are made in the first few hours following the administration. During this initial period you may not use the toilet so that practically all of the administered radioiodine is still present in you. This is necessary since the initial whole body measurement is used to scale all of the later measurements as a fraction or percentage of the first value, which should represent 100 percent of the administered ^{131}I. Furthermore, if your ^{131}I is administered as a capsule, then we need to wait one or two hours to allow the capsule to dissolve and for most of the radioiodine to be absorbed from your stomach. (Absorption of ^{131}I in liquid form is faster.) Additional measurements and blood collections will then be repeated approximately once every 24 hours for the next four days. If the removal of the radioiodine is slower than usual, then these measurements might be extended an additional one to three days. In general, most patients with thyroid cancer who have been treated previously with radioiodine will have less than 4 percent of the administered ^{131}I still remaining in their body after a period of four days.

What about my tumor?

Nowhere in this discussion of dosimetry was there any mention of the thyroid cancer that is being treated. Unfortunately, this is one of the limitations of this form of dosimetry. The underlying premise of this approach is simple: "Deliver the maximum radiation dose possible to the cancer while minimizing any serious side effect elsewhere." This approach will result in a treatment that will achieve the best therapeutic outcome that is possible. Whether or not the dose of ^{131}I will be sufficient to kill the tumor is not known. To address this issue a few institutions have attempted to calculate how much of the administered radioiodine would actually be taken up by the thyroid cancer. This poses a real challenge but represents what we might refer to as "lesion dosimetry," that is, a measurement of the amount of radiation dose that would be delivered to your tumor (also called a lesion) from the radioiodine treatment. This involves not only additional measurements and tests using nuclear medicine equipment but also requires a CT or MRI exam to measure the size of each lesion. Furthermore, it turns out that it is frequently not even feasible to perform such a calculation for many patients. This is because with the typical dosage of ^{131}I used for dosimetry, the lesions in many instances cannot be visualized on the nuclear medicine scan at these low levels of radioactivity. If the lesion cannot be detected, then it cannot be evaluated. The advantage of this approach is that it would provide your physician with some information beforehand

TABLE 2
Method of Determining Treatment Dosage

	Advantages	Disadvantages
Empiric (standard dosages)	• Simple, less time commitment • Shorter period of time required to remain off thyroid hormones • Generally less risk of side effects since treatment dosages are typically $1/2$ to $1/3$ of that based on dosimetry	• May not result in an adequate radiation dose to destroy the thyroid cancer • In a few cases the dose might exceed a "maximum permissible dosage,"* and the patient may be at higher risk of side effects • Some variability remains in the selection of empiric doses depending on the policies of the treatment facility
Bone Marrow Dosimetry	• Able to determine the "maximum permissible dosage"* that is specific for you • Allows your physician to treat with a higher dosage • Radiation dose delivered to the thyroid cancer increases with increasing dosage • In a few patients, the risk of side effects may be lower	• In most patients the risk of side effects may be greater • You must remain in a hypothyroid state for approximately 1 week longer • Multiple blood samples required • Additional visits to the clinic required
Lesion Dosimetry	• Can provide some indication of the chance that the treatment will be successful • Could possibly guide your physician in decreasing or increasing your treatment dosage	• Additional imaging time required • Can be performed only for moderately sized lesions with uptake of radioiodine

*Based on the Memorial Sloan-Kettering protocol limit of a maximum of 200 rads to the blood.

regarding the likelihood of success of a radioiodine treatment. Your physician might be able to use this information to modify your planned radioiodine treatment. It should also be pointed out that bone marrow dosimetry would also be performed at the same time because this information is used to determine the maximum amount of radioiodine that could be administered for your therapy.

Summary

There are two approaches to arrive at the dosage of radioiodine to use for your treatment for thyroid cancer: (1) a standard value which all patients receive (also called *empiric dose*) or (2) a value determined from how your body and your thyroid cancer handle the radioiodine (i.e. dosimetry). The purpose of dosimetry is to determine how much radiation dose you would receive from your treatment and to adjust the amount accordingly. As a consequence, the amount of radioiodine used for your treatment might be two to four times (or more) greater than what would be prescribed on the basis of an empiric value. Larger dosages would in turn result in a corresponding increase in the radiation dose that is delivered to your thyroid cancer. However, the increased radioiodine dosage may also result in a somewhat elevated risk of other side effects (see chapter 18). On the other hand, in as many as 20 percent of patients the dose determined by dosimetry may be less than the empiric value, and these patients would have a reduced risk of bone marrow suppression. You should discuss with your physician the risk of the side effects, the seriousness of the side effects, and whether the potential benefit of the treatment outweighs the risk and seriousness of the side effects. The advantages and disadvantages of these different approaches to determining an appropriate radioiodine dosage are listed in Table 2 on the previous page.

CHAPTER 16

Additional Diagnostic Imaging Studies

Douglas Van Nostrand, M.D., James Jelinek, M.D.,
Alexander Mark, M.D., Robert Bridwell, M.D.,
Lalitha Shankar, M.D.

Introduction

Many diagnostic imaging tests are available and may be used to evaluate your thyroid cancer. Although this book cannot address every available imaging study, this chapter will review those diagnostic imaging tests that are more commonly used and several that are less commonly used. These are noted in Table 1. For each diagnostic study, most of the subjects listed in Table 2 will be reviewed as applicable.

TABLE 1
Computer Tomography (CT Scan)
MR (Magnetic Resonance Imaging)
Ultrasonography
Positron Emission Tomography (PET scan)
^{201}Thallium and ^{99m}TcSestamibi (Cardiolite® or Miraluma®)
^{111}In-pentetreotide (Octreotide) (Octreoscan®) and ^{99m}Tc depreotide (Neotech®)

TABLE 2
Nicknames
Overview
Special notes
Indications
What to expect
How is the study done
What type of information may be obtained
Example(s)
Advantages and disadvantages
Reimbursement

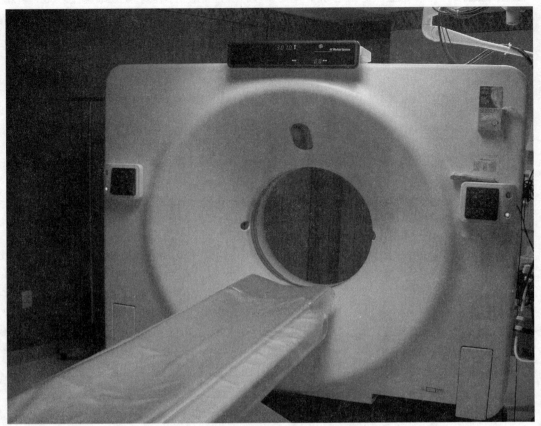

FIGURE 1: Computer Tomography scanner

Computer Assisted Tomography

Nicknames: CT, CAT scan

Overview: Computer Tomography is a valuable scan, which is widely available (see figure 1). CT scans first became routinely used in the 1970s, and the quality of CT images continues to improve.

Special Note: A CT scan is frequently performed with an injection of a material called "contrast." Before receiving the contrast injection, check with your endocrinologist, nuclear medicine physician or nuclear radiologist to assure that you are permitted to receive the contrast. If you are not sure, do not take the contrast. In most cases, you may assume that your endocrinologist does not want you to be given contrast if you have well-differentiated thyroid cancer.

Contrast contains large amounts of iodine, which may block or significantly reduce the uptake of radioiodine by thyroid tissue. This could affect the quality of your radioiodine whole body scan or effectiveness of your treatment.

Indications: CT scans may be performed in patients with thyroid cancer to evaluate many areas. One of the more frequent areas evaluated with CT is the lung and chest area. Your physician will decide when you need a CT scan and in what area.

What to expect: Typically you will not receive any injection. As noted above, if the CT technician or radiologist wishes to give you an injection, make sure that your referring physician has approved this injection.

The CT technologists will give you all the instructions for your CT scan. The total time to perform the CT scan (excluding waiting for your turn on the scanner and registration) is usually less than 30 minutes. In brief, you will lie on a table, and the table will be positioned within the CT scanner's opening. Then, automatically, the table will move in order for images to be obtained of the entire area of interest. There is no pain. After completion of your images but before you leave, a radiologist will usually review your images in order to determine whether any repeat or extra images are needed. However, do not be concerned if repeat or extra images are performed. Repeat or extra views are frequently necessary, and they do not necessarily mean that the radiologist has found something of concern. After completion of the images, the CT technician will release you. As a rule, the radiologist does not review the results with you but will send a report to your physician.

How is the study done? A small amount of radiation is passed through the patient, and a small X-ray image is obtained and stored on a computer. By performing this same process many times around the outside of the body in a circular arc, the computer obtains an "image-in-the-round" of the body. Through computer processing, these images allow the construction of highly detailed cross-sectional images of many of the organs and structures in the area imaged. This would be the same if one took multiple little X-rays around a loaf of bread, and then with computer processing, an image is displayed showing you the details of one of the slices of bread in the loaf. The image of that one slice of bread from the middle of the loaf is a cross-sectional image. Although this analogy is not completely accurate, it does convey a general concept of how CT scans obtain cross-sectional images. As noted, CT scans use X-ray; however, the amount of radiation is low.

What type of information may be obtained: A CT scan obtains high quality images of many of the organs and other structures inside your body and displays these structures in cross-section. As noted above, CT scans are frequently used in patients with thyroid carcinoma to evaluate the lungs and chest. Specifically, the CT is looking for any small masses or abnormal spots in the lungs or in the center of the chest between the lungs. The latter is called the mediastinum and hilum. Examples of CT scans are shown in figures 2, 3, and 4.

Advantages and Disadvantages: The advantages of CT scans are that they can be obtained relatively fast, are widely available, show excellent anatomy, and

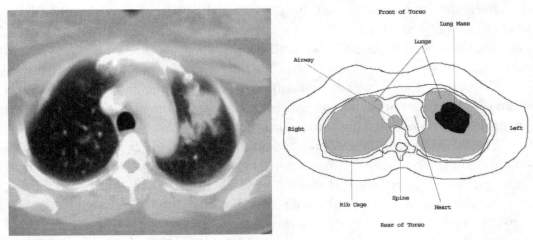

FIGURE 2: CT scan through the mid-upper chest. The right lung is normal. In the left lung, there is a mass.

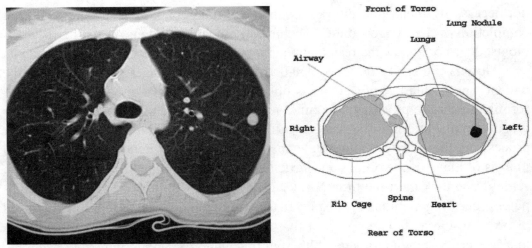

FIGURE 3: CT scan image performed at the level of the upper chest. The right lung is normal. The left lung shows a small pulmonary nodule (tumor).

offer an excellent way to look inside the body without surgery.

A disadvantage of CT scans in the evaluation of thyroid cancer is that better images are often obtained with injection of contrast, but you usually cannot take the contrast as discussed above. The inability to use contrast reduces the information obtained from the CT scan in the mediastinum and hilum, but the CT scan is still very useful, especially in the lungs, without the contrast. Another disadvantage of a CT scan is that although good at detecting masses or spots in the lungs or mediastinum, the CT scan cannot determine with certainty whether a mass or spot is cancerous or non-cancerous.

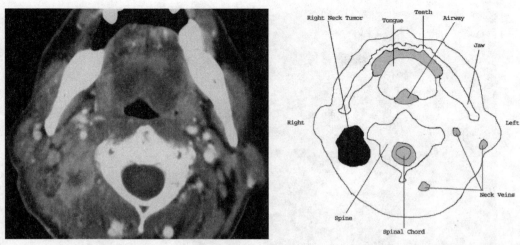

Figure 4: A CT image through the neck at the level of the jaw. On the right side of the neck, beside the spine, there is a poorly defined tumor, which is against the spine and just behind the right angle of the jaw.

Reimbursement: CT scans are usually reimbursed by Medicare and by most insurance plans. Nevertheless and as always, every insurance plan can be different, and you are strongly encouraged to check with your insurance company to make sure that costs for the CT scan will be paid.

Magnetic Resonance Imaging

Nickname: MRI, MR

Overview: MR is a relatively new imaging study, which is also widely available in hospitals and outpatient radiology facilities. An MR unit is very similar in appearance to a CT or PET scanner, although there are some differences. MR does not use radiation, and it allows superior images of soft tissue structures such as in the neck (see figure 5).

Indications: Although your physician may order an MR to evaluate many different areas of your body, the most frequent area your physician will evaluate with MR is your thyroid bed area and neck area.

Special note: A "contrast" agent called gadolinium may be injected as part of an MR study. Unlike the "contrast" agent administered for a CT scan, this contrast agent does not contain iodine and does not block or reduce the uptake of radioiodine into thyroid tissue, and thus you may receive this "contrast" agent.

What to expect: The MR technologists will give you all the instructions for your MR scan. The total time to perform the MR scan excluding waiting for your turn on the scanner and registration is approximately 30 minutes. In brief, you will lie on a table, and the table will be positioned within the MR scanner's opening. Then automatically, the table will move in order for images to be obtained of the

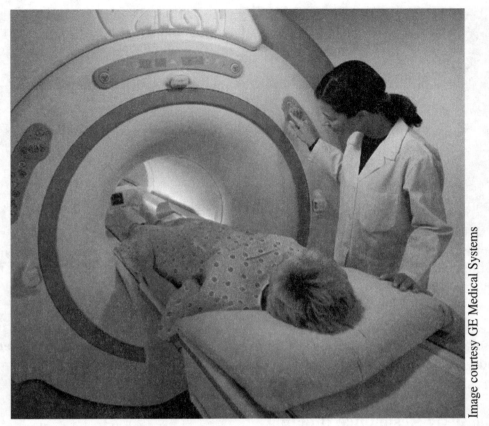

Image courtesy GE Medical Systems

FIGURE 5: A Magnetic Resonance scanner.

entire area of interest. During the images, you will hear a knocking sound, which is normal. There is no pain. After completion of your images but before you leave, a radiologist will usually review your images in order to determine if any repeat or extra images are needed. However, do not be concerned if repeat or extra images are performed. Repeat or extra views are frequently necessary, and they do not necessarily mean that the radiologist has found something of concern. After completion of the images, the MR technician will release you. As a rule, the radiologist does not review the results with you but will send a report to your physician.

How is the study done? By placing a high-strength magnetic field around the area of the body to be imaged, certain atoms such as hydrogen "align" to the magnetic field. When the magnetic field is removed, the atoms go back to their previous state, and as they return to their normal state they emit radio signals. These radio signals can be detected and allow high-resolution tomographic images.

What type of information may be obtained: MR can be used to image many areas of the body including the brain and spine. In patients with thyroid cancer, MR is especially useful in imaging the thyroid bed area and the neck such as for enlarged lymph nodes or other soft tissue masses. An example of an MR scan is shown in figure 6.

Advantages and disadvantages: MR scans have many advantages. They do not use radiation, are widely available, show excellent anatomy inside the body without having to undergo exploratory surgery, and show structure, which other scans show poorly or cannot show at all.

MR also has disadvantages. A major disadvantage of MR scans is that patients with metallic objects such as an aneurysm clip or a pacemaker may not be able to have an MR scan. The MR technologist will review this with you to determine if you can have an MR scan. MR scans are also more expensive. Another disadvantage is that some patients may feel claustrophobic within the chamber, and often a physician may order an oral Valium® tablet or other sedative before the exam. Finally, although MR may demonstrate lymph nodes and may demonstrate the size of the lymph nodes, the MR scan cannot determine with certainty whether a lymph node is cancer or not. However, like CT, MRI scans are extremely valuable imaging studies.

Reimbursement: Medicare and most insurance plans usually reimburse for MR scans. Nevertheless and as always, every insurance plan can be different, and

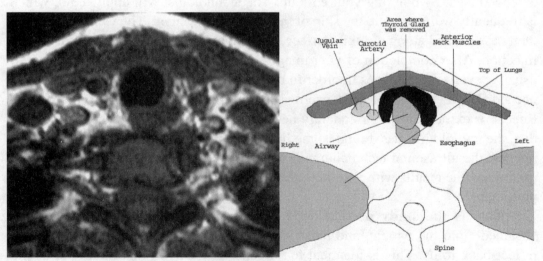

FIGURE 6: MR cross-section through the lower neck. The thyroid gland has been removed. However, in the above illustrations, the location of where a normal thyroid gland would be is drawn. The thyroid is a horseshoe-shaped gland that fits around the lower part of the trachea in the neck. The thyroid gland is directly in front of the esophagus, which is the upper part of the digestive tract. Just to the side of the thyroid gland are the carotid arteries, which are the major arteries to the head. Just lateral and next to the carotid arteries are the jugular veins, which return the blood from the head. CT and MR are complementary in evaluating neck tumors.

you are strongly encouraged to check with your insurance company to make sure that costs for the MR scan are paid.

Ultrasonography

Nicknames: Echo, ultrasound, sonogram

Overview: Ultrasound is also a valuable, widely available imaging study, which uses "sonar" (sound waves) to evaluate various areas of the body. It does not use radiation, and it can also be used to help guide fine needle aspirations.

Indications: Ultrasound is used predominately in three areas for patients with or suspected of having thyroid cancer. First, ultrasound is frequently used to help determine and to characterize any mass (nodule) within the thyroid gland. Second, it is frequently used to evaluate the thyroid bed and neck area for recurrence of thyroid cancer. Third, ultrasound is frequently used to help guide a biopsy or fine needle aspiration of a mass in the thyroid or neck, or in a lymph node.

What to expect: The ultrasound technologists will give you all the instructions for your ultrasound scan. The total time to perform the ultrasound scan excluding waiting for your turn on the scanner and registration is usually less than 30 minutes. In brief, you will lie on a table, and usually your head will be slightly extended back by pointing your chin up. The technologist will apply a gel, which is frequently warmed, onto the skin of the area to be scanned. The technologist will then pass a wand along the skin surface, obtaining images. There is no pain and no injection. After completion of your images but before you leave, a radiologist will usually review your images in order to determine if any repeat or extra images are needed. However, do not be concerned if repeat or extra images are performed. Repeat or extra views are frequently necessary, and they do not necessarily mean that the radiologist has found something of concern. After completion of the images, the ultrasound technician will release you. As a rule, the radiologist does not review the results with you; however, the radiologist will send a report to your physician.

How is the study done: Sound waves above our hearing frequency are "beamed" into the patient, and these sound waves hit an object deep within and reflect back to us. This is identical to an echo in a canyon in which your sound waves hit the opposite wall of the canyon and return to you as an echo. Based on the speed of sound and the time it took from sending the sound wave until its return, the computer calculates how deep the tissue structure (canyon wall) must be. Because not all sound waves are reflected at the first structural interface, many sound waves penetrate successive layers with echoes returning from each interface to give us a two-dimensional image.

What type of information may be obtained? Ultrasound may demonstrate masses or lymph nodes in the thyroid bed or neck area. If a mass or lymph node is found, ultrasound can further demonstrate the size, shape, and possibly internal features. When first evaluating a mass in thyroid, ultrasound can determine if it is fluid-filled or solid. Examples are demonstrated in figure 7.

Advantages and disadvantages: Ultrasound has many advantages. It is widely available, does not use radiation, is relatively inexpensive, and is simple to perform. Its disadvantages are that it requires more skill of the operator, may not see all masses or lymph nodes, and if a mass or lymph node is seen, it cannot determine if it is cancer or not. However, there are some characteristics of the ultrasound images of lymph nodes that are suggestive of malignancy.

Reimbursement: Ultrasound scans are usually reimbursed by Medicare and by most insurance plans. Nevertheless and as always, every insurance plan can be different, and you are strongly encouraged to check with your insurance company to make sure that costs for the ultrasound scan will be paid.

Positron Emission Tomography

Nickname: PET scans

Overview: A PET scan is a "Positron Emission Tomography" scan, which helps evaluate your body for any sites of spread of your cancer. PET imaging is one of the most advanced non-invasive imaging techniques that allows detection of tumors frequently earlier and sometimes more reliably than other imaging methods (see figure 8). It involves the injection of a small amount of radioactive sugar

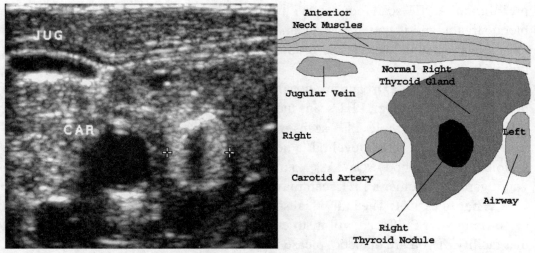

FIGURE 7: Ultrasound image of the neck. The images of the neck show the blood vessels toward the patient's right side with the jugular vein a little more to the front and further to the side. The carotid artery is located immediately next to and slightly toward the back of the thyroid gland. A thyroid nodule is present in the middle of the thyroid gland.

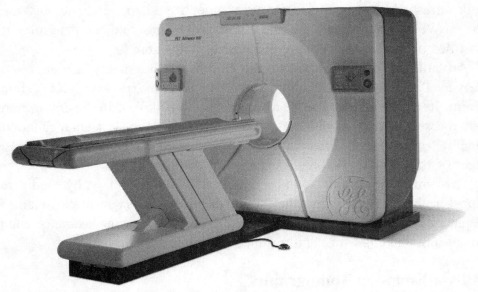

Image courtesy GE Medical Systems

FIGURE 8: GE Advance NXi PET system.

called FDG into your vein followed by obtaining "pictures" of your body. Because tumor cells are typically very active and need sugar, the tumor cells will take up the radioactive sugar, which in turn allows the PET camera to image the radioactivity. This is discussed in further detail below.

Special notes: If you have diabetes, please inform the individual who is scheduling your PET scan and obtain any special instructions regarding your preparation. A PET scan requires the injection of a radioactive substance into your blood stream, and if you are a woman and of childbearing age you may be asked to take a pregnancy test. These tests do not interfere with a therapeutic dose of radioactive iodine.

Indications: PET scans are not indicated on a routine basis in patients with thyroid cancer. However, PET scans may be indicated in selected patients with thyroid cancer. For example, PET scans may be valuable in patients who have a positive thyroglobulin blood level but a negative physical exam as well as a negative radioiodine whole body scan. Ask your endocrinologist or the physician managing you regarding whether a PET scan may be valuable for you.

What to expect: The individual scheduling your PET scan or the technologist performing your PET scan will instruct you regarding preparation for your scan at that facility. If you are diabetic, please inform the individual scheduling your scan. Upon arrival for your PET scan, you will receive an injection of radioactive sugar (FDG) into your vein, which is similar to having a tube of blood drawn. The amount of radioactivity is low. You will then be asked to lie still on a reclining chair without talking for about one hour in order for the sugar to distribute in your body.

Afterwards you will be taken into the PET scanner room for imaging. The PET scanner is a doughnut-shaped device with a padded examination table similar in appearance to the examination table for a CT. You will be asked to lie flat on the scanner table, which is designed to move you slowly through the center of the scanner ring. The scanning procedure will last approximately 60 minutes. The entire procedure including registration will take approximately 2 to 3 hours.

For preparation for your PET scan, you should be well hydrated. On the day before your PET scan, drink plenty of fluids (any beverage), and on the morning of your scan, drink several extra glasses of plain water.

How are images obtained: Sugar (glucose) is an important source of energy for most cells including tumor cells, and because many tumor cells are very active, these cells require even more energy and thus more glucose. By tagging a small amount of radioactivity (fluorine) onto the glucose, injecting the radiolabeled glucose into your blood, and waiting about one hour, the physician can then obtain images, which demonstrate where the glucose has localized. By knowing the normal distribution of glucose and by looking for intense areas of radiolabeled glucose accumulation, one can identify areas of possible thyroid cancer metastasis.

What type of information may be obtained: PET scans are valuable in helping to localize sites of spread of your thyroid cancer that may or may not have been identified on other imaging studies. This information could then modify your physician's recommended diagnostic studies or therapy. For example, localization of the radioactive glucose may encourage fine needle aspiration of lymph nodes that were considered normal on ultrasound or MR. If your lymph nodes are enlarged on ultrasound or MR and your physician is considering fine needle aspiration, a PET scan may help direct where the fine needle aspiration should be performed. If surgery is being considered, a PET scan may demonstrate possible spread of your cancer in areas not previously known, which may alter the approach or type of surgery. Again, these are only several examples describing how a PET scan may alter the diagnostic evaluation or therapy. For your specific situation, consult with your endocrinologist or the physician managing your case regarding the utility of a PET scan for you.

Example: Examples of PET scans are shown in figures 9 and 10.

Advantages and disadvantages: The major advantages of PET scanning are threefold. First and foremost, PET scans assess your body by looking at the metabolism of the cells such as in a mass and not the structure of a mass. The metabolism may suggest that the mass is malignant rather than benign. Second, by looking at metabolism the FDG PET scans may identify sites of cancer that were not see on CT, MR or ultrasound. And third, the amount of radiation is low. The major disadvantage of PET scans is that they are expensive, and many insurance companies still do not reimburse for them.

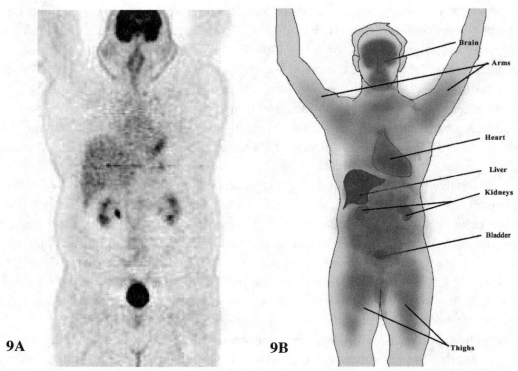

9A **9B**

FIGURE 9A: Normal PET scan. See figure 9b for identification of some of the structures in the scan.

FIGURE 9B: Identification of some of the structures in figure 9a.

Reimbursement: At the time of the printing of this book, PET scans were just approved by Medicare for reimbursement for patients who (1) are being restaged for recurrent or residual thyroid cancer of follicular origin (not including medullary or anaplastic thyroid carcinoma), (2) have a positive thyroglobulin blood level greater than 10ng/ml, *and* (3) have had a negative radioiodine whole body scan.

The reimbursement of PET scans for thyroid carcinoma by other medical insurance plans is variable, and many insurance plans require pre-authorizations. Contact your medical insurance company regarding coverage and the requirement for pre-authorization. If you are covered or if you have been given pre-authorization, you are encouraged to get this in writing. If you are not able to obtain this in writing then at a minimum you should record the name and telephone number of the individual who told you that your medical insurance would cover the cost of the PET scan or gave you pre-authorization for the PET scan. Also, record the day and time of the telephone conversation. If the medical insurance representative cannot answer your question, ask for a supervisor.

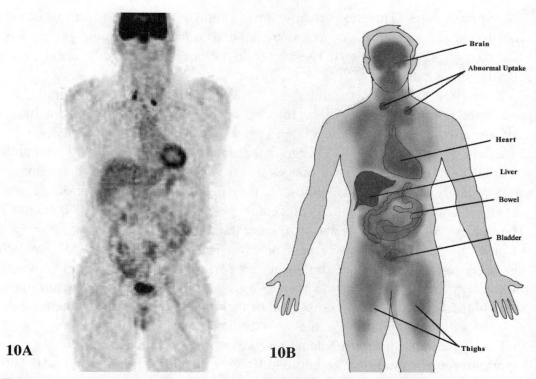

10A   **10B**

FIGURE 10A: Abnormal PET scan demonstrating two abnormal areas of glucose uptake in the neck area, which suggests recurrent thyroid cancer in lymph nodes. See figure 10b for identification of some of the structures in the scan.

FIGURE 10B: Identification of some of the structures in figure 10a.

[201]Thallium and ^{99m}Tc-Sestamibi

Nickname: Thallium, Sestamibi, MIBI (pronounced "mibby")

Overview: [201]Thallous chloride and ^{99m}Tc-Sestamibi (Cardiolite®, Miraluma®) are two radioactive scanning agents that are routinely used for cardiac imaging. However, research studies have demonstrated that these agents will localize in many cancers and specifically in thyroid cancer. As a result, some nuclear medicine and radiology facilities will use these agents in order to evaluate for thyroid cancer in specific clinical situations.

Indications: Although the indications for the above agents remain controversial, they may have utility in the evaluation of patients with negative radioiodine whole body scans and positive thyroglobulin blood tests and help by identifying potential areas of metastatic thyroid cancer not identified on any other study. The study may also be of potential value in demonstrating the extent of disease, which might affect the diagnostic or therapeutic approach.

Special notes: These tests require the injection of a radioactive substance into your blood stream, and if you are a woman and of childbearing age you may be asked to take a pregnancy test. These tests do not interfere with a therapeutic dose of radioactive iodine.

What to expect: With either ^{201}Thallous chloride or ^{99m}Tc-Sestamibi, the procedure is similar. You will be injected with either radioactive agent into a vein. Approximately 1 to 6 hours later, you will be asked to lie flat on the scanner table, and the technologists will program the camera to pass slowly over your body or to take individual sequential images down your body. Although these images are frequently called a whole body scan, they may stop at the mid-aspect of your lower extremities. The scanning procedure will last approximately 60 minutes. The nuclear medicine physician or nuclear radiologist will review your images in order to determine if any repeat or extra images are needed. However, do not be concerned if repeat or extra images are performed. Repeat or extra views are frequently necessary, and they do not necessarily mean that the physician has found something of concern. After completion of the images, the nuclear medicine technologist will release you. As a rule, the physician will not review the results with you; however, the nuclear medicine physician or nuclear radiologist will send a report to your physician. The entire procedure including registration will take approximately 2 to 3 hours.

How does ^{201}Thallous chloride or ^{99m}Tc-Sestamibi (Cardiolite®, Miraluma ®) localize in thyroid carcinoma? The exact mechanism for the localization of either radio-agent is not known. However, ^{99m}Tc-Sestamibi may localize in special structures in the cell, which are called mitochondria. These structures are related to energy production for the cell. Nevertheless and despite our lack of knowledge of the precise mechanism(s) of localizations, these radio-agents are useful because they can localize in thyroid cancer.

What type of information may be obtained? As noted above, scans using these radio-agents can help localize possible sites of spread of your thyroid cancer that were not identified on any other imaging study.

Advantages and disadvantages: The advantage of these agents is the ability to image a metabolic process within cells. This is in contrast with studies such as CT, MRI, and ultrasound that predominantly image structure (anatomy). Another potential advantage of these agents relative to radioiodine is that they image a different metabolic process of thyroid cancer cells. Radioiodine permits imaging of the "metabolism" of iodine, whereas these agents image "metabolism" such as energy production. The disadvantage of these agents is that neither one of these agents can be used to prove or disprove that a lymph node or mass is cancer. They just help identify sites that have a high potential to be cancer.

Reimbursement: Reimbursement varies with Medicare and medical insurance companies. Your nuclear medicine or radiology facility may already know whether your insurance company will reimburse for this study.

In regard to Medicare, you might assume that the policy for Medicare would be the same throughout the United States; however, this is not necessarily true. The Center for Medicare & Medicaid Services (CMS) oversees the entire Medicare program and may contract the local oversight to a non-governmental company. These non-governmental companies may have different policies in different geographical areas. As a result, different areas may have different policies regarding the reimbursement of ^{201}Thallous chloride or ^{99m}Tc-Sestamibi. Likewise, the policies of reimbursement of ^{201}Thallous chloride or ^{99m}Tc-Sestamibi by medical insurance companies will vary. As always, check with your insurance company.

^{111}In-pentetreotide (Octreotide) (Octreoscan®) and ^{99m}Tc Depreotide (Neotech®)

Nicknames: Octreotide, somatostatin scan, Neotech scan

Overview: Every cell has different chemicals as part of the cell wall, to which other chemicals can attach. In one sense, these chemicals on the cell wall are like an electrical *"receptacle"* on the wall in your house and are called **receptors.** One type of receptor is called a somatostatin receptor. Although a full discussion of somatostatin receptors is beyond the scope of this book, there are five known types of somatostatin receptors (types 1, 2, 3, 4, and 5). Various types of somatostatin receptors are found on all normal cells, and most cancer cells have an excess amount of certain somatostatin receptors. For example, normal thyroid tissue has a normal amount of predominantly somatostatin receptors types 3 and 5, and well-differentiated thyroid cancer has an excess amount of predominantly types 1 and 3.

Pentetreotide and depreotide are two chemicals that can attach to some of the various types of somatostatin receptors. These chemicals can be tagged with radioactive labels (^{111}In onto pentetreotide and ^{99m}Tc onto depreotide). When tagged, these radiolabeled chemicals can be injected into a patient to get an image of tissue that has an excess amount of somatostatin receptors. ^{111}In-pentetreotide (octreotide) will attach predominantly to tissue that has an excess amount of somatostatin types 2 and 4 receptors while depreotide attaches predominantly to tissue that has an excess amount of types 2, 3, and 5.

Indications: Both octreotide and depreotide scanning are not indicated on a routine basis in patients with thyroid cancer. However, selected patients with certain cancers like medullary thyroid cancer, or those individuals with well-differentiated thyroid cancer who have rising thyroglobulin blood levels, a negative physical exam, a negative CT scan, a negative MRI scan, and a negative radioiodine whole body scan may benefit. You physician will determine when these scans may be useful.

Special notes: These tests require the injection of a radioactive substance into your blood stream, and if you are a woman and of childbearing age you may be asked to take a pregnancy test. These tests do not interfere with a therapeutic dose of radioactive iodine.

What to expect: ^{111}In-pentetreotide (Octreotide) (Octreoscan®): There is no preparation for an octreotide scan. The radio-agent will be injected into a vein usually in your arm. Four hours after the injection, the technologist will obtain images of your whole body. To obtain these, you will lie on a table similar to those used for radioiodine whole body scans. The camera taking the pictures moves over your body for approximately 30 to 50 minutes. Frequently, additional 3-D images are taken, and the camera will slowly spin around your body. These "special" images are called SPECT (single photon emission tomography images) and usually take thirty to forty-five minutes to perform. The nuclear medicine physician or nuclear radiologist will then review your images. Your physician may order additional delayed images at 48 hours, which may be very helpful. However, do not assume that because you are getting extra views that there is something worrisome. This can be part of the clinic's standard routine or an attempt by your nuclear medicine physician or nuclear radiologist to get the very best images possible.

^{99m}Tc-depreotide (Neotech®): The imaging procedure for ^{99m}Tc-depreotide (Neotech®) is very similar to the procedure for octreotide; however, there are differences. ^{99m}Tc-depreotide (Neotech®) (1) attaches to different types of somatostatin receptors than octreotide, (2) is a smaller molecule that clears the body more rapidly than octreotide, and (3) uses a different radioelement, which disappears faster. As a result, depreotide images are performed earlier (between 30 minutes to two hours after injection). In addition, no additional delayed images are obtained.

What type of information may be obtained: These agents may be used for the same indications as ^{201}Thallous chloride and ^{99m}Tc-Sestamibi, which is the evaluation of patients with negative CT and MRI, negative radioiodine whole body scans, and positive thyroglobulin blood tests. The goal as discussed above is to try to help identify potential areas of metastatic thyroid cancer not identified on any other imaging study (see figure 11). Likewise, these scans may also be of value in demonstrating the extent of disease, which might affect the therapeutic approach. Finally, research studies have suggested that some thyroid cancers such as medullary thyroid cancer may be treated with non-radioactive somatostatin drugs. The demonstration of significant somatostatin radioactivity on these scans has been proposed as a way to identify patients who may benefit from treatment with non-radioactive somatostatin drugs. However, further research is still needed.

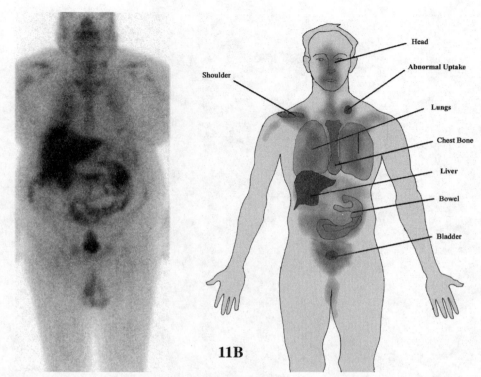

11A   **11B**

FIGURE 11A: The above image is a ^{99m}Tc depreotide. The patient had a negative ^{131}I whole body scan; however, the above scan demonstrated the thyroid cancer in the left neck area. The patient was treated with radioiodine, and on the ^{131}I whole body scan performed after the treatment, uptake was seen in this area. See figure 11b for identification of some of the structures in the scan.

FIGURE 11B: Identification of some of the structures in figure 11a.

Advantages and disadvantages: Imaging with these radio-agents has a number of advantages compared with other types of imaging. First, utilizing these types of scans may allow your doctor to "see" tumor deposits when they could not be seen by other means. As discussed above, visualizing the tumor deposits may allow your treatment plan to be tailored to your specific clinical situation.

A disadvantage of these radio-agents is that they are new and further experience is needed to assess their utility. However, in individual patients scans performed with these radio-agents may be beneficial.

Reimbursement: Octreotide scans may be reimbursed by Medicare and by some insurance plans, but as always, every insurance plan can be different. You are strongly encouraged to check with your insurance company to make sure that costs for the octreotide scan are paid. Medicare or most insurance plans do not cover Depreotide scans for thyroid cancer.

CHAPTER 17

Radioiodine Ablation and Treatment
For Well-Differentiated Thyroid Cancer
Douglas Van Nostrand, M.D.

Introduction

R adioiodine ablation and treatment are very important in the management of well-differentiated thyroid carcinoma. This chapter is divided into six sections, the first of which is a compilation of "Frequently Asked Questions" concerning radioiodine ablation and treatment. The second discusses steps you will need to take before your radioiodine ablation, and the third covers steps to be followed on the day of your treatment. The fourth section describes what you may expect if you are admitted to the hospital for your treatment, and the fifth describes what steps you need to take after your treatment including radiation safety precautions. The chapter concludes with a section discussing immediate and long-term follow up after your ablation or treatment.

Radioiodine ablation and treatment are performed with ^{131}I and are frequently called RAI.

I. Frequently asked questions

What is radioiodine ablation?

Radioiodine ablation is radiation therapy in which radioactive iodine is administered to destroy or ablate residual healthy thyroid tissue remaining after thyroidectomy.

What is radioiodine treatment?

Radioiodine treatment is radiation therapy in which radioactive iodine is administered to destroy or ablate thyroid cancer by irradiating that tissue.

What is the difference between ablation and treatment?

Many physicians use "ablation" and "treatment" interchangeably. Other physicians use "ablation" to mean the administration of radioiodine to eliminate any normal thyroid tissue remaining in the neck after initial surgery and "treatment" to mean the subsequent administration of radioiodine for the elimination of metastatic disease in the neck or elsewhere. Although we believe the terms can be interchanged, we will use the above definitions to avoid confusion.

Why do I have any thyroid tissue left after my surgery? I thought my surgeon took it all out.

Although your surgeon removed your thyroid gland, most surgeons leave behind small amounts of thyroid tissue to minimize any damage to the nerve that controls your voice box. This nerve is called the recurrent laryngeal nerve and runs behind your thyroid tissue. Your surgeon may also leave some thyroid tissue behind to make sure some of your parathyroid glands remain intact. These glands control your body's calcium levels and are usually located within or behind your thyroid tissue.

Why do I need an initial radioiodine ablation when my physician believes he has removed all of my thyroid carcinoma?

Most physicians will recommend that patients with thyroid carcinoma undergo at least one ablation radiation therapy with radioiodine. Research and fifty years of experience suggest that the combination of surgery, radioiodine ablation, and thyroid hormone replacement can reduce the chances of your thyroid carcinoma recurring. There are some situations, however, in which your physicians may not recommend an initial ablation with radioiodine. This is briefly discussed below and in more detail in chapter 4.

What are the criteria for not receiving an ablation with radioiodine?

Radioiodine ablation may not be recommended depending on several factors. These include the size of the original thyroid cancer, the number of sites involved, the lack of any involvement of the borders of the thyroid or adjacent tissues, and a lack of evidence that the cancer has spread. Your physician will review all of your medical information to decide whether radioiodine ablation is necessary for you.

If radioiodine ablation is recommended, what is its goals?

Radioiodine ablation has four goals.

First, and for most patients, it will reduce the chance of the thyroid cancer recurring. Although the exact reason is not known, the most likely possibility is that the radioiodine helps kill any thyroid cancer cells that may be present in the remaining thyroid tissue.

Second, destroying the remaining thyroid tissue will improve the ability of the radioiodine whole body scan to monitor you for evidence of any recurrence of the cancer. If any healthy thyroid tissue remains in your neck, that tissue may take up a significant amount of the radioiodine, making it difficult to detect any cancerous tissue. If the healthy thyroid tissue is destroyed, a radioiodine whole body scan will be better able to detect any spread of thyroid cancer. Thus the ablation of any remaining normal thyroid tissue improves the ability of future radioiodine whole body scans to detect spread of your cancer.

The third goal is to facilitate the use of the blood levels of thyroglobulin to monitor you for metastasis. Normal thyroid tissue also produces thyroglobulin, and thus, in the presence of normal thyroid tissue, changes in your blood thyroglobulin levels are not as reliable for indicating spread of your cancer. The use of thyroglobulin as a marker for well-differentiated cancer has been discussed in more detail in chapter 3.

The fourth goal is to enhance the effectiveness of future radioiodine treatments, if needed, by allowing you to receive a higher dosage of radioiodine, which has the potential to deliver more radiation to your cancer cells. Any significant normal thyroid tissue remaining may restrict the amount of radioiodine that could be used for your treatments.

If I had only one lobe of my thyroid removed, do I need to have the other lobe removed also? If so, should it be removed by surgery or destroyed by radioiodine treatment?

The decision to remove the other lobe will depend on many factors: the size of your original primary tumor; any spread into the walls of the thyroid, adjacent tissue or lymph nodes; your age; and your health. Your physician will advise you based on your clinical situation. Further information is also present in chapters 4 and 6.

Surgery or radioiodine treatment may be used if the decision is to remove the other lobe. The advantages and disadvantages of each are controversial. Supporters of surgery argue that there is a chance of cancer being present in the remaining lobe and that removal of this lobe improves the prognosis. Supporters of radioiodine treatment argue that surgery does not affect the overall prognosis and that the risks of a second surgery should be avoided whenever possible.

Physicians who recommend radioiodine treatment also say that the dosage of radioiodine needed to destroy the remaining lobe is usually smaller than that needed to destroy any small area of thyroid tissue left after removal of that lobe. While we prefer complete thyroidectomy by surgery to radioiodine, you should discuss these options with your physicians.

What dosage of radioiodine should I receive for ablation?

The dosage for your first-time ablation will typically range from 29 mCi up to 150 mCi. You should speak with your endocrinologist, nuclear medicine physician or nuclear radiologist on their rationale for a given dose and particularly if the planned treatment dosage is not in this range.

In deciding what dosage between 29 and 150 mCi should be administered, there are many factors to consider and many advantages and disadvantages that must be weighed. These factors include federal or state radiation regulations, insurance coverage, your physicians' treatment objectives and your clinical situation. Patients who have a small, single site of cancer and no evidence of spread may not even require a radioiodine ablation. Patients who have a large amount of thyroid tissue that takes up a lot of radioiodine may—paradoxically—receive smaller dosages. Patients and physicians who wish to avoid hospitalization may also use lower dosages while those who want to reduce the chance of a repeat ablation or treatment may use higher dosages. Some facilities may use dosimetry to determine the dosage, which will deliver an estimated, pre-determined amount of radiation exposure to the tissue (see chapter 15).

II. Preparation for ablation or treatment prior to the day of ablation or treatment

This section discusses the preparation for radioiodine ablation prior to the day of your treatment.

Summary Checklist:
☑ 1. **Obtain lemons, candies or other foods that will make you salivate**
☑ 2. **Have your favorite drinks available**
☑ 3. **Find out whether you will be treated as an outpatient or if you will be admitted to the hospital**
☑ 4. **Verify your insurance coverage and, if required, obtain pre-authorization**
☑ 5. **Have all required laboratory tests performed at the scheduled times**
☑ 6. **Follow your physician's instructions if he or she is withdrawing your thyroid hormone**
☑ 7. **Start on a low-iodine diet as recommended by your physician**

1. Obtain lemons, sour candies or other foods that will make you salivate.

One of the side effects of radioiodine ablation or treatment is salivary gland pain, swelling, and subsequent dry mouth (xerostomia), which is discussed further in chapter 18 entitled "Side Effects of Radioiodine." Radioiodine localizes not only in your thyroid tissue but also in other organs including your salivary glands. While the goal is to deliver enough radiation to destroy your thyroid tissue, every effort should be made to minimize radiation damage to your salivary glands. Lemons or sour candies will cause you to salivate and therefore help flush the radioiodine out of your salivary glands. This, in turn, will reduce the radiation exposure to your salivary glands. You will need enough candies to be sucking on continuously while awake or at a minimum of every 15 minutes while you are awake for the first two days after treatment and several times during the night. (If you are on a low iodine diet and your physician wishes you to continue this diet while in the hospital, do not eat candies that contain the color additive Red #3, which contains iodine.)

2. Have your favorite drinks available

Drinking plenty of fluids will help keep you hydrated and help your kidneys urinate out the radioiodine that your thyroid tissue did not take up. Hydration not only reduces radiation exposure to your other body tissues but also dilutes the radioiodine in your urine, which decreases the radiation exposure to your urinary bladder. Also by drinking plenty of fluids, this may help lead to early release from the hospital.

We encourage you to bring your own non-alcoholic drinks to the hospital, if permissible, so you will not need to depend as much on the nurses to provide your liquids. Easy access to fluids also will encourage you to drink more frequently.

3. Find out whether you will be treated as an outpatient or if you will be admitted to the hospital.

The rules requiring hospitalization for radioiodine treatment have changed in some states. Ask your physician whether you will be treated as an outpatient or inpatient.

4. Verify your insurance coverage and, if required, obtain pre-authorization.

Make sure your insurance company will cover the expenses of all of the necessary laboratory tests, physician visits, X-rays, whole body scans and radioiodine ablations and treatments. Keep track of any expenses that will be your responsibility.

Some insurance companies require pre-authorization before agreeing to pay any of your expenses. If so, you must first contact the insurance company for approval before having any of the tests, scans or treatments. Once you receive approval you will be given a pre-authorization number. If you fail to verify that you have appropriate medical insurance coverage or to obtain any necessary pre-authorization from your insurance company, your diagnostic tests and treatment may be delayed significantly, and you may be liable for the entire medical bill.

If your insurance company does require pre-authorization but will not grant it at your request, then contact your endocrinologist or primary care physician and have them obtain it for you. The nuclear medicine physician or nuclear radiologist may be able to obtain pre-authorization, but some insurance companies may grant these requests only from your referring endocrinologist or primary care physician. In addition, while you may be able to gain verbal pre-authorization from your insurance company, it is best to get this information in writing. If written pre-authorization is not possible, then at least record the date and time you received the pre-authorization and the name of the person who provided it along with the pre-authorization number. Dealing with an insurance company can be frustrating, but it is critically important to do so and to know whether you may be responsible for all or a portion of the bill. More information on insurance and pre-authorizations may be obtained through websites listed in appendix C.

If you do not have insurance, meet with a financial representative of the facility from which you will receive your care. Find out about standard fees and any reduced fees for self-pay patients. You should get these fees in writing and record the name of the individual who gave you the information.

5. Have all required laboratory tests performed at the scheduled times.

Your physician will determine which laboratory tests you need before your treatment. The most common laboratory tests are TSH (thyroid stimulating hormone), TG (thyroglobulin), TGab (thyroglobulin antibodies), CBC with ANC (complete blood count with absolute neutrophil count), comprehensive medical profile (such as Chemistry 20), spot urine iodine level, and a serum pregnancy test for women of childbearing age. Many specimens used for these laboratory tests must be drawn at specific times before your radioiodine treatment. Your physician will tell you which laboratory tests are necessary and when these need to be performed.

6. Follow your physician's instructions if he or she is withdrawing your thyroid hormone.

The preparation for your radioiodine treatment may require either withdrawal of your thyroid hormone or Thyrogen® injections. If your treatment requires withdrawal of your thyroid hormone, either your referring physician, nuclear medicine physician or nuclear radiologist will give you instructions that must be followed leading up to the day of your treatment. Most facilities use a schedule similar to the following:

Discontinue your thyroid hormone (e.g. thyroxine, Synthroid®, L-thyroxine, etc.) and immediately initiate Cytomel®. More information is in Chapter 9 entitled "Withdrawal of Thyroid Hormone."

Discontinue your Cytomel® after two to four weeks and then wait approximately 10 days to two weeks to have your radioiodine whole body scan performed. (As discussed elsewhere, some institutions may not perform this scan.)

Shortly after the scan, you will have your radioiodine ablation (treatment).

7. Start on a low-iodine diet if recommended by your physician.

Some physicians recommend patients follow low-iodine diets for two to four weeks. This subject is discussed in more detail in chapter 8. Contact your physician if you did not receive instructions regarding a low iodine diet.

III. Preparation for ablation or treatment on the day of the ablation or treatment

Summary Checklist:
☑ 1. **Bring your photo identification**
☑ 2. **Follow the instructions given to you regarding eating prior to treatment**
☑ 3. **Discuss the need for anti-nausea medication**

Additional items if you are going to be treated as an inpatient:
☑ 4. **Bring lemons, sour candies or other foods that will make you salivate**
☑ 5. **Bring drinks**
☑ 6. **Bring a two- to three-day supply of your medications**
☑ 7. **Bring only the clothes that are necessary**
☑ 8. **Leave jewelry, watches, and other unessential items at home**
☑ 9. **Ask about an early release program**
☑ 10. **Anticipate a lot of waiting**

1. Bring your photo identification.

You likely will need to show at least one photo identification (ID) card at the hospital, and some facilities may require two photo ID cards before administering the radioiodine. Check with the physician or technologist who will administer the radioiodine for clarification.

2. Follow the instructions given to you regarding eating prior to treatment.

Your physician will advise you regarding what you may eat or drink, including any medications, on the day of your radioiodine treatment. Usually these instructions will include taking all of your regular medications (other than thyroid hormone) along with a small amount of fluids. Diabetics should notify their physicians for any further instructions.

Patients should not eat or drink anything for two to six hours before receiving the treatment dose. The physician treating you should give you an approximate time for the treatment so you will know when to stop eating. Estimating the time may be more difficult regarding inpatients because of various factors out of the physician's control. These include waiting for the previous patient to vacate the room and for the hospital staff and radiation safety personnel to clean and prepare the room for you. Thus to reduce your expectations and frustrations, expect a "hurry up and wait" situation. You may wish to bring something to read or do in case you have to wait.

3. Discuss the need for anti-nausea medication.

Most people will not experience any side effects from their first radioiodine ablation. For further information, see chapter 18 entitled "Side Effects of Radioiodine." Patients prone to nausea and vomiting, however, should notify their admitting physician who can order medication to reduce the likelihood of these side effects. Anti-nausea medication generally is recommended for patients preparing for a radioiodine dosage of 200 mCi or more. Also, if you are nauseated, then you are less likely to take your candies and to drink fluids.

Additional items if you are going to be treated as an inpatient:

4. Bring lemons, sour candies or other foods that will make you salivate.

Remember to bring a supply that will last for at least two days to help you flush any excess radiation out of your salivary glands.

5. Bring drinks.

Staying hydrated will benefit you in many ways. Among them, it will help your kidneys urinate out the radioiodine that your thyroid tissue did not take up and reduce radiation exposure to your other body tissues.

6. Bring a two- to three-day supply of your medications.

Unless your facility requires the hospital staff to administer all of your medications, you may be allowed to bring your own medications to take as if you were at home. Discuss this with your admitting physician.

7. Bring only clothes that are necessary.

We typically recommend that you bring only the clothes you are wearing. Once you are assigned a room at the hospital, you will change into a hospital gown and store your belongings in a nearby closet. If you wear your own clothes, they may become contaminated and may have to remain at the hospital even after you are discharged. Generally these items will be returned to you after the contamination has reduced to a safe level, which can take several months.

Check with your treating physician or technician if you want to bring anything you cannot leave behind.

8. Leave jewelry, watches, and other unessential items at home.

We strongly recommend that you do not bring any personal belongings such as jewelry, watches, books or radios. Before you leave the hospital, the technologist will check your personal belongings for radioactive contamination. If there is contamination, the technologist may be required to keep your belongings, and you will not be able to take them with you. Usually the facility will return these items after several months. Check with the technologists. For reading material, we recommend magazines or newspapers that you can leave behind. You may bring eyeglasses. Although you will usually be able to take your eyeglasses home with you after cleaning them, we recommend bringing an old pair of eyeglasses just in case these need to be left at the hospital. Televisions and telephones are usually provided in the rooms.

Check with your physician regarding contact lenses and hearing aids. At Washington Hospital Center, we permit the patients to bring these and to take them home.

9. Ask about an early release program.

Some patients are being discharged from the hospital earlier than in years past, thanks to new federal and, in some cases, state regulations that have increased the radiation levels for hospital release after radioiodine ablations or treatments. If your facility and state use these new regulations, then you will be asked specific questions or given a questionnaire to determine whether you are a candidate for early release. Ask your treating physician or technologist to find out whether your facility has an early release program.

Our hospital does offer an early release program for patients depending on how they will be cared for after they leave the facility. As an example our "Early Release Form" is enclosed in appendix E.

10. Anticipate a lot of waiting.

Although the people servicing you strive to do everything in a timely manner, they often are unable to eliminate long waiting periods. Patients often are asked to wait to ensure that the many steps necessary for their radioiodine treatment occur in sequence. To help you appreciate the number of people who may be involved in your care, the following list is provided:
- You,
- The hospital admissions and registration staff,
- The patient in your assigned room, who must be discharged,
- The housekeeping staff, who must clean your room,
- The radiation safety staff, who must prepare your room for your treatment,

- Your referring physician, endocrinologist, nuclear medicine physician, or nuclear radiologist, who must admit you,
- The nursing staff, who must coordinate all other aspects of your admission,
- The commercial company, which manufactures the radioiodine,
- The airline company, which flies your dose to your city,
- The local radiopharmaceutical company, which delivers your dose to your facility,
- The nuclear medicine or nuclear radiologist technologist who administers your dose, and
- The radiation safety staff or nuclear medicine technologist who will monitor you to determine when you can be released.

IV. What you may expect during hospitalization

Summary checklist and sequence of events
☑ 1. **Waiting**
☑ 2. **Admissions and registration**
☑ 3. **Room preparation**
☑ 4. **Informed consent**
☑ 5. **Visitor restrictions (very few or even none allowed)**
☑ 6. **Radioiodine administration (liquid versus capsule)**
☑ 7. **Radiation level monitoring**

1. Waiting.

Long waits at the hospital often cannot be avoided due to the many physicians, technicians, and procedures involved in your treatment. As noted above, anticipate waiting and please be patient.

2. Admissions and registration.

Your physician will either ask you to visit him or her first or go directly to the admissions or registration desk, where you will complete the necessary forms. Once you have registered, the hospital staff will escort or direct you to your room.

3. Room preparation.

Since your treatment involves radioiodine, your room must be specially prepared. Each facility has its own approach for room preparation, and the extent of this preparation will depend on various factors: how soon your room will be used for another patient after your discharge and how easy the team, who cleans up the room, wishes that process to be.

If a quick turn-around of your hospital room is required, then you may find extensive preparations with coverings on the floor, bed, telephone, bathroom fixtures, and just about every place that you might touch and possibly contaminate. If you happen to be in such a room, your first impression may be that the radioiodine treatment is more dangerous than you thought. However again, the degree of preparation of the room is not because the radioiodine is so harmful but rather because of the staff's desire for easy decontamination and the need to release the room quickly for the next patient.

Radiation safety staff will be the only medical staff to enter your room routinely to monitor your radiation level. The nursing staff will not usually enter your room during your stay unless there is some medical reason, and your food will most likely be placed on a table just inside your door, along with disposable eating utensils and cups. Remember, you are not admitted to the hospital because your health requires it. Rather you are admitted only to prevent the spread of radioiodine to others.

4. Informed consent.

Your physician will ask you to sign an informed consent form before your treatment. It is your decision alone whether to receive the radioiodine. By signing the consent form, you are stating that: (1) an informed consent discussion was carried out, (2) all your questions were answered to your satisfaction, and (3) you give your physician permission to treat you with radioiodine.

5. Visitor restrictions.

Some facilities will not permit any visitors while others will restrict visitation by minors and pregnant women. Even if visitors are permitted, they usually are not allowed to enter your room and may remain for only a short period of time. If the patient is a child and requires the presence of a parent, then the parent may be permitted to remain in the room with the child. Your physician or technologist will inform you of your facility's policy.

6. Radioiodine administration (liquid versus capsule).

Radioiodine is taken by mouth and administered either as a liquid or a capsule, as determined by the facility. If you have a preference for either a capsule or liquid, you should let your physician know at least several days in advance of your admission so that he or she will have time to try to accommodate you.

7. Radiation level monitoring.

Shortly after the administration of the radioiodine, a technologist or physician will measure you with a special radiation counter. This measurement, along with others that will be taken periodically, will be used to determine when you can be released from the hospital.

V. Steps to take after your treatment

Summary Checklist:
- ☑ 1. **Re-start your thyroid hormone**
- ☑ 2. **Reinitiate your routine diet**
- ☑ 3. **Initiate your radiation safety precautions at home**
- ☑ 4. **Schedule a follow-up appointment with your referring physician or endocrinologist**
- ☑ 5. **Have your blood drawn (if necessary)**
- ☑ 6. **Schedule your post-treatment scan**
- ☑ 7. **Verify that you have authorization from your insurance company for a post-treatment scan**
- ☑ 8. **Have your post-treatment scan performed**

1. Re-start your thyroid hormone.

Re-start your thyroid hormone according to the instructions from your referring physician or endocrinologist. If you do not have instructions, immediately call your physician's office to get them. Generally you will start taking this medication before you are discharged or at the time you leave the hospital. This is discussed in more detail in chapter 9.

2. Re-start your routine diet.

The low-iodine diet is finally over! You should re-start your routine diet according to the instructions of your referring physician or endocrinologist. Indeed, some physicians may already have started you on a regular diet during your hospital stay. If you do not have instructions regarding your diet, then call your physician's office to get them.

3. Initiate your radiation safety precautions at home.

Radiation safety guidelines vary primarily because of the different amounts of radioiodine administered and of the numerous different, but reasonable, approaches to minimizing radiation exposure to others. Your physician or technologist will give you specific instructions, but the **objective** and the **methods** for achieving radiation safety are the same for all facilities. Quite simply, the goal is to limit the radiation exposure to your family and anyone else who might come in contact with you. The methods are threefold: (1) increase the **DISTANCE** between you and others, (2) reduce the **TIME** you spend near others, and (3) **CONTAIN** the radioiodine that comes out in your saliva, perspiration, and urine.

Radiation safety precautions at home are discussed in more detail in chapter 20; however, an additional example of a radiation safety guideline with recommendations for patients just released from the hospital is included below. We are not proposing that this is the only or best guideline, and as always, you should follow the instructions from your facility. The guidelines and recommendations may also be different if you are not admitted to the hospital for your radioiodine treatment.

GENERAL SAFETY GUIDELINES AND RECOMMENDATIONS AFTER DISCHARGE FROM HOSPITAL

After your radioiodine treatment and after you have been discharged from the hospital, you will still be slightly radioactive. Although the radiation exposure you received is hopefully beneficial to you, the radioactivity remaining within you will expose other individuals. Although this exposure is usually minimal, it provides no benefit to them. To reduce the radiation exposure to others, please follow the general safety guidelines noted below.

I. During first three to five days after discharge practice the following three basic principles:

Principles 1 and 2: Time & Distance
The radiation exposure given to your family, friends, and caregivers depends on how long you stay close to them and how close you are to them. A few feet can make a big difference. So, minimize prolonged close contact with any individual (more than one hour at less than 3 feet).

For example:
- Do not sleep in the same bed as your spouse or significant other.
- Do not sit next to someone in a movie theater or other enclosed close space for more than one hour.
- Do not take a trip requiring more than one hour of travel time during which you would be sitting next to someone such as in an airplane, train or car.
- Many physicians advise not driving while hypothyroid. So, if somebody is driving you home and to reduce the radiation exposure to the drive, sit in the rear seat on the passenger side.

Principle 3: Hygiene
Radioiodine comes out in your saliva, urine, and perspiration. Proper hygiene decreases the likelihood that anyone else will be exposed to any of your body fluids. Good toilet hygiene and thorough hand washing are essential to reduce the possibility of exposure to others.

For example:
- Avoid kissing and sexual intercourse.
- Wash your eating utensils and clothes separately.
- Avoid contamination with urine (e.g. wash your hands well and flush the toilet twice after each use).
- Bathe or shower frequently.
- Use ONLY YOUR OWN towels and washcloths.
- Do not prepare food for others. If you must prepare food for others, then use disposable gloves.
- Contact your physician if you vomit within the first four hours after your discharge.

II. With regard to potential exposure to children less than two years of age and pregnant women:

Practice all of the above basic principles of time, distance, and hygiene for THREE DAYS, and if you want to be very cautious, SEVEN DAYS. In addition, children should sleep in a separate room.

III. Nursing mothers MUST stop breast-feeding their babies as the iodine is secreted in breast milk and WILL damage the children's thyroid glands.

Any additional questions regarding restrictions for work or personal lifestyle should be directed to your nuclear medicine physician or nuclear radiologist.

4. Schedule a follow-up appointment with your referring physician or endocrinologist.

If your referring physician or endocrinologist did not give you a follow-up appointment, then contact the physician's office and ask when you should have the appointment and schedule it.

5. Have your blood drawn (if necessary).

Your physician may have ordered certain laboratory tests to be performed before your follow-up appointment. Contact your referring physician or endocrinologist for clarification if you did not receive instructions regarding these tests. We encourage you to have a CBC blood test with platelet count and absolute neutrophil count (ANC) at approximately four to six weeks after your radioiodine treatment. In case you ever do need another treatment with radioiodine, this CBC result may be useful in helping to determine an appropriate dosage. As noted in chapter 18 on side effects, your CBC values may drop for a short period of time, with the lowest point occurring between four and six weeks after your treatment. If you were to receive another treatment dose of radioiodine, it may be helpful to know whether and how far your CBC dropped.

6. Schedule your post-treatment scan.

It is important to set a date for a post-treatment scan. These scans are usually done seven to 14 days after your treatment, but some facilities will perform them within three to five days after your treatment.

Post-treatment scans can be valuable. It is well known that the higher the dose of radioiodine used for scanning, the better that scan is at detecting small areas of normal or abnormal thyroid tissue. The radioiodine dosages used for ablation and treatment are significantly higher than those used for routine scanning, and thus scanning after a treatment dose may better detect small areas of normal or abnormal thyroid tissue. Although identification of additional areas of normal or abnormal activity will not immediately alter treatment, this information may be valuable for your follow–up, for interpreting subsequent whole body radioiodine scans, and for determining additional treatments at some point in the future.

7. Verify that you have authorization from your insurance company for a post-treatment scan.

Make sure that your medical insurance will cover post-treatment scans and that you have obtained any necessary pre-authorization.

8. Have your post-treatment scan performed.

You will not receive another dose of radioiodine for this scan, which you should have performed as scheduled. Rather, the post-treatment scan will image the radioiodine that still remains in you from your treatment.

V. Long-term follow-up after your ablation or treatment

Summary Checklist:
- ☑ **1. Self exam**
- ☑ **2. Follow-up laboratory tests**
- ☑ **3. Follow-up appointment**
- ☑ **4. Follow-up whole body radioiodine scan**

1. Self exam.

Self-examination of your neck and thyroid area is valuable, and we encourage this on a routine basis. Self-examination is not difficult and simply involves rubbing your neck and thyroid area with your fingers using modest pressure. You are feeling for any lumps or bumps. If you need help, ask your physician. Although there is no strict guideline regarding the frequency for self-examination, we recommend every month.

2. Follow-up laboratory tests.

Your physician will determine and order any long-term follow-up laboratory tests you will need. These may include tests for thyroid hormone levels, TSH (thyroid stimulating hormone), TG (thyroglobulin), and TGab (thyroglobulin antibodies).

3. Follow-up appointment.

Your physician should have given you a long-term follow-up appointment or a time to call in order to schedule the long-term follow-up appointment. The length of time between your treatment and follow up will vary depending on your specific situation but typically is no later than one year after your treatment. It may be sooner in order to monitor and, if necessary, adjust the amount of thyroid hormone replacement you are taking.

4. Follow-up whole body radioiodine scan.

Your physician will advise you regarding whether you will need a follow-up radioiodine whole body scan, which is frequently called a surveillance scan. Although surveillance scans have been performed in the past as a matter of routine, some facilities no longer perform them for all patients. Instead, they monitor patients on the basis of a physical exam, thyroglobulin blood levels, and other diagnostic studies. If the evaluation suggests recurrence of the thyroid cancer, then a radioiodine whole body scan is considered. Facilities that still routinely perform radioiodine surveillance whole body scans do so as an additional method to monitor for recurrence of your thyroid cancer. The first surveillance scan may be performed as early as six months and as long as one year after the initial treatment with subsequent surveillance scans performed annually, but this frequency is highly variable depending upon the clinical circumstances. Your physician will advise you.

CHAPTER 18

Side Effects of Radioiodine

Douglas Van Nostrand, M.D.

Introduction

The nuclear medicine physician or nuclear radiologist is responsible for recommending dosages of radioiodine for scans and therapies, writing, if you will, a "prescription" for your treatment. Whenever we have a prescription filled at a pharmacy, we receive the medication that our physician has prescribed, along with a flyer, brochure or instruction sheet that lists the potential side effects of the medication. However, information presented this way is not sufficient for radioiodine, because many other questions also must be addressed (see Table 1). Although it is not practical to list and discuss all potential side effects in detail, the goal of this chapter is to help the reader have a more complete understanding of the potential side effects of radioiodine.

Potential side effects will vary depending on the dosage of the radioiodine administered. To make it easier for you to understand the side effects, this discussion is separated into three sections based on the three possible dosage types: (1) low diagnostic dosages for scanning purposes only, (2) ablation dosages used for first-time treatments shortly after the initial surgery, and (3) multiple dosages, high-dosages or both used to treat thyroid cancer that may be resistant to treatment or may have spread. You should consider the side effects that you might experience based on the specific type of dosage that is being given or considered.

In regard to selecting dosages for radioiodine ablation or treatment, three points should be remembered. First, the type, frequency, and severity of side effects must be weighed against the benefit of the dosage for ablation or treatment. Second, although your physicians may know the potential risks and benefits of the various dosages, they cannot predict what will happen in a given patient. Everyone responds differently to radioiodine ablation or treatment, which often makes it difficult for a patient to decide which dosages might be best for him or her. Your personal physician is likely your best resource to help you make this decision. He or she has the experience caring for many patients with thyroid cancer and is able to consult with other specialists as needed. Your physician also has the latest information on new developments regarding your illness and the training necessary to advise you on a reasonable plan for your specific situation.

TABLE 1
Questions Involving Side Effects of Radioiodine

- What are the potential side effects?
- What is the likelihood that you will have a specific side effect?
- If you have the side effect, what is the likelihood that it will be mild, moderate or severe?
- If you have the side effect, how long will the side effect last and when might it occur?
- Will the side effect be temporary or permanent?
- How will the side effect affect your well-being or long-term health?
- What, if anything, can you do to minimize the likelihood and severity of the side effect?

Even with all this information and advice, some patients become frozen into inaction and may opt to do nothing rather than make a decision. However, doing nothing is still a decision. With the help of your physician, we strongly recommend that you make an active decision—-even if that decision is indeed to do "nothing." But when you decide to do nothing, you must be aware of the possible consequences.

I. Side effects from low diagnostic dosages for scanning

No more than a trace of radioiodine is used in the doses for scanning or dosimetry. Therefore, side effects resulting from these doses are extremely unlikely. Some patients claim to have experienced a side effect, such as nausea, vomiting or dry mouth that resulted from a scanning dose of radioiodine, but the "side effect" most likely resulted from other causes. For example, some symptoms seen at the time of radioiodine therapy are due to other medications, health issues, hypothyroidism that may result from the withdrawal of your thyroid hormone, or even your emotional state for that particular day.

An allergic response to radioiodine is also highly unlikely. Although some patients report a history of an allergy to iodine based on their body's reaction to seafood or contrast dyes used for X-ray studies, this allergic response actually is to other chemicals within the seafood or the contrast dyes—not to the iodine. Iodine is in many foods, and a list is noted in the chapter 8 on low iodine diets. The amount of iodine in these foods far exceeds the amount of iodine administered for a radioiodine scan or treatment. If you are not certain whether you should take radioiodine in light of an apparent history of allergy to iodine, consult with your physician.

II. Side effects from radioiodine ablation dosages used for first-time treatments

Boredom

Most patients will experience no side effects whatsoever after their first ablation (treatment) of residual thyroid tissue. In fact the most frequent complaint following the first treatment is boredom—a reality new patients often respond to with disbelief. Of course boredom is not truly a side effect but a consequence of hospitalization and the radiation safety precautions, which must be followed to protect those around you. Of course, boredom can be managed with sleeping, pacing the room for exercise, television, a telephone, magazines, and books.

Fear

The second most frequent side effect is fear. While this, again, may not be a side effect in the strictest sense, it can be frequent and painful. The fear may be of the unknown or from all the attention paid and precautions used in the handling of the radioiodine. On seeing almost everything in their room covered with plastic or other materials, patients hospitalized for their first ablation (treatment) may conclude: "this radioiodine must really be bad." This preparation is intended simply to help contain the radioiodine and help assure that even small amounts of radioiodine from your ablation do not affect anyone else. This preparation also permits easier and faster clean up of your hospital room for the next patient. In addition, patients are not admitted to the hospital because of concerns of the side effects of the radiation. They are admitted to help contain the radioiodine.

Hypothyroidism

Regardless of whether you receive radioiodine ablation, you will most likely be hypothyroid after your initial surgery. However, radioiodine ablation will destroy any thyroid tissue remaining after surgery. Thus during any future withdrawal of thyroid hormone, you will be even more hypothyroid. Hypothyroidism and its consequences are discussed in more detail in chapter 9.

Nausea and vomiting

Although nausea and vomiting might occur after the first radioiodine ablation, most patients do not experience nausea, and vomiting occurs even less frequently. Any nausea or vomiting that does occur typically is mild, begins several hours to one day after the ablation and resolves shortly thereafter. Nausea that lasts longer than 24 hours is unusual.

Several factors may lead to nausea and vomiting. These include mild inflammation of your stomach and intestines, anxiety over the unknown, and the power of suggestion such as from this book or chemical changes that occur in your body when you are hypothyroid. In addition, the large volumes of liquids that you must drink after the radiation may worsen the chemical changes. Anyone who experiences "car sickness" or "sea sickness" or is otherwise prone to nausea and vomiting should inform their physician ahead of time. Anti-nausea medication, which is also known as anti-emetic medication, may be given before the treatment. This medication may reduce or eliminate the nausea or vomiting, and it may encourage you to drink the necessary fluids to help eliminate the unused radioiodine from your body. However, regardless of whether you easily become nauseated, there is no benefit from enduring unnecessary discomfort. If you have any concerns about nausea or vomiting, talk with your physician.

If you decide not to take anti-nausea medication before the radioiodine, you may want to talk to your physician about taking the medication at your discretion after the radioiodine should you experience these symptoms later. If you are an outpatient, your physician may give you a prescription, which can be filled at a pharmacy. If you are admitted to the hospital, your physician can instruct hospital staff to give you the medication at your request.

It is very important that you notify your treating physician immediately if you have any vomiting within two to three hours after your radioiodine dose.

Early onset of salivary gland swelling and pain (within several days)

Before even discussing this side effect, we must emphasize that it is very important that you follow your physician's instructions or those found in this guide in order to limit the radiation exposure to your salivary glands from your radioiodine ablation. By following several simple precautions for your first ablation (treatment), you will not only reduce the chances of these side effects after your first ablation but the likelihood of these side effects after any additional treatments. Do not wait to implement these instructions for subsequent or high-dose radioiodine treatments. We cannot overemphasize this, and the reasons will be come clear as you read further in this and subsequent sections.

You have two major pairs of salivary glands in your face region. One pair is called your parotid salivary glands, and these lie in front of each ear. The second pair lies just under your jawbone on each side, and these are called the submandibular salivary glands. These glands as well as other smaller salivary glands produce saliva, which makes it easier to chew, swallow, and digest food.

Although the salivary glands are not endocrine glands and have no direct relationship to the thyroid gland, radioiodine accumulates in these glands. The irradiation that results from this accumulation of radioiodine may inflame your salivary glands (called sialoadenitis), which is accompanied by pain, swelling or both. Although most patients will not have any swelling or pain after their first dose of radioiodine, as many as a third will experience some of these symptoms. The pain and swelling may begin as soon as six hours after treatment or not for another several days. In a minority of cases the pain and swelling will be severe and persistent. But for most patients, the side effects last less than two weeks and almost always disappear completely. You should notify your physician of any swelling or pain.

There are several important ways you can minimize the radiation exposure to your salivary glands: (1) eat sour candies or other foods that will make you salivate, (2) drink plenty of fluids to stay well hydrated, (3) massage your salivary glands, and (4) take medications. Although medical data is not available to confirm the effectiveness of these various precautions, they are reasonable and simple to perform.

• Candies

Follow your physician's instructions or within one hour after administration of your radioiodine, begin eating sour candies or any other foods that will make you salivate. Sour lemon drops are an excellent choice. The use of chewing gum is controversial. Although chewing gum may help you salivate, some physicians suggest that the chewing gum concentrates the radioiodine. Nevertheless and but whatever method, by salivating you are helping your salivary glands get rid of some of the accumulated radioiodine, thereby reducing radiation exposure to these glands. This strategy will be effective only if you take the candies or lemon drops frequently or continuously while awake. (Some patients prefer fresh lemon slices as even sour lemon drops can be sweet enough to cause mild nausea.) Shortly after you salivate and secrete the radioiodine, your salivary glands start to re-accumulate additional radioiodine. Although no one has determined the optimum frequency for eating candies, we recommend that patients take a new candy at least every 15 minutes since the radioiodine can re-accumulate that quickly. This recommendation may seem overly cautious, but it is harmless and should minimize the salivary side effects.

Patients should continue to suck on the lemon drops or slices throughout the day the radioiodine treatment was administered. We also strongly recommend that the nurses wake you up at least twice, and preferably three or four times, during that first night to take candies to salivate. It is perhaps during your sleep that your salivary glands receive their greatest radiation exposure. As noted below, you should also drink fluids and urinate throughout the night.

Any benefits to continuing this regimen the day after your radioiodine treatment are unknown. Consequently, there is no right or wrong recommendation. We prefer to err on the side of caution and recommend continued use of stimulants for salivation, but perhaps at reduced frequency.

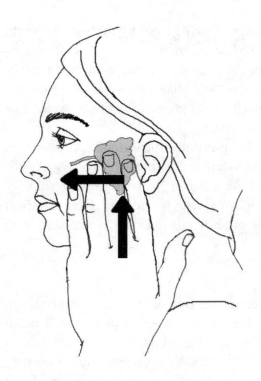

FIGURE 1: Your parotid gland (the gray area) lies just in front of your ear. To help your gland eliminate radioiodine, take your fingers and move them upward until you reach the palm of your hand, and then also push your fingers toward your face. Although difficult to convey visually, this is all one circular–like motion.

- **Massage**

While scientific evidence demonstrating the benefit of massage is not available, it cannot hurt and may facilitate secretion of the radioiodine. We suggest that you massage your salivary glands on a schedule similar to taking the lemon drops, which includes throughout the day and each time you wake up during the night. Your physician can instruct you on how to do this (see figure 1.)

- **Fluids**

Drink plenty of fluids—non-alcoholic of course. Drinking helps you remain well hydrated, which helps your kidneys remove unused radioiodine from your body. We suggest you drink fluids frequently throughout the day, starting shortly after your radioiodine treatment, and at multiple times during the night.

- **Medications**

Five types of medications might also be taken with your treatment, although most physicians treating thyroid cancer do not administer them routinely. These medications are categorized as: (1) pain, (2) anti-inflammatory, (3) parasympathomimetics, (4) anti-cholinergics, and (5) salivary gland radiation protectors. Significant medical information verifying the use of these medications is not available, but we believe they may be of value. None of these drugs should be taken if other health reasons prohibit their use.

1. **Pain medication:** In the event of severe salivary gland inflammation, medications such as acetaminophen (Tylenol®) may help relieve pain. Tylenol®, however, has little to no effect in reducing the inflammation from the radiation.

2. **Anti-inflammatory medication:** Medications such as aspirin, or ibuprofen (Advil® or Motrin®) have not been proven to reduce the radiation-induced inflammation of the salivary glands, but we believe it is reasonable to take these anti-inflammatory medications. These drugs may also help reduce pain. Steroids such as prednisone can be used to treat severe inflammation but are not routinely given for mild pain and swelling. Steroids may reduce radioiodine uptake in thyroid tissue and therefore are not given before radioiodine ablation or treatment.

3. **Parasympathomimetics:** Because these drugs are infrequently used and because of the complexity of the topic, it is beyond the scope of this book to discuss in detail parasympathomimetic drugs and how they work. However, one such drug is pilocarpine (Salagen®). This drug stimulates the parasympathomimetic nerve system in the salivary glands, which increases salivation. This drug has been given to promote the release of radioiodine from the salivary glands, but medical reports of the success of pilocarpine remain unconvincing and controversial. To our knowledge, most facilities do not routinely give pilocarpine. Consult your physician for more information.

4. **Anti-cholinergics:** For the same reasons noted above for parasympathomimetic drugs, it is not the goal of this book to discuss in detail anti-cholinergic drugs or their mechanisms. However, some facilities have used these types of medications to try to reduce the uptake of radioiodine in the salivary gland by blocking the parasympathomimetic nerve system. The success of these drugs has not been proven, and thus far these drugs are rarely used.

5. **Radiation protectors:** Amifostine is a radiation protector, which means that it can reduce the effects of radiation on some tissues. Amifostine has been demonstrated to help protect salivary glands in patients who have been treated with external beam irradiation for non-thyroid cancers in the head and neck. Although some medical data suggest that the amifostine will help protect the salivary glands from the radiation effects of radioiodine, it is not known whether the amifostine also "protects" the thyroid cancer. If this were the case, the results of the entire radioiodine treatment would be undesirably reduced. Thus the use of amifostine in patients with thyroid cancer who are going to be treated with radioiodine is controversial. To our knowledge, most facilities are not routinely administering amifostine. You should discuss this with your physician.

Delayed salivary gland pain and swelling

While pain and swelling of the salivary glands can occur within days of a radioiodine treatment, some patients may not experience it until several months later. The most likely cause for this appears to be a blockage of the flow of the saliva out of the glands caused by a narrowing of the ducts. This narrowing is the result of scarring due to inflammation caused by the radiation. Thus, as one begins to eat, the volume of saliva increases but cannot pass through the narrowed duct into the mouth. The gland then rapidly swells, which can be painful. In some people, discomfort can result simply by looking at appetizing food. The pain and swelling usually are not permanent but may last for several weeks to a few months. Chronic pain and swelling also is possible. The presence or absence of swelling and pain of your salivary glands within the first week after your treatment does not necessarily mean you will or will not experience this side effect months later.

Gently massaging your salivary glands may help reduce the swelling or pain. Depending on the severity and persistence of the symptoms, your physician may refer you to an otolaryngologist, also called an ear, nose, and throat specialist. This physician can evaluate the swelling and pain to make sure they are not due to other causes. If the radiation turns out to be the likely cause, the physician may consider other diagnostic tests to see if any of the main ducts are narrowed and could be reopened.

If you have experienced problems with your salivary glands following a previous radioiodine treatment, notify your physician before undergoing any additional radioiodine treatments. This side effect should not necessarily prohibit you from having additional radioiodine treatments.

Dry mouth (xerostomia)

Occasionally a patient may experience a dry mouth, a condition known as xerostomia, which is a result of reduced saliva production. Dry mouth also is a result of inflammation in your salivary glands caused by radiation exposure from your radioiodine treatment. It may occur several weeks to months after your treatment but tends to last only several weeks or months, and usually goes away completely. This side effect is rarely severe or permanent after only one radioiodine treatment. You should let your physician know if you experience any persistent dry mouth.

Change in taste

As many as a third of all patients will experience changes in taste after their first radioiodine treatment. Food may taste metallic or like cardboard, or it may not have any flavor at all. This side effect may begin a few days to weeks after the radioiodine treatment and lasts typically for several weeks and rarely for several months. Permanent changes in taste after the first radioiodine treatment are rare, but the risk increases with higher individual or total accumulated doses.

Conjunctivitis, inflammation of the lacrimal gland and obstruction of the nasolacrimal duct

The conjunctiva is the mucous membrane that lines the inside surface of the eyelid and the front part of the eyeball. The lacrimal gland secretes tears and lies above and toward the outside of the eyeball. The nasolacrimal duct is a channel that drains excess tears into the nasal cavity and is located on the inside of the lower aspect of the "lower" eyelid on each side of the nose. Radioiodine treatment has been associated with inflammation (1) of the conjunctiva, which is called conjunctivitis, (2) of the lacrimal glands, which may result in dry eyes, and (3) of the nasolacrimal duct, which may result in obstruction of the lacrimal duct and then in excess tearing. The latter is called epiphora. The frequency of these side effects is not well known and may depend on how hard one looks for them. In one report, conjunctivitis occurred in about 1 out of 5 patients. Chronic conjunctivitis has been reported. These side effects rarely require additional care from an ophthalmologist, or eye specialist.

Hypoparathyroidism

The parathyroid glands are four pea-sized glands that normally lie behind the thyroid gland (see figure 2). Their product, parathyroid hormone, regulates the body's calcium levels. Underactivity of the parathyroid glands is called hypoparathyroidism. This side effect of radioiodine treatment is very rare but is a well-recognized complication of thyroid surgery.

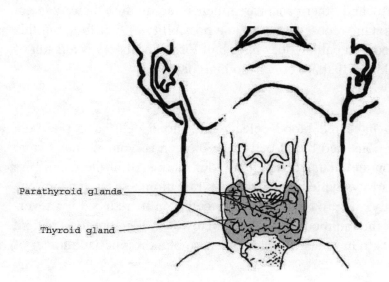

FIGURE 2: The typical location for four parathyroid glands is illustrated. These glands are usually located on the back side (posterior aspect) of the thyroid gland.

Parathyroid glands

Thyroid gland

Vocal cord paralysis

Your vocal cords may become paralyzed following any injury to the recurrent laryngeal nerve, which controls your voice box and is usually located behind your thyroid gland. However this side effect due to radioiodine is very rare, with only a handful of cases ever reported in the medical literature after tens of thousands of radioiodine treatments. If damage does occur, it probably happened during earlier operative trauma to the nerve during thyroidectomy.

Swelling and pain in your thyroid area

For your first treatment, you will receive radioiodine to destroy (ablate) any normal or abnormal thyroid tissue that remains after your initial surgery. Swelling or pain in this area may result from the intended radiation injury and subsequent destruction of the remaining thyroid tissue (radiation thyroiditis). The swelling or pain may begin several hours to several days after your treatment, may last just a day or two and should go away completely. Although the pain and swelling usually do not require treatment, pain or anti-inflammation medications such as aspirin or ibuprofen (e.g. Advil® or Motrin®), or pain medication such as acetaminophen (Tylenol®) may ease any discomfort. Your physician may prescribe other medications if the symptoms are severe or persistent.

Nose pain

Pain in the nose is not likely to occur after the first dose of radioiodine but may occur with larger or repeated doses. This side effect is discussed later in this chapter.

Loss of hair (alopecia)

Unlike chemotherapy and other cancer treatments, radioiodine therapy is not associated with hair loss. One report suggested the possibility of hair loss, but this has not been substantiated. If a patient does have hair loss, it probably is a result of thyroid hormone blood levels that are either too high or too low.

Drop in blood counts

In your blood you have red blood cells, white blood cells, and platelets. Among their many functions, red blood cells take oxygen to your tissues, white blood cells fight infection and platelets help clot your blood. All of these cells are made in your bone marrow, which does receive radiation exposure from the radioiodine. Consequently, the production of these cells can be reduced for several weeks or months after the radioiodine treatment. However, it is rare for a patient with normal blood counts to have any problem because of a drop in the number of red cells, white cells or platelets after the first radioiodine treatment. If the blood counts do drop, they usually return to approximately the levels that they were before the treatment, and the drop of blood counts is rarely associated with any consequences.

We recommend a complete blood count (CBC) before any treatment to help your physician decide how much radioiodine to use. An additional CBC is recommended between four and six weeks, because this is the time that the lowest blood counts will occur. This information may help demonstrate the response of the bone marrow to the treatment and be valuable in the event that a future treatment is necessary. We advise a final count after one year.

Fertility

Fertility in women does not seem to be affected by the first radioiodine treatment, although studies are ongoing. However, it is unclear how long women should wait after their ablation or treatment with radioiodine before becoming pregnant, and recommendations range from not waiting at all to waiting several years. We believe women should wait at least one year based on the following arguments: First, one report suggested a possible increase in the frequency of miscarriages occurring within the first year after treatment. The study, however, was inconclusive as to whether the increase was due to the radioiodine or hypothyroidism and poor control of the thyroid hormone replacement. Still, waiting one year might reduce the potential for a miscarriage. Second, waiting one year will allow for a one-year follow-up visit to determine, based on lab tests, X-rays or radioiodine whole body imaging, whether further treatments are needed. And third, the time may help you deal with other issues that naturally arise with a diagnosis of cancer.

Limited information is available regarding the effects of therapeutic radioiodine on testicular function. However, the data to date suggest that radioiodine treatment will affect the testicular function and fertility in as many as one third of the men treated with radioiodine. The sperm count may drop for as long as 12 to 24 months. Permanent reduction of sperm count is unlikely with the first treatment but has been reported. The drop in sperm count appears to be at least in part related to the dose of radioiodine as well as to whether sperm counts were normal prior to the treatment.

While permanent sperm count reduction is not likely, men hoping to have children may want to take precautions. One option is to "bank" sperm, or place it in storage, before the radioiodine ablation. A second option, depending on the stage of your disease, would be to postpone treatment until after conception. Patients should consult with their endocrinologist, nuclear medicine physician or nuclear radiologist for more information.

Congenital Abnormalities

Here the concern is whether possible radiation injury to either the sperm in a man or to the eggs (ova) in a woman may have resulted from the treatment. The first radioiodine treatment will not lead to a significant increase in the risk of having a child with a congenital abnormality. This statement does not mean that you will not have a child with a congenital abnormality. Every developing unborn baby has some risk of having a genetic defect. However, the radioiodine treatment will not significantly increase those risks.

Miscarriages

The risk of having a miscarriage does not appear to increase significantly after a radioiodine treatment. As noted above, one study that found a possible increase in miscarriages within one year after the treatment was inconclusive as to whether the rise was due to the radioiodine or the hypothyroidism and poor control of the thyroid hormone replacement.

Other cancers

Studies to date suggest there is no significant increased risk of developing other cancers as a result of the first radioiodine treatment.

Any significant increased risk of developing other cancers after multiple or higher doses of radioiodine is discussed in the next section entitled "Side effects from repeated or large dosages of radioiodine." Although the scientific data are not conclusive that there is an increased risk of developing another cancer, we believe it is prudent to take precautions with the first radioiodine treatment and any subsequent radioiodine treatments to minimize radiation exposure to the bladder, colon, and bone marrow. These precautions are easy to do and cause no harm unless restricted by your physician for other health reasons.

To reduce the radiation exposure to the bladder and the risk of bladder cancer, drinking a lot of fluids and frequently voiding throughout the day and night can reduce the radiation exposure to the bladder. Radioiodine kept in your bladder for a shorter period of time will lower the radiation dose to that organ. We realize waking up at night to void can be inconvenient. But we strongly encourage either the nurses waking you or setting your alarm to force yourself to get up during the night to drink more fluids and to empty your bladder. Some physicians have prescribed diuretics, which are drugs that increase your urine production and make you urinate more frequently. Your physician will advise you regarding this option.

To reduce the radiation exposure to the bowel and the risk of colon cancer, some physicians prescribe laxatives. Since significant amounts of radioiodine can be excreted into your stomach and intestines, precautions to reduce the time that the radioiodine remains in your intestines should reduce the radiation exposure to your intestines. Although it is unclear how long laxatives will be effective, we recommend taking them for at least one day after treatment and preferably for several days.

To reduce the radiation exposure to your bone marrow and the risk of leukemia, drink a lot of fluids. Staying well hydrated will help your body eliminate the radioiodine not taken up by thyroid cells, which will reduce unnecessary radiation exposure to the bone marrow as well as to all your organs. As already discussed, some physicians may prescribe diuretics. In addition to the benefits described above for the urinary bladder, diuretics may help clear the radioiodine from your blood faster. This also reduces the total radiation exposure to your bone marrow. Finally, some facilities have proposed a longer time interval between treatments in order to allow more time for the bone marrow to heal. This has not been proven; however, if the situation permits, time does allow healing of more of the radiation damage to the bone marrow. Again, your physician will advise you regarding these options.

III. Side effects from multiple or high dosages of radioiodine

As a general rule, side effects increase in frequency and severity with repeated or larger dosages of radioiodine. However, as discussed in the introduction of this chapter, the increased frequency and severity of the side effects must be weighed against the severity of your thyroid cancer.

Nausea and vomiting

Patients are more likely to experience nausea and vomiting after radioiodine in dosages of 200 mCi or more. Not all patients experience nausea or vomiting, but we recommend speaking with your physician about taking an anti-nausea medication before the treatment. Contrary to the usual recommendation that you do not eat or drink before or within two hours after the treatment, we suggest that you drink some water. We believe that the additional water taken with your radioiodine liquid or capsule may reduce the radiation exposure to your stomach and intestines, thereby reducing the likelihood and/or severity of any nausea and vomiting without affecting the absorption of the radioiodine. However, this has not been proven, and your physician will instruct you regarding ways to minimize nausea and vomiting.

Notify your physician immediately if vomiting occurs within two or three hours after your radioiodine dose.

Early onset of salivary gland swelling and pain

Pain and swelling of the salivary glands may be one of the most frequent complaints associated with radioiodine treatment. As discussed earlier in this chapter, radioiodine accumulates in your salivary glands, and as radioiodine accumulates with repeated and larger doses, the salivary glands are exposed to more and more radiation. This results in a higher risk of inflammation, swelling, and pain, which are usually more severe than those symptoms experienced after the initial treatment.

Steps you can take to reduce the radiation exposure to the salivary glands are discussed earlier in this chapter. We cannot emphasize enough that every reasonable effort should be made to decrease the amount of radiation exposed to the salivary glands beginning with the *first* treatment.

Delayed salivary swelling and pain

As with the first treatment, salivary pain or swelling may suddenly occur several months after a radioiodine ablation or treatment (see above). It is unclear whether these symptoms occur more frequently with larger doses than after the initial dose.

Dry mouth (xerostomia)

Larger doses and repeated treatments of radioiodine increase the risk of dry mouth, possibly to a point where saliva flow is severely reduced. These symptoms could lead to thicker mucous, especially in the morning, and an increase in tooth decay. If severe dry mouth (xerostomia) does develop, you are encouraged to meet with both your dentist and an ear, nose, and throat specialist. Your dentist will help you develop a more extensive dental hygienic plan, and the ear, nose, and throat specialist may prescribe medications to help increase saliva production. These medications include Salagen® (pilocarpine HCL) and Evoxac® (civimeline).

Change in taste

As the number of treatments increases, so does the likelihood of a change in the sense of taste. Depending on the dosage, these changes could be permanent. You should discuss these possible symptoms with your physician.

Conjunctivitis, inflammation of the lacrimal gland and obstruction of the nasolacrimal duct

No extensive study has been reported that evaluates the frequency and severity of these side effects with repeated or higher dosages of radioiodine. Although one study does suggest that changes are very frequent in the conjunctiva, the changes in the conjunctiva, lacrimal glands or nasolacrimal duct do not typically appear to cause any problems or to be noticed by the patient.

Swelling and pain in thyroid bed

Radioiodine doses of 200 mCi or greater do not necessarily lead to an increased likelihood of swelling and pain in the thyroid bed. These larger dosages typically are used only after an initial ablation has destroyed all or most of the normal thyroid tissue. Since little thyroid tissue remains to be destroyed, swelling or pain does not usually occur.

However, since you are receiving another radioiodine treatment, your physician must be trying to treat an area or areas of cancer. In these areas, you may experience swelling, pain or both. If you do experience swelling, pain or both, then these imply the treatment is working.

Nose pain

Glands located in the tip of the nose can take up radioiodine and thus be exposed to radiation, which can cause inflammation and be painful. This rarely occurs, except in patients who have received larger radioiodine dosages. Any pain localized in the nose usually lasts no more than a few days to a few weeks and then resolves completely. Occasionally a patient will have slight bleeding from the nose (epistaxis). Your nuclear medicine physician or nuclear radiologist can help you determine whether you are likely to experience these side effects based on a review of your pre-treatment radioiodine scan for uptake of radioiodine in the tip of your nose.

Loss of hair (alopecia)

General hair loss does *not* result from repeated treatments using large dosages of radioiodine.

Drop in blood counts

Repeated doses or larger dosages of radioiodine almost always lead to some drop in blood count levels. The drop typically begins one to two weeks after the radioiodine treatment with the lowest values occurring within four to six weeks after the treatment. The blood counts will then rise, usually returning to their pre-treatment values or just below their pre-treatment values.

In the unlikely event that the blood counts do drop significantly, the blood cells most likely affected are the white blood cells and platelets. If the white blood cells are too low, then the patient will be more susceptible to infection, and if the platelets are too low, the patient will be more susceptible to bleeding. Again, these complications are unlikely, but if they occur an additional treatment is available with agents to stimulate the bone marrow to make more white blood cells and platelets. Blood transfusions are also possible but rarely necessary. A significant drop in red blood cells requiring any treatment is also uncommon.

Patients who have either low pre-treatment blood counts or have already received several large doses of radioiodine can still receive additional radioiodine treatments. Factors that should be considered include (1) the actual blood counts,

(2) the degree to which your thyroid cancer has spread, (3) the amount of radioiodine uptake in the areas of the thyroid cancer, and (4) options available to stimulate or supplement your low baseline blood counts. If treatment is warranted, procedures are also available to save cells from your bone marrow prior to the administration of the radioiodine treatment dose. These cells are called "stem" cells, which can be placed back into your bone marrow at a later date (bone marrow transplant). Your physician can discuss these options with you.

Fertility

Although the risk of infertility in women does not appear to increase significantly after an initial radioiodine treatment, large clinical studies assessing the risk of infertility in women after large or repeated doses of radioiodine have not been conducted. However, studies have shown that there is a higher risk of a reduction of sperm count after larger or repeated doses. Accordingly, men who anticipate receiving repeated or large dosages of radioiodine and hope to have children may want to discuss with their doctors the options of banking sperm or postponing treatment until after conception.

Congenital Abnormalities

Theoretically, repeated, larger dosages of radioiodine could lead to a greater risk of congenital abnormalities in offspring, but clinical studies linking such an increase are not available. You should discuss your interests in conception with your physician.

Lung inflammation (pneumonitis) and lung scarring (fibrosis)

If your thyroid carcinoma has spread to your lungs, lung inflammation and fibrosis are possible side effects of repeated or high dosages of radioiodine. If the thyroid cancer in your lung(s) takes up radioiodine, then some adjacent normal lung tissue will be irradiated. This can lead first to inflammation (pneumonitis) and then to scarring (fibrosis) of this lung tissue. However, several factors determine whether the irradiation will lead to inflammation (pneumonitis) and then scarring (fibrosis) of the lung tissue. These include whether the thyroid cancer is distributed in just a few or many areas of your lungs, whether it is focal (well localized) or diffuse (widespread), the size of the areas, and how much radioiodine is taken up in each area. Your physician can assess these situations to determine whether the side effects of lung inflammation or scarring are important concerns. If so, some facilities might restrict the dosage of radioiodine while others might recommend dosimetry, which is discussed in detail in chapter 15. Although dosimetry determines a maximal allowable dose of radioiodine based on an estimated radiation exposure to the bone marrow, previous experience with dosimetry in patients who have thyroid cancer in the lungs has established additional restrictions to reduce the likelihood of lung inflammation and scarring.

For more information on the spread of cancer to the lungs, we recommend you discuss your situation with your team of physicians.

Bone pain

Some types of thyroid cancer may spread to various bones, which can lead to bone pain after radioiodine treatment. Pain that existed before the treatment may become more intense for several weeks after the treatment. Some physicians have suggested that increased pain indicates a better therapeutic outcome, but this theory has not been proven. Other side effects are possible depending on which bones are involved and should be discussed with your physician.

Other cancers

With repeated or larger dosages of radioiodine, an increased risk of developing other cancers is possible but not known. These cancers include, but are not limited to, bladder cancer, colon cancer and leukemia. At this point, the natural question is "If there is an increased risk, what is the risk of developing these cancers?" Unfortunately, determining the increased risk is very difficult to do, and there are many factors that enter into this. These factors include the age of the patient at the time of diagnosis, the present age of the patient, the total amount of radioiodine administered from all treatments, the amount of each individual dose, and the time between doses, to name only a few. This is further complicated by (1) different populations of patients studied, (2) how the data are reported in the literature, and (3) contradictory results among different studies. In addition and as mentioned previously, how well you adhere to the regimens prescribed to reduce the body burden of radioactivity (fluids, lemon candies, getting up at night, diuretics, laxatives, etc.) will also affect your risk for other cancers. As a result, patients may hear many different and often contradictory statements from their physicians, media pundits or acquaintances regarding the amount of increased risk or a lack of increased risk of developing other cancers.

So, what can we say regarding this very difficult and serious subject? We believe the following generalizations are reasonable:

1. There is either no increased risk or the risk of developing another cancer from one treatment of radioiodine is so small that it is not a valid reason to refuse the first radioiodine treatment. The only exception to this would be patients who have occult cancers (see chapter 4).
2. As individual and cumulative dosages of radioiodine increase, we believe that there is an increased risk of developing other cancers. Although this

risk is difficult to quantify, we believe it is still small and must be weighed against the risk of your thyroid cancer affecting your health. Of course, the latter is also difficult to quantify. This is especially a problem in patients who have no evidence of thyroid cancer except for persistently elevated thyroglobulin levels and who are being considered for large or repeated dosages of radioiodine for treatment.

3. We do not believe that any strict upper limit of total cumulative dosage such as 1 or 2 curies (1000-2000 millicuries) should be used. We believe that many factors must be weighed including but not limited to (1) the severity of the disease, (2) the location of the disease, (3) whether the metastasis takes up radioiodine, (4) how the patient has previously responded to radioiodine, (5) how long ago the last treatment was administered, (6) the total blood counts, (7) what was the response of the blood counts to the last radioiodine treatment, (8) the age of the patient, (9) the patient's other health problems, if any, and (10) other options available to the patient.

4. All reasonable efforts should be made to minimize any real or imagined risk of other cancers, and this should be initiated at the *first* treatment.

Other side effects

Other side effects may occur depending on where the thyroid cancer metastasis may be located. Although it is beyond the scope of this book to discuss side effects based on each location, a metastasis to the brain warrants further discussion with your physician regarding the risks and benefits of radioiodine. This discussion should also include consideration of potential modification of the dosage of radioiodine and the use of drugs, such as steroids, glycerol, and mannitol, to reduce side effects of the treatment of brain metastasis with radioiodine.

Summary

As with most treatments or drugs, radioiodine has side effects, and these generally increase in frequency and severity with increasing dosage of radioiodine. In this chapter, we have tried to give a reasonable and honest overview of the side effects based on diagnostic dosages, first-time ablative dosages, and repeated or high dosages. Unfortunately, such a list of side effects and everything that could possibly go wrong is always disheartening. However, keep in mind three things:

- Many of these side effects are infrequent,
- Most of the side effects are manageable, and
- The risk of the frequency and severity of the side effects must be weighed in light of the severity of your thyroid cancer.

CHAPTER 19

Radioactivity and Radiation

John E. Glenn, M.D.

Radioactivity and radiation are two closely related concepts, but the distinction between them is very important for determining methods to protect you and your loved ones from the effects of either.

Radioactivity is "stuff" made up of atoms, as are you, your house, your food, and everything else that you can see, feel, taste, smell or touch. You can get radioactivity in or on you. Unwanted radioactivity on a person or thing is called contamination.

Radioactive atoms are different from other atoms in that they can decay and release energy in the form of radiation. Radiation is a means of transporting small bundles of energy from one place to another. Light from a flashlight is radiation. The microwaves that cook your food are radiation. The heat that warms your face in front of the fireplace is radiation. The atomic particles released by the sun as solar wind are radiation. The energy from radiation often is emitted in waves, such as X-rays, gamma rays or alpha or beta particles. You can be exposed to radiation but not contaminated with radiation. In other words, radiation exposure is an event, not a substance.

Ionizing radiation

Radiation comes in many forms. Ionizing radiation is emitted from radioactivity and may exist as tiny moving particles or electromagnetic waves similar to light. Ionizing radiation has enough energy to get inside objects and alter the number of electrons within the atoms that make up those objects. Those affected atoms are called ions because they have either lost or gained one or more electrons. The number of ions that are created within matter, including your body, depends on the amount of energy given off by the ionizing radiation. This amount is called the radiation dose. A high radiation dose, usually about 50 rem or 50,000 millirem, means an extremely large number of ions (about a billion trillion) have been created in your body. Although the number of ions is very large, the energy absorbed by your body is about one million times smaller than the energy required to light a bulb for one hour.

Hazards of radiation

Too much of any kind of radiation can be harmful, although in moderate doses radiation can be welcomed and even comforting. A bright light can help you read, but if you look right at the light, it can blind you. Heat from the sun can feel good on your skin, but too much exposure can burn and cause skin cancer. Too much microwave radiation can cook you, and too high a dose of ionizing radiation can cause burns, hair loss or a reduced numbers of blood cells.

Ionizing radiation and cancer

As radiation enters your cells and converts atoms into ions, it causes chemical changes in the cells. Too many changes can kill the cells or cause other long-term effects such as cancer. But so far scientists have detected just minor effects in people exposed to levels of ionizing radiation lower than 50 rems or 50,000 millirems.

In the first day or two after your radioactive iodine cancer treatment, anyone coming near you is at risk of receiving a radiation dose greater than 500 millirem but less than 5,000 millirem. They can receive it directly, from the radiation emitted from your body, or by ingesting or inhaling radioactive iodine that you shed through breath or body fluids.

To keep cancer risks to friends and family members As Low As is Reasonably Achievable—a concept radiation health experts refer to as ALARA—hospital staff will send you home with instructions based on "radiation protection standards" set by the Nuclear Regulatory Commission (NRC).

These instructions are intended to establish a level of risk one half to one tenth of the annual accident rate from falling, fire or other hazards typical in an office environment or manufacturing plant. Thus the most exposed individual coming in contact with you should receive a radiation dose with a maximum estimated risk of 0.002 percent of developing a fatal cancer sometime in the next 10 to 60 years. In other words, fewer than two out of every 100,000 people exposed to you would develop a fatal cancer later in life. The average exposure friends and family members receive annually from thyroid cancer patients is normally one fifth to one tenth of the maximum permitted.

Over time, your risk of contaminating anyone else with radioactive iodine decreases. Table 1 shows how the dose rate drops off for measurements made at one meter, or slightly more than three feet, from your body. This table is calculated from the [131]iodine retention assumptions in the NRC's Regulatory Guide 8.39, prepared to help hospitals determine the conditions appropriate for the release of patients receiving [131]iodine and other radioactivity. The guide lists assumptions that can be made to keep radiation doses to family and friends at less than 500 millirem and preferably less than 100 millirem. The radioactivity you are given initially is often 100 millicuries or larger. The millicurie is a measure of how many radioactive atoms decay and emit radiation in a given time. One hundred millicuries represent a quantity of radioactivity decaying and emitting radiation 3.7 billion times a second.

There is a potential risk of injury to another individual's thyroid if he or she ingests or inhales more than 0.03 millicuries as a result of exposure to radioactive iodine that comes from you. As long as you wash your hands and stay at least one meter away from everyone else, no one around you will receive an unhealthy dose of radiation. Certain intimate contacts could transfer more than 0.03 millicuries in the very early days after you receive your radioactive iodine. Of particular concern are breast milk and pregnancy. Women of childbearing age must avoid pregnancy during their treatment, and mothers must not nurse infants.

The amount of radioactivity you shed through breath, saliva, urine, and perspiration drops rapidly over time. Intimate contact needs to be avoided for only days rather than weeks. Table 2 shows estimates of the amount of radioactivity you will release, through your perspiration, saliva, breath, and urine, during each day following dosage. Other than radioactivity excreted in urine, by day four the levels are

TABLE 1*
Dose rate at 1 meter in millirem/hour (mrem/h)

Dosage	100 mCi	150 mCi	200 mCi
Time (days)	Dose Rate		
0	50 mrem/h	75 mrem/h	100 mrem/h
0.25	30	45	60
0.5	18	27	36
0.75	11	16.5	22
1	7	10.5	14
2	2.5	3.8	5
3	1.6	2.4	3.2
4	1.5	1.8	3.0
5	1.3	19.5	2.6
6	1.2	1.8	2.4
7	1.1	1.7	2.2
14	0.6	0.9	1.2
21	0.3	0.45	0.6

*This table does not show rates for dosages greater than 200 millicurie (mCi). These larger dosages are usually calculated based on measurements showing that you will eliminate the radioactive iodine from your body at a much faster rate than assumed in the NRC guide. If you received a larger dosage, you may use the estimates for a dosage of 200 millicuries after the first two days.

much smaller than 30 microcuries and by day seven are extremely small. Table 2 was calculated using an average of measurements made at 24 and 48 hours by the Medical College of Wisconsin and assuming that the measured levels after 48 hours would drop as predicted using the NRC Regulatory Guide 8.39 retention model. The measurements indicated that the levels (except for urine) are greatest at 24 hours.

Myths about radioactivity

1. **Radiation exposure will make me radioactive.**

   You do not become radioactive. You are a source of radiation exposure only as long as radioactive iodine remains in your body. More than 99 percent of the radioactive iodine is eliminated in the first several days.

TABLE 2*
Amount of radioactive iodine excreted by various pathways during days following dosage. The excreted activity is millicuries per 100 millicuries administered.

Day	Perspiration Activity on whole body	Saliva Per cubic centimeter	Breath Per cubic centimeter	Urine Per day
1	0.025	0.046	0.045	80.000
2	0.013	0.008	0.011	8.600
3	0.002	0.0009	0.0013	1.000
4	0.0002	0.0001	0.0002	0.100
5	0.00002	0.00001	0.0002	0.013
6	0.000002	0.000001	0.000002	0.002
7	0.000000	0.000000	0.000000	0.0002

*Iodine-131 Contamination from Thyroid Cancer Patients. Erkan Ibis, Charles R. Wilson, B. David Collier, Gur Akansel, Ali T. Isitman, and Robert G. Yoss, The Journal of Nuclear Medicine, Vol. 33, No. 12, p 2110–2115, (1992).

2. **Most radiation exposure results from human activities.**

   In fact, most radiation exposure comes from nature.

   Natural sources:

   - RADON gas—55 percent
   - Natural radioactivity in your body—11 percent
   - Natural radioactivity in the Earth—8 percent
   - Radiation from outer space—8 percent

   Man-made sources:

   - Medical therapy and diagnosis—15 percent
   - Consumer products—3 percent
   - Nuclear power—< 1 percent

3. **Living near a nuclear power plant exposes me to a large amount of radiation.**
   - The amount of radiation exposure you receive leaving near a nuclear power plant is equivalent to the radiation exposure received while flying in a high-altitude airplane.
   - Nuclear Power Plant (at plant boundary)—0.6 millirem/year.
   - Coast to coast airplane roundtrip—5.0 millirem.

4. **Radiation exposure can turn people and animals into monsters.**
   A large radiation dose can cause injury or death, smaller doses can increase the risk for cancer and exposure of the developing fetus can cause deformations and deficiencies. But exposure to radiation will not change people or animals into monsters as depicted in the movies.

CHAPTER 20

Radiation Safety Precautions During Your Hospital Stay and at Home

John E. Glenn, M.D.

The medical staff, support staff, other patients, visitors, and the next patient to occupy your room must be protected from unnecessary exposure to radiation and radioactive material. The methods of achieving protection are:

- Isolation
- Containment of any contamination
- Measurement and release of anything entering the room
- Good hygiene

Isolation

Perhaps the biggest sacrifice you will make is isolation from all but a few hospital staff. The hospital staff will be instructed to have as little contact with you as possible given your medical condition. Visitors are not permitted unless the physician in charge of the iodine administration believes that your condition requires family members or close friends to assist you. An example would be a young child receiving radioiodine treatment and needing assistance. Your isolation is not required because of immediate danger to people coming in close contact but in order to assure that each exposure is kept as low as is reasonably achievable (ALARA principle). In an emergency, the medical staff will give you all the necessary medical attention you need. Proximity to you, even right after your treatment, should not expose them to more radiation than a member of the public gets in a year from natural background radiation. However, that kind of radiation exposure 20 to 40 times a year would result in unreasonably high radiation exposure and an unnecessary but small risk of cancer later in their life.

Containment

Everything that enters your room will be left in the room unless cleared by radiation safety personnel. As long as the radioactive material stays in your room, other people in the hospital will be protected from exposure. You should limit personal belongings to clothes, disposable materials or things that easily can be cleaned. Personal belongings that cannot be cleaned and are contaminated with ^{131}iodine above a certain limit will be disposed of by the hospital or kept until the radioactivity decays.

Measurement and release

Everything in your room, including you, will be measured for radiation before it can leave. There are three possibilities:

- Release— if not contaminated above the release limit
- Held for later release after radioactive decay
- Disposal as radioactive waste such as utensils or property

Your room likely will be specially prepared before you arrive to make measurement and release of the radioactivity in the room as quick and simple as possible. Floors, door handles, telephones and other things you touch will be covered with paper or plastic. These coverings will be treated as waste to assure that measurements of the uncovered areas will not reveal contamination after you leave.

Hygiene

Good hygiene practices will help make sure that your belongings and the fixtures in your room will not be contaminated with radioactive material. Frequent showers and washings will reduce skin contamination. The most likely area to be contaminated in the room is the toilet. Men are encouraged to sit when urinating to minimize contamination.

Radioactive iodine safety

From 1973 until 1997, the NRC required that all patients receiving more than 30 millicuries of radioactive material for therapy remain in the hospital until the radioactivity dropped below 30 millicuries. Patients also could go home as long as the radiation dose measured at 1 meter from their bodies dropped below 5 millirem per hour. These criteria were intended to make sure friends and family members would not be exposed to more than 500 millirem from any patient receiving ^{131}iodine. The criteria were released under some rather cautious assumptions:

1. None of the radioactive material would be eliminated except by natural decay (that is, no radioactivity is eliminated in urine).
2. The patient's body would not absorb any of the energy from the radiation.

3. The most exposed individual family member or friend would spend no more than 25 percent of his or her time within three feet of the patient until all of the radioactive material was gone due to natural decay.

Based on comments from physicians treating patients with radioactive material, the NRC changed its patient release criteria in 1997 (62 FR 4120, Jan. 29, 1997).

Instead of a mandated 30 millicuries or 5 millirem/hour at one meter, the NRC-regulated hospital now is required to demonstrate that friends and family will not receive a radiation dose in excess of 500 millirem in one year from the released patient. (The NRC may relinquish its regulatory program to a state if there is a similar program in place for regulating radioactive material. More than half of the states meet these criteria; therefore; the descriptions of the NRC's requirements discussed here may vary slightly from one state to another.)

The hospital has two choices:

- Base the estimated radiation dose on the administered dose and the three cautious assumptions discussed above.
- Base the estimated dose on the activity at the time of release and more realistic assumptions on the actual circumstances of the patient. The default release limit for ^{131}iodine, based on only the administered or remaining radioactivity in the body and the three cautious assumptions, is the same as the NRC's previous release criterion adjusted to be slightly more accurate.

Advantages and disadvantages of hospitalization

Your hospital will ask you questions to document that you are a suitable candidate for early release. If you are planning any activity that hospital staff do not raise, bring that activity to their attention.

Of particular concern is your potential to contaminate the people around you during the first 24 to 36 hours. After two days, you won't emit, through breath, urine or sweat, any radioactive contamination of consequence (see Table 2 in the previous chapter). During the first 24 hours, urine, saliva, breath, and blood will contain concentrations of radioactive iodine that could harm another person's thyroid. Both you and the releasing hospital must seriously evaluate both the probability and the consequences of an accident that could result in another person's uptake of radioactive iodine. An 18-hour hospital stay or longer significantly reduces the risks associated with any accidental exposure to your bodily fluids.

Earlier release

A patient's agreement to limit close contact with family and friends to three hours a day for the first few days often is enough for an NRC licensee to justify early release. Under certain circumstances, an NRC licensee may immediately release a patient who has been given hundreds of millicuries of radioactive material based on that patient's ability to isolate himself or herself from other people. Most hospitals will release all but a few patients within 18 to 30 hours after administration of radioactive iodine.

Some hospitals may encourage even earlier releases. Considerations for release earlier than 18 hours should include:

- Almost total isolation at home for the first day
- Separate eating, bathing, and toilet facilities for the first few days
- No use of public facilities or transportation for the first few days
- No trips longer than an hour in a private automobile or in contact with other passengers during the first day after administration
- Ability of the patient to care for himself or herself with no assistance
- No medical need to observe the patient the first day
- Absolutely no intimate contact for several days
- High confidence that the patient will not become sick in the first several hours from [131]iodine remaining in the stomach. Vomiting may significantly contaminate a home or public place, putting untrained cleaning personnel at risk.

Precautions at home

The main protection for family and friends is for you to avoid close contact for about 3 days. If you review the dose rates and contamination levels in Tables 1 and 2, you will note how quickly the levels drop.

There is one critical person who is at potential great risk of harm. Nursing an infant or small child after receiving radioactive iodine will transfer the radioactive iodine from the mother to the child in the milk. Radioactive iodine ingested by the child will expose the thyroid of the child to potentially harmful levels of radiation. Lifelong medication may be required to prevent serious effects both mentally and physically if the child's thyroid receives a high dose of radiation.

Although there is no evidence that the amount of radiation received by those people coming close to you will do harm, it is reasonable (ALARA) to take certain precautions for at least three days following release, and four days if you are released in less than 24 hours.

Once you get home:

1. Keep a safe distance from other people
   - Sleep alone for three nights.
   - Avoid kissing and sexual intercourse for three days.
   - Stay at least three feet away from anyone you will be in contact with for more than an hour during your first three days home.

2. Minimize time in public places including public transportation, theaters, and sporting events for three days.

3. Feel free to eat meals with your family and care for your children, but time spent holding a child on a lap or lying next to you should be minimized.

4. Avoid breast feeding because it could seriously harm the infant.

5. Wash your hands frequently for several days as sweat contains a minuscule amount of radioactive iodine.

6. Wash your bed linens and clothes separately for three days before resuming normal care.

7. Use a separate bathroom for three days, if possible, and flush twice when using the toilet, as urine contains excreted radioactive iodine. If separate facilities are not available, good hygiene habits are more than adequate to minimize exposure.

These guidelines will limit other people to radiation exposure at far below the acceptable levels. Radioactive iodine will disappear completely through your own body excretions and as part of the physical process that makes it radioactive. If you wish to be very cautious, maintain these restrictions for up to seven days.

CHAPTER 21

External Beam
Radiation Therapy

James D. Brierley, BSc, MB

Introduction

This chapter discusses (1) what external beam radiation is, (2) how radiation works, (3) the objectives of external radiation, (4) what a radiation prescription is, (5) a description of what is involved in radiation and therapy, (6) indications for treatment, and (7) side effects of external radiation. The chapter concludes with several frequently asked questions.

I. What is external beam radiation?

External beam radiation is a form of radiation therapy used to treat cancer. There are two types of radiation therapy that may be used in thyroid cancer: external radiation therapy, often abbreviated as XRT, and internal radiation, which is radioactive iodine. External radiation therapy is called such because the radiation is produced by a machine outside (external to) the body.

The most frequently used machine to produce the radiation is called a linear accelerator (see figures 1 and 2). A linear accelerator uses microwaves to accelerate electrons. These electrons then hit a target and produce X-rays, and then the X-rays enter your body to irradiate your cancer. Sometimes electrons themselves are used for radiation therapy instead of X-rays. These electrons have a much higher energy than those produced by the decay of radioiodine so the machine can be some distance away from the area to be treated.

An alternative to a linear accelerator is a Cobalt machine, which is less commonly used. These machines contain radioactive cobalt (^{60}Co), and when the cobalt decays, high-energy gamma radiation is produced, which can be used as external radiation. This gamma radiation has a much higher energy than that produced by the decay of radioiodine.

Although X-rays and gamma rays have different names, X-rays are identical to gamma rays except for how they are produced. X-rays are produced from electrons hitting a target, and gamma rays are the result of the decay of a radioactive material such as ^{60}Co and ^{131}I.

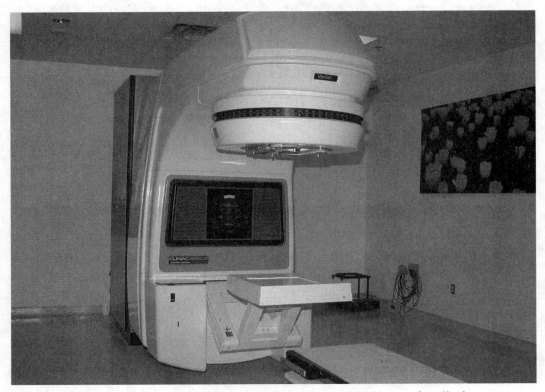

FIGURE 1: Linear accelerator in the usual position at the start of radiation and to deliver radiation from above.

II. How does radiation work?

Unlike radioiodine, which you take internally, XRT is directed to a specific area of the body. In thyroid cancer this is usually to the neck. XRT works like any other type of radiation in damaging the DNA of cells, and the cells then die when they try to divide or multiply. Both normal and cancer cells are affected by radiation, but radiation works because cancers cells usually divide more frequently than normal cells, and thus cancer cells are affected more than normal cells. In addition, normal cells are not only better than cancer cells in repairing any damage from radiation, but normal cells outside the area irradiated can also grow into the areas affected and help replace the damaged cells. Thus, radiation therapy works by damaging cancer cells more than normal cells.

III. The objectives of external radiation

There are three distinct goals of XRT: adjuvant radiation, radical radiation, and palliative radiation

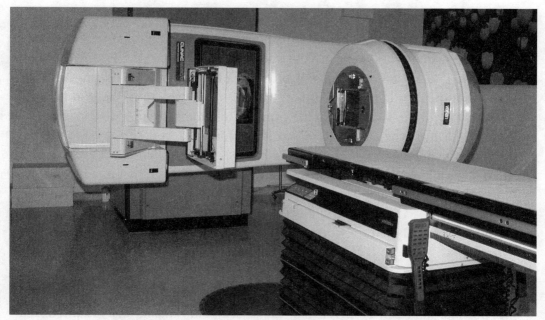

FIGURE 2: Linear accelerator in position to deliver radiation to the left side.

Adjuvant radiation

Adjuvant radiation is radiation that is given as an addition to the primary or main treatment. The primary treatment in all types of thyroid cancer is surgery. As noted in the other chapters, typically radioiodine ablation (treatment) is given after the surgery for well-differentiated thyroid cancer, which is papillary or follicular cancer. However, radioiodine is not used for medullary or anaplastic thyroid cancer. This radioiodine ablation (treatment) is considered to be adjuvant to surgery. XRT is rarely given as adjuvant radiation after the first ablation (treatment) with radioiodine. However, if your physician thinks that there may be a high risk of the cancer returning in the neck despite surgery and radioiodine, XRT may be recommended as adjuvant therapy after the radioiodine. In medullary thyroid cancer and anaplastic thyroid cancer XRT can be given after surgery and is considered adjuvant therapy. This XRT is given to help reduce the risk of the cancer recurring in the neck.

Adjuvant radiation is usually given with many small fractions over a long time, and a typical adjuvant radiation prescription is "50 Gy over 5 weeks, given as 25 daily fractions of 2 Gy per day, 5 days a week." Another adjuvant radiation prescription is "45 Gy over 5 weeks, given as 25 daily fractions of 1.8 Gy per day, 5 days a week." More information is presented in section III entitled "What is a radiation prescription" in this chapter. If your physicians are particularly concerned about a specific area, then a boost of radiation may be given.

B. Radical radiation

Rarely in differentiated thyroid cancer and medullary thyroid cancer, but more often in anaplastic thyroid cancer, your surgeon cannot remove the cancer because it is invading vital tissues or organs. If surgery cannot remove the cancer, XRT may be given as radical or curative treatment to try and destroy the cancer in the neck. The radiation in these situations is the primary treatment. A high dose of radiation is needed to destroy the cancer in radical radiation.

Like adjuvant radiation, radical radiation is usually given with many small fractions over a long time, but it achieves a higher total dose than in adjuvant therapy. A typical radical radiation prescription is "60 Gy over 6 weeks, given as 30 daily fractions of 2 Gy per day, 5 days a week." Another typical radical radiation prescription is "50 Gy over 4 weeks, given as 20 daily fractions of 2.5 Gy per day, 5 days a week."

C. Palliative radiation

If no treatment can be given that may cure your cancer, any radiation treatment given is palliative, and its aim is to improve your quality of life and reduce or alleviate any symptoms you have from your cancer.

Palliative radiation can be given to the original site of the cancer in your neck or to sites of spread (metastasis) when your physicians believe that the cancer cannot be completely removed by surgery and or destroyed by radical radiation.

The palliative radiation may be given to the neck to control pain or to relieve obstruction if the cancer is pressing on the esophagus or trachea. It may be given to bone metastases to reduce pain or prevent fractures. It may also be given to large lung metastases that are causing pain or bleeding or causing obstruction in the lung. Unfortunately, the lung and liver do not tolerate radiation well, and therefore XRT cannot be given to widespread metastases throughout the lung or liver without destroying too much normal lung tissue or liver. However, it can be safely given to a small area of lung if a metastasis in that volume is causing specific symptoms.

Palliative radiation is usually given with a small number of large fractions over a short time, as a high dose often is not needed to reduce symptoms. A typical palliative radiation prescriptions is "30 Gy over 2 weeks, given as 10 daily fractions of 3 Gy per day, 5 days a week." Two other typical palliative radiation prescription are "20 Gy over 1 week, given as 5 daily fractions of 4 Gy per day, 5 days a week" and "8 Gy given as single daily fraction of 8 Gy."

IV. What a radiation prescription is

A radiation treatment is prescribed like a drug treatment. The radiation prescription describes the total dose of radiation to be given, the number of fractions (the number of daily treatments), the size of each daily treatment, and the overall length of the treatment course. Sometimes more than one fraction per day may be prescribed. Treatments are usually given daily 5 days a week.

What is a Gy?

The unit dose of radiation is the Grey abbreviated to Gy. Most prescriptions are given in centiGrey or cGy. One Gy = 100 cGy. Occasionally the radiation dose is described in rads, which is an older term. One rad equals 1 cGy. One hundred rads equals 100cGy, which equals 1Gy. Your radiation oncologist will prescribe the radiation appropriately for what is needed.

What is a radiation fraction?

A fraction is the amount of radiation delivered to the target at any one time. For a radical course of radiotherapy the fraction size is usually small, such as 1.8 cGy or 2 cGy. This is because large fraction sizes result in more late toxicity, and if the radiation oncologist plans to give a high total dose, then giving small fraction sizes results in less risk of late radiation damage.

This, however, means that the course of radiation is long. If the cancer is growing rapidly, then it may be better to give the radiation quickly over a short time. Increasing the fraction size can do this, but this is at the risk of more late toxicity. Another possibility is to give more than one fraction a day, which is called accelerated fractionation. Because this also results in more damage to the normal rapidly dividing tissues such as the skin and mucosa, it is important to ensure that there is a long enough time period between each daily fraction to allow the normal tissue to repair some of the damage from radiation. Usually, therefore, there is a 6- to 8-hour period between fractions if more than one fraction is given each day.

To reduce the risk of toxicity further, even smaller fractions than 1.8 Gy or 2 Gy may be given. This is called hyperfractionation. If more than one small fraction is given each day, then this is called accelerated hyperfractionation. This is sometimes prescribed in anaplastic thyroid cancer.

An example of accelerated hyperfractions would be giving 60 Gy over 4 weeks for 40 twice-daily fractions of 1.5 Gy for 5 days a week. This is instead of 60 Gy over 6 weeks, for 30 daily-fractions of 2 Gy per day for 5 days a week.

How is the radiation prescription chosen?

The examples of radiation treatment prescriptions given above are just that—examples. There are many factors that go into deciding what is the appropriate radiation prescription for you. There is no evidence that a different particular prescription that another patient received is better or worse than the prescription you received. Your physician takes into account your type of cancer, the extent of cancer, the extent of surgery, your symptoms, your age, your general health, your wishes, and the radiation therapy physician's experience with different radiation prescriptions. Thus, if radiation is recommended for you, you may be prescribed a course of radiation that is different than the examples given above or different than a prescription described for another individual with thyroid cancer.

V. What is involved in radiation therapy?

A course of radiation therapy involves (1) an initial consultation with a radiation oncologist with a decision to treat or not, (2) the development of a treatment plan, (3) the administering of the radiation treatment, (4) treatment assessment, and (5) follow up.

1. The initial consultation

If your endocrinologist or surgeon thinks that you might benefit from XRT you will be referred to a radiation oncologist for an opinion on the role of XRT for your case. For this consultation and appointment, either you will call the radiation oncologist's office or the radiation oncologist's staff will call you. At your first visit and as with any first visit to a physician, the radiation oncologist will obtain a history from you and examine you. The radiation oncologist will also review other information such as operative, pathology and diagnostic imaging study reports. Occasionally, an additional appointment to see the radiation oncologist and more time may be required because he or she needs more information or investigations such as CT scan or needs to discuss your case with your referring physicians before he or she gives you a recommendation.

2. The development of a treatment plan

If radiation therapy is recommended, then the next stage is to plan the radiation treatment. The aim of the treatment plan is to ensure that a precisely measured dose of radiation as prescribed by your radiation oncologist is delivered to a volume defined by your radiation oncologist with minimal dose to the surrounding healthy tissues. There are two components to planning: first, "treatment simulation" and second, "plan development and calculation."

Treatment simulation

Simulation is a process in which the radiation oncologist and dosimetrist assess how the radiation treatment plan is going to be given. This assessment may take 30 minutes, but occasionally this may take longer.

One frequent aspect of simulation, which is especially important for high-dose radiation to the neck, is to ensure that you do not move your head or neck

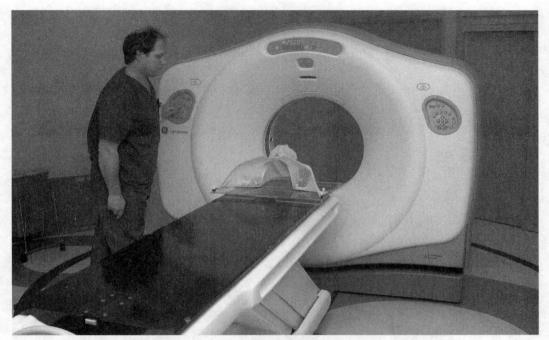

FIGURE 3: CT Simulator, with immobilization device (mask) on couch.

during the radiation treatment. Obviously, if you do move your head, then the radiation may end up being directed to the wrong area. To prevent movement, an immobilization device or mask may be made to keep your neck immobile during treatment. There are many different types of masks, and examples are shown in figures 3 and 4. Making the mask may take an additional 30 minutes or more.

At simulation you will be asked to lie very still on an X-ray table, just like the one that will be used during your treatment, and in the same position that you will be treated in. The radiation oncologist will assess the area to be treated, and an X-ray machine will take X-ray films. The difference between the X-ray machine used in simulation and an ordinary X-ray machine is that the simulation X-ray machine moves and rotates about you in exactly the same way that the treatment machine will so that it can simulate the treatment. The center of the area to be treated will be marked on your mask or sometimes on you. If marked on you, indelible ink may be used, in which case it is very important that it does not get removed or washed off. If indelible ink is not used, then a tiny tattoo forming a dot on your skin is made with ink and a sterile needle. These marks are used to make sure you are in the same position every time you have a radiation treatment. When you are in the correct position, X-rays will be taken. Your radiation oncologist will use these X-rays to determine the area to be treated. In addition to these X-rays, the

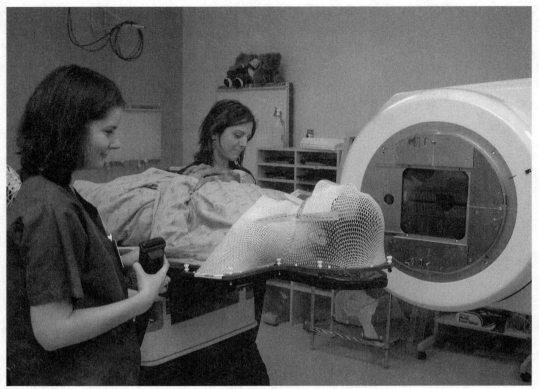

FIGURE 4: Patient in immobilization device (mask) being set up for treatment to the right side of the neck.

dosimetrist may take additional specific measurements while you are still in the same position. These measurements may be needed to plan your treatment.

In many centers a CT (computer tomography) simulator is used instead of a simulator using conventional X-rays. A CT simulator is similar to a diagnostic CT scan, which you most likely have had before, but like the conventional simulator, you will be in exactly the same position you will be in for treatment, including the mask, if used (see figure 4).

Plan development and calculation

By using either the X-rays or the CT scans obtained during simulation, your radiation oncologist will mark the exact volume of tissue, which will include both known cancer and nearby normal tissue that may contain microscopic cancer that needs to be irradiated. This is called the clinical treatment volume, which is abbreviated as CTV. The normal tissues that need to be spared as much as possible, such as the spinal cord, are also identified. Using this information and additional measurements taken at the time of simulation, the dosimetrist will develop the treatment plan in consultation with your radiation oncologist.

The treatment plan is a combination of radiation treatment "fields," and each treatment "field" is a beam of radiation directed at the cancer, but from different positions around the body. Thus, when all of the doses of radiation deposited in the cancer from each field of radiation are added together, the dose of radiation to the cancer will be high in the clinical treatment volume (CTV), but very low outside the CTV. This reduces the radiation exposure to the normal tissues that the radiation must pass through to get to the cancer, but ensures that the cancer is effectively treated.

3. Administering the radiation treatment

Most radiation treatments last only for 1 to 5 minutes; however your, appointment may be for 15 to 30 minutes. This extra time is for you to get into the correct position for treatment. Your treatment therapist will help you get into the correct position, which is identical to the position established during your simulation. The treatment therapist adjusts the position of the treatment table and the machine so that the center of the radiation field is correctly aligned with the marks on the mask, other immobilization device, or the tattoos. When you are correctly aligned the therapist will leave the radiation room and close the door. Although no one else will be in the room with you, you will not be alone during the actual treatment. You will be closely monitored and in contact with the therapist by camera, windows, a communication system, or all three. When the machine is turned on there may be some strange noises, but you will not see or feel anything. Once the first field of treatment is completed the machine will move to the next treatment position ("field"), and the process is repeated until all treatment fields are completed. The first treatment session usually takes longer than others, as it takes longer the first time to ensure that you are in the correct position.

During your first treatment, X-ray films will also be taken and reviewed by your radiation oncologist to ensure the treatment is correctly directed. These X-rays may be taken at the same time as the treatment, and you may not be aware they are being taken. They may be repeated several times during your treatment.

4. Treatment assessment and follow up

Throughout your treatment, your radiation oncologist will regularly see you, ensure the treatment is going well, and if you develop any acute side effects, discuss them with you and give appropriate advice and treatment. If you have any concerns, you should not hesitate to discuss them with your radiation oncologist during your assessments. You may also bring these issues to the attention of your radiation nurse or radiation therapist. Once you have completed your radiation treatments, your doctor will monitor the results of your therapy at regularly scheduled visits and monitor and treat any radiation side effects.

VI. The indications for XRT

The reasons for using XRT vary depending upon the type of thyroid cancer and the goals of the treatment. The types of thyroid cancer are (1) well-differentiated thyroid cancer-papillary and follicular, (2) medullary, and (3) anaplastic. The goals of XRT have been previously discussed and include radical, adjuvant and palliative treatment.

1. Well-differentiated thyroid cancer (papillary and follicular)

Radical XRT

Occasionally in well-differentiated thyroid cancer, the surgeon cannot remove all the cancer and radioiodine cannot control residual tumor left behind after surgery. In this situation you may be advised to have radical XRT in addition to radioiodine.

Adjuvant XRT

The role of adjuvant XRT is controversial. Some experts do not think that there is a role for XRT. Others believe that in situations in which there is a high risk of the cancer recurring in the neck, adjuvant XRT can reduce that risk. Risk factors have been discussed in chapter 4, and the option of adjuvant XRT should be discussed with your endocrinologist.

Some experts also believe that adjuvant XRT can reduce the risk of recurrence in the neck in patients with extensive involvement of the lymph nodes, especially if there is local extension of the cancer with invasion through the capsule of the node into the surrounding tissue. Again, you should discuss this option with your endocrinologist.

Palliative XRT

If your cancer comes back in the neck, surgery is usually performed. However, if surgery is not an option and if the cancer does not take up radioiodine, then XRT alone should be strongly considered to treat the recurrence. XRT may also be used in addition to the surgery and/or radioiodine to reduce the risk for further recurrence.

1. Medullary thyroid cancer

Because medullary thyroid cancer does not take up radioiodine, surgery alone is the main treatment. As in well-differentiated thyroid cancer, the role of XRT is controversial, but if there is gross tumor left behind after surgery or if the tumor cannot be removed by surgery, then radical XRT should be considered. Similarly, if there is a high risk of recurrence in the neck because of either extension outside of the thyroid or extensive lymph node involvement, then adjuvant XRT may be recommended.

2. Anaplastic thyroid cancer

In most cases of anaplastic thyroid cancer, the cancer cannot be removed surgically, and XRT is usually recommended. Sometimes chemotherapy is given with the XRT, which is called concurrent chemoradiation. Occasionally XRT alone or with chemotherapy is given prior to surgery with the goal of attempting to shrink the cancer before the surgery. Even if the anaplastic cancer can be removed surgically, the risk of recurrence is high, and XRT may be advised after surgery.

VII. The side effects of radiation therapy

Although every attempt will be made to reduce the frequency or severity of side effects from radiation, side effects are still expected. The side effects also vary in frequency, severity, and rate of healing, depending on whether the normal tissue, which was irradiated, has cells that multiply quickly or slowly or never multiply. For example, normal tissues that have cells that are multiplying quickly such as the skin and the mucosa (the lining of the mouth and throat in the esophagus, larynx, and trachea) show the effects of radiation quickly and often during the course of radiation. However, these tissues rapidly repair themselves because normal cells not only repair damage from radiation, but they also can increase the rate they multiply. Tissues that have cells that do not divide, such as muscles and nerves, are resistant to radiation, and thus side effects directly due to the radiation are less frequent. However, these tissues can have side effects indirectly due to the radiation. These tissues rely on oxygen delivered by blood vessels, and the blood vessels contain dividing cells that can be damaged. If these cells are damaged, then the blood vessels are damaged, and the oxygen supply to these radiation-resistant tissues is reduced. This in turn indirectly results in injury. This process of damage to the blood vessels takes time and may occur three months or more after the radiation.

Side effects can be divided into "early" and "late." Early side effects are those that occur within three months of treatment, and late side effects are those that occur three months or more after treatment.

Whether you will experience any side effects from XRT is difficult to predict. Everyone is different. Some people get very few side effects, while others find the experience of XRT very difficult with significant side effects. Below is a list of possible side effects. You may experience none or all in varying degrees. Apart from fatigue, all other radiation toxicities are due to the local effect of radiating the normal tissues within the radiation field, and this will depend on the site and size of the area being treated.

A. Early Side Effects (occurring within three months of the treatment)

Fatigue

Fatigue is one of the common side effects of radiation. Not only is the stress of radiation therapy, coping with cancer, and the daily travel for radiation fatiguing, but the actual radiation therapy itself is also fatiguing. Some patients feel especially tired an hour or two after their radiation treatment. Like most early side effects of radiation, fatigue improves about two weeks after completion of treatment. However, in a few patients it may last for many weeks.

To help manage the fatigue, it is important during your radiation that you do not overexert yourself. Continue your usual activities if you can, including exercise, but do not push yourself. Stop and rest when you get tired. Try and sleep well at night and nap during the day if you can.

In regard to your ability to keep working during your treatments, this is difficult to predict. This will depend partly on the type of job you perform and the type of radiation you are receiving. If you are undergoing a prolonged course of adjuvant or radical radiation and have a physically demanding job, then you may not be able to return to work. However, you may be able to continue other occupations, especially if you can work part time or at home. If your voice box is in the field of radiation treatment and if you have a job where the use of your voice is very important, then you may not be able to work until your voice returns to normal. You should discuss this with your radiation oncologist and your employer before your radiation starts.

Skin

Many patients have no skin toxicity, especially if the radiation course is short. However, if you are having a prolonged course of radiation to the neck, then toxicity of the skin in the area of the radiation field is inevitable. The toxicity is typically mild and includes the skin feeling warm, itchy, and dry with some redness, which is called erythema. The skin may peel and flake, and this is called dry desquamation. If the toxicity gets worse, then the skin may break down and weep, and this is called moist desquamation. The skin usually heals within a few weeks after treatment, and when the healing begins, the healing is usually quick. To minimize any skin toxicity, the following is recommended:

- Avoid wearing tight clothing over the treatment area such as buttoned shirts, tie or both;
- Wear loose clothing;
- Don't rub or scrub your skin;
- Don't use soaps or detergents or anything with deodorants or alcohol on your skin;

- If you shave, use an electric razor;
- Wash the area with lukewarm water, pat the area dry, and do not rub;
- Avoid the sun on the area being treated;
- Do not put anything very hot or cold on the area being treated; and
- Apply a light dusting of baby powder or cornstarch.

Finally, if the skin becomes moist, stop using baby powder or cornstarch. Switch to salt-water soaks on the area. If you develop a moist-skin reaction, tell your treatment therapist or nurse or radiation oncologist.

Throat

Apart from skin toxicity, the most significant toxicity during a course of radiation for thyroid cancer is to the throat. The throat includes the esophagus (the gullet), the larynx (voice box), and the trachea (windpipe). Just as the skin gets red and sore, the same happens to the mucosa or lining of the esophagus, larynx, and trachea. This usually starts during the second or third week of treatment. It may start to improve before the radiation has finished or start two to four weeks after the radiation treatment has been completed. The toxicity to the throat has usually resolved by a month after completion of treatment.

In regard to the esophagus, it may at first become sore when swallowing foods and later when swallowing your saliva. You may need a diet of soft and pureed food or liquid food. Your radiation oncologist can prescribe painkillers and other medications to help. A dietitian may give advice on foods that are easy to swallow and on ways to ensure that you get adequate nutrition. With high doses of radiation to the neck, rarely your swallowing may become so difficult that you cannot get fluids down at all. In this situation you may need to be admitted to the hospital and given intravenous fluids.

In regard to the larynx, this also may become red (erythema) and swell. This, along with dryness due to reduced saliva production, may cause hoarseness. Your voice quality may also change to a grating or harsh sound, and the tone may deepen. Hoarseness may start two weeks into your treatment, and you may lose your voice for two to four weeks after the treatment is complete.

Mouth, teeth, and salivary glands

If the goal is to irradiate all the lymph nodes in your neck, the floor of your mouth may be also be irradiated. This can result in reduced volume of your saliva as well as thickening of your saliva. This usually occurs in the first and second week. Your mouth may feel sticky and dry, and it may make swallowing difficult. This may be made worse if you already have some dryness following your radioiodine treatment. However, it is unlikely that the main salivary glands (the parotid glands) will be affected.

If the lining of the mouth is included in the volume being treated, then the lining of the mouth may also become dry, red, and possibly break down with blisters. Mild discomfort and sometimes pain in the mouth area along with difficulty in swallowing may occur.

To help with these side effects, the following are recommended:

- Keep your mouth and throat moist;
- Carry water with you to sip frequently;
- Drink eight to ten glasses of water a day;
- Keep the air moist at home;
- Eat small amounts of food and chew thoroughly;
- Moisten food with sauces, gravy, butter, margarine, mayonnaise or yogurt;
- Eat soft or pureed food;
- Avoid rough-textured food such as chips, popcorn, and dry toast;
- Avoid hot and cold food and drinks;
- Avoid spicy food;
- Use liquid diet supplements; these can be blended with ice cream;
- Discuss your diet with a dietitian;
- Use a mouthwash without alcohol or use salt or baking soda solution (mix 1 teaspoon of salt or baking soda with 2 cups of warm water);
- Avoid smoking and alcohol, especially spirits, during you radiation as they can worsen a radiation reaction in your mouth or throat; and
- If necessary, speak with your physician for a prescription for analgesic or local anesthetic solutions.

Weight Loss

Because your mouth and throat are sore and because you may also lose your sense of taste and appetite, you may eat less and lose weight. Thus, if eating becomes difficult, it is important to maintain an adequate diet. A dietitian or nutritionist can discuss your diet with you and ensure that you have an adequate intake. Soft, pureed food may help, and you may need liquid supplements.

Dentition/teeth

Although it is unlikely that your teeth will be in the area treated with radiation, your teeth can still be affected indirectly. Saliva is important to maintain good dental health, and the radiation may damage your salivary glands thereby reducing the production of saliva. This is turn may increased dental cavities and gum disease. However, there are things that you can do to maintain good dental health, and these are listed below:

- Have any dental work performed before the start of radiation;

- Brush after all meals and at bedtime with a soft brush;
- Floss your teeth; and
- Rinse with a salt or baking soda solution after brushing your teeth (mix 1 teaspoon of salt or backing soda with 2 cups of warm water).

Neck swelling (edema)

A few weeks after completion of your radiation treatments, swelling of the neck may occur. This is called edema or a "dewlap."

In your neck as well as most parts of your body, there are lymphatic ducts, and these ducts help drain away extra fluid within your tissue. However, the radiation may cause irritation of the lymphatic ducts, which results in the ducts becoming obstructed and the inability of the ducts to drain the extra fluid from your tissue resulting in edema or dewlap. Edema of the neck is more common when previous surgery removed lymph nodes. You should not be concerned about the edema, and it usually resolves slowly.

B. Late Side Effects

Skin

After the skin has healed, it may be thicker and a little darker than before. If the dose to the skin is high, small, red, curvy marks may develop. These are called telangectasias and are small blood vessels on the surface of the skin. After radiation, the skin may also be sensitive to the sun, and it is therefore important to either avoid sun exposure to any skin that has received radiation or to use a sunscreen with a high skin protection factor (spf).

Esophagus

The radiation may cause scarring in the esophagus, and this scarring may cause narrowing and difficulty swallowing. However, this is extremely rare. If you develop any difficulty swallowing, you should notify your physician. Options are available to treat this, and these options include stretching or dilating the esophagus.

Frequently asked questions

If I have had radiation, can I have it again?

This depends on what dose you have had and what areas were irradiated. If you had adjuvant or radical radiation, then it is extremely unlikely that you can have additional radiation to the same area. However, if you had a short course of palliative radiation, then it may be possible to receive additional radiation. Of note, radiation to one area does not prevent radiation to another area that has never received any radiation.

If I have had radiation can I have surgery again?

Yes. If the cancer returns in an area that was previously irradiated, it is still possible to have surgery. However, because of the changes that radiation causes in the tissue, it is important that your surgeon is experienced in operating on previously irradiated tissues. This should be further discussed with your endocrinologist and surgeon.

When I had radioiodine I was radioactive for a period of time and had to protect others from radiation. Do I have to do the same after external radiation?

No. You cannot expose anyone else to radiation after treatment with XRT. The radiation for XRT comes from the treatment machine. It does not come from you.

If XRT is effective in reducing the risk of my cancer recurring in my neck, then why don't I use it instead of radioiodine?

XRT is only a local treatment whereas radioiodine is a systemic treatment. Because radioiodine is administered internally and because radioiodine is taken up specifically by cells of well-differentiated thyroid cancer, these cancer cells anywhere in the body can take up the radioiodine and be irradiated.

As a local treatment, XRT should be considered in well-differentiated thyroid cancer when the cancer cells do not take up enough radioiodine or the size of the tumor is large and cannot be removed by surgery.

Who will be involved in my care?

There are many different professionals involved in the planning and delivery of your care before, during and after your course of radiation therapy. These include a radiation oncologist, radiation therapist, radiation nurse, dosimetrist, radiation physicist and dietician. These people are described in the glossary.

Where can I get additional information?

For additional information such as Web sites and books see appendixes C and D.

CHAPTER 22

Additional Modalities of Treatment for Well-Differentiated Thyroid Cancer and Future Directions

Matthew D. Ringel, M.D.

Introduction

Well-differentiated thyroid cancer cells typically grow in response to thyroid stimulating hormone (TSH) and also take up iodine. For most thyroid cancers, following surgery, treatment with thyroid hormone to reduce TSH levels will reduce the growth of any remaining thyroid cancer cells, and thyroid cell-specific radiation therapy using radioactive iodine will either cure or control the disease. In some cases these treatments are ineffective and alternative approaches are needed. Two types of thyroid cancers, papillary and follicular, account for about 80 to 90 percent of all thyroid cancers. This chapter will focus on those papillary and follicular thyroid cancers that are not responsive to our usual treatments. Anaplastic thyroid cancer and medullary thyroid cancer, both unusual tumors that also do not typically respond to TSH suppression or radioactive iodine, will be reviewed in chapters 24 and 25, respectively. Examples of the more commonly considered alternatives, including re-differentiation therapy, non-iodine forms of radiation therapy and chemotherapy, will be discussed below. Certain promising areas of laboratory and clinical research also will be reviewed.

Thyroid cancer is a cancer

At the time of diagnosis, many patients are told that "thyroid cancer is the best type of cancer to have." While this may be true from a statistical standpoint, thyroid cancer, like any cancer, has the potential to be aggressive and spread through lymphatic channels and blood vessels, and to distant locations. This movement is what makes cancer cells different from normal cells. While metastasis is not a common event in thyroid cancer, if you are a patient in whom this occurs, thyroid cancer clearly is not a benign disease.

Like all cancer cells, thyroid cancer cells develop from what were originally normal tissues. Scientists believe that this change occurs when a single cell within the thyroid gains mutations in genes that allow it to divide and grow in an uncontrolled manner, known as clonal expansion. Thus all cells in a cancer are derived from the same parent cell. As these cells grow, they retain some, but not all, of the characteristics of the normal cells that surround them. In thyroid cancer, these characteristics are the abilities to respond to TSH, take up iodine and produce thyroglobulin. The ability to respond to TSH is important for TSH suppression therapy, the iodine uptake is important for treatment and scanning with radioiodine, and the thyroglobulin is important as a marker in the blood for the presence of thyroid cancer.

In most cases, thyroid cancer cells do not change much over time. They sometimes are able to penetrate the thin walls of lymphatic channels or spread throughout the thyroid, but they rarely invade through the wall of the thyroid or into larger blood vessels. Even when thyroid cancer does spread, it often still retains some TSH responsiveness and ability to take up iodine. Such tumors usually can be controlled with standard treatment methods. In some cases, the thyroid cancer cells become less like normal thyroid cells and grow in a more uncontrolled manner, losing the ability to respond to TSH or take up radioiodine. This process, called dedifferentiation, is usually associated with thyroid cancers that behave in a more aggressive manner. Research has shown that these thyroid cancers develop many more genetic changes and that their growth becomes controlled by biologic pathways different from those common to usual thyroid cancer. For patients with these more aggressive tumors, alternative therapies are needed.

Who develops more aggressive thyroid cancer?

It is not easy to predict which patients will develop thyroid cancers that are unresponsive to radioiodine and TSH. These aggressive cancers do appear to be more common in older patients or those who, at the time of surgery, have larger cancers that penetrate into the tissue around the thyroid gland. Patients previously exposed to large amounts of radiation, such as from nuclear test sites or external beam radiation for Hodgkin's disease, also are more likely to develop thyroid cancer, but the prognosis does not appear worse for these people. Thyroid cancer in young patients more frequently metastasizes to the lymph nodes. Although these patients may have recurrent disease, the nodes seem to have little impact on the long-term prognosis, which is generally very good.

Under the microscope, some changes in the appearance of thyroid cancer cells may predict a more aggressive course. Some of these tumors, called thyroid cancer variants, derive from papillary cancers while others appear to derive from follicular cancers. Some variants are related to the appearance of the cells, such as tall or columnar, while others are related to the growth pattern of the cells, such as solid, insular or trabecular. Other variants, such as Hurthle cell cancers, can derive from either follicular or papillary cancer and are not as clearly associated with a more aggressive course. The most aggressive form of thyroid cancer, anaplastic thyroid cancer, loses all thyroid cell characteristics and is sometimes found in tumors that are otherwise classified as either well-differentiated or variant thyroid cancer. This type of complete transition to anaplastic thyroid cancer is rare.

In the future, rather than rely on the eye of the pathologist, it may be possible to evaluate the DNA of cancers to determine which ones are more likely to be aggressive and thus tailor therapy more appropriately. Many research groups are analyzing thyroid cancers to prepare a genetic profile of each tumor. Several genes appear to be related to thyroid cancer progression. One gene, p53, has been particularly well studied in thyroid cancer. In the research setting, detection of p53 mutations has been used to predict aggressive behavior. More general, or global, changes in a cell's DNA seem to occur in aggressive thyroid cancer, and this is called genomic instability. In the future, it may be possible to determine the degree of genomic instability within all cancers to offer better therapies.

Re-differentiation therapy

The goal of re-differentiation therapy is to convert a "dedifferentiated tumor"—one that loses all recognizable signs that it derived from thyroid cells—into one with more differentiated features. For thyroid cancer, the goal is to increase the amount of radioiodine a tumor will take up and to slow its growth rate. The most well studied drugs, not all of which have been FDA approved, are the retinoids and demethylating agents. Retinoids are similar to vitamin A and bind to one of several retinoic acid receptors. In cell culture, activation of some of these receptors results in increased iodine uptake by thyroid cancer cells. The current retinoid approved by the Food and Drug Administration is all-cis retinoic acid (Accutane®), which is used to treat acne but also has anti-tumor effects and can induce iodine uptake. Accutane® has been used in some studies with varying success, probably related to its ability to be broken down into other forms of vitamin A that bind to nearly all of the retinoic acid receptors. Studies with more specific receptor–binding drugs are ongoing in animals and in clinical trials. Because Accutane® is well tolerated, some centers are using this agent as treatment before the administration of radioactive iodine.

A second form of re-differentiation therapy is the use of demethylating agents. Methylation, a natural occurrence in the body in which methyl groups are added to genes, is one mechanism by which cancer cells can turn genes on or off. One gene, the sodium iodide (NaI) symporter, NIS, is frequently turned off by methylation and is the one responsible for transport of iodine into thyroid cells. In the laboratory, FDA-approved demethylating agents such as 5-azacytidine are able to increase expression of NIS by thyroid cancer cells and, in some cases, increase iodine uptake. These agents are now being studied in clinical trials.

One additional form of re-differentiation therapy is gene therapy. Several research groups have used viruses to carry the gene for NIS into thyroid cancer cells, resulting in increased iodine uptake. Other genes that slow down cancer cell growth, kill the cancers or re-differentiate the cancers (e.g., the p53 gene) also have been added to viruses and used to treat thyroid cancer cells. This gene therapy approach has worked well in the laboratory and in animals when the virus has been directly injected into tumors. However, systemic therapy in which a whole animal or person is treated with the virus, through inhalation or injection, has not been successful, as the body's immune response fights off the virus quite effectively. This may someday become a more viable option.

Alternative forms of radiotherapy for thyroid cancer

For the past five decades, radiation treatment of thyroid cancer has primarily involved the use of radioactive iodine, ^{131}I, and external beam radiation therapy. During the past 10 to 20 years several new agents have been developed, and ^{131}I has also been "tagged" to a variety of other tumor markers for use as potential radiotherapy agents. The best studied of these new agents is labeled octreotide, an analog of somatostatin. Somatostatin is a hormone that binds to a family of receptors that are frequently expressed on cancer cells. The activated somatostatin receptors act to reduce the growth of cells. Thus, treatment with octreotide coupled with radioactive agents could block the growth of cancer cells directly and also be used to provide cancer-specific radiation therapy. While initial reports looked promising, the published studies so far have been disappointing.

Radioactive agents also have been used as possible treatment for medullary thyroid cancer, which frequently expresses a protein called carcinoembryonic antigen (CEA). Radioactive iodine linked to CEA was made and used both to monitor and treat patients with medullary thyroid cancer. Again, after initial promising results, this method has not yet proven effective. Further studies are planned.

These types of therapies, adding nuclear isotopes to proteins that will be taken up specifically by the cancer cells, are very exciting, and significant research is being performed in this area. This therapy may someday be quite useful for treating patients with thyroid cancer.

Chemotherapy for aggressive thyroid cancer

The decision to use chemotherapy to treat patients with metastatic differentiated thyroid cancer is often difficult and requires open and honest discussions between patients and their families and care providers. The typical forms of chemotherapy used for other cancers are associated with side effects that can impact on quality of life, and the risk-benefit ratio of treatment must be seriously considered. Classic chemotherapy agents used for other solid tumors, such as breast and colon cancer, have not been well studied for well-differentiated metastatic thyroid cancer. This limited knowledge can be attributed to the fact that thyroid cancer progresses slowly and that most patients with metastatic thyroid cancer enjoy an excellent quality of life and survive often for decades. Thus, it often is difficult to recommend chemotherapy to a patient with metastatic thyroid cancer in the absence of rapid progression, as many will have a relatively stable disease for many years. Determining the genetic profile of each cancer (see above) may help physicians identify patients who might respond best to early intervention with chemotherapy.

Chemotherapy has been studied for the treatment of anaplastic thyroid cancer, the most dedifferentiated of thyroid cancers. Again, these studies are described in more detail in chapters 24 and 25. A variety of other agents have been shown to kill anaplastic thyroid cancer cells in the laboratory and in animal models but have not been studied in patients with thyroid cancer. Some drugs, including gemcitabine and taxitere, are FDA-approved for other cancers, and it is likely that agents that have shown an ability to fight anaplastic thyroid cancer also may be effective against more well-differentiated but progressive tumors. For anaplastic thyroid cancer, response rates showing at least a 50 percent reduction in the tumor have been reported in about 30 percent of the cases for doxorubicin (Adriamycin®) alone or with cis-Platinum and paclitaxel (Taxol®).

Approaches to new therapies

Over the past decade, there have been tremendous advances in understanding how cancer cells grow in their primary sites, evade cell death and the immune system, spread throughout the body, and implant into new tissue and grow in those areas. The mechanism for these processes is similar for many different types of cancer, including thyroid cancer, and new agents designed to block each of these functions are under development in the laboratory or are already being tested in clinical trials.

Cell growth inhibitors

Most thyroid cancer cells develop, in part, through mutations in genes that result in unregulated cell growth. For thyroid cancer, the best understood of these are the *ret*/PTC anti-B-Raf genes in papillary thyroid cancer and the *ras* and PPM/PAx8 genes in follicular thyroid cancer. These mutant genes produce proteins that cause uncontrolled activation of cell-signaling pathways, resulting in the uncontrolled growth of cancer cells. New drugs have been designed to block the *ras, ret, B-Raf* and other similar pathways at the outer membrane of the cancer cell or deep within the cell. For all of the agents, the goal is the same: to see if blocking these pathways kills or inhibits the growth of cancer cells. This approach has been used successfully in the past few years to dramatically improve the treatment of patients with chronic myelogenous leukemia (CML), non-Hodgkin's lymphoma and gastro-intestinal stromal tumors (GIST). A wide variety of pathway inhibitors are now in pre-clinical and clinical trials with the side-effect profiles varying among the different agents. Several of these agents that are in clinical trials are logical choices for thyroid cancer patients based on our knowledge of thyroid cancer cell biology.

Cell death activators

As cells age, they undergo an orderly process of programmed cell death, called apoptosis. Apoptosis and other types of cell death can also be initiated by outside factors, such as activation of the immune system. Thyroid cancer cells, however, are resistant to apoptosis and can also evade immune–mediated cell death. Thyroid cancer cells also have a slowing of their internal "biological clock" by activation of a protein called telomerase that is able to keep old cells young, thereby delaying apoptosis.

Researchers are exploring a variety of methods to sensitize thyroid cancer cells to both cell aging apoptosis and immune mediated cell death. These treatments are designed to boost the body's ability to kill the cancer cells and make the cells age more normally. This approach is attractive as it takes advantage of the body's own very efficient systems, but it is still in the basic research phases.

More classic immunotherapies using tumor vaccines and agents to boost the body's immune response against tumor cells also have been evaluated in thyroid cancer. Tumor vaccines have been disappointing, but new approaches using special immune activating proteins called interleukins hold great promise. The use of vaccines in conjunction with interleukins, most prominently interleukin 12, is now in clinical trials.

Inhibition of metastases

Blocking the ability of cancer cells to spread to distant sites has become an important area of laboratory research that is quite promising for developing new therapies. For most cancers, including thyroid cancer, patients who develop distant metastases are more likely to have an aggressive clinical course. Prevention or reversal of metastases is an obvious goal for therapy. Several recent studies have clarified the "homing" mechanism for cancer cells to metastasize in specific locations.

For example, it has long been known that when follicular thyroid cancers metastasize, they tend to go to the bone or lungs. Why is that the case? It is now known that tumors that metastasize have specific proteins on them that direct them to certain tissues. These proteins, called chemokines, are very important in the development of metastatic cancer. Several proteins that function to inhibit tumor metastases have also been described and are made by some thyroid cancer cells and lost in others. The treatment importance or prognostic importance of these proteins is uncertain but is under active investigation.

Inhibitors of cancer blood vessel formation (anti-angiogenesis)

Once cancer cells implant in a tissue or grow as a primary tumor beyond their usual blood supply, they must find a way to obtain nutrients for growth. For many years, it has been known that cancer cells have the ability to form new blood vessels and connect to existing blood supplies to survive and grow. Proteins, several of which have recently been identified, regulate this process. The proteins that block angiogenesis could be used to treat cancers while those that stimulate blood vessel formations are potential targets for new therapies. Two naturally occurring blockers of angiogenesis, endostatin and angiostatin, were recently used in clinical trials. Scientists noted activity against several cancers, including thyroid cancer. Larger studies demonstrated significant problems with the drug, but new variations on these agents are under careful evaluation.

One of the principal activators of angiogenesis in thyroid cancer is vascular-endothelial growth factor (VEGF). Researchers believe that the thyroid cancers respond to VEGF, secrete VEGF and induce the local cells around it to secrete it—all acting together to result in the development of new blood vessels. Several blockers of the VEGF pathway have been manufactured and appear to be active against the growth of human thyroid cancer cells both in cell culture and in animal models. Clinical studies with this agent such as combretastatins are under way.

A word about clinical trials

Cancer therapy clinical trials are classified as Phase 1, 2 or 3 studies. Each phase serves a specific purpose on the pathway to determining whether a drug is safe and effective in the treatment of a particular disease. It is important to remember that, by definition, these trials are research. Thus, it may not be possible to predict whether an individual patient will respond to the agent(s) or will have adverse side effects. In all cases, an institutional review board (IRB) will have reviewed the study, and informed consent documents must be reviewed and obtained. A participant can terminate his or her involvement at any time. A drug trial will be discontinued if it fails to show safety in any phase or efficacy in phases 2 or 3. Some drugs are dropped as solitary agents but re-studied later in combination with other agents.

Phase 1 studies

These are the first to be performed in humans and intended to determine safety rather than efficacy. Typically they are designed to test several different doses of a new drug in nearly any type of cancer to determine the maximally tolerated dose and the clearance rate of the drug from humans. These studies carry the highest risk to the patient but also may be beneficial if one chooses logically and carefully for a specific cancer. Patients in these studies usually have very aggressive cancers, or doctors have identified an important biological reason to anticipate a possible response to therapy.

Phase 2 studies

Once the maximum tolerated dose is determined, a more focused study evaluating several different dosing regimens is designed. These may be directed at a particular tumor or family of tumors (e.g., endocrine tumors or solid tumors) based on pre-clinical laboratory data or information from the phase 1 study. These studies are often optimal for thyroid cancer patients.

Phase 3 studies

These are even more focused but usually much larger than the phase 2 trials. In these studies, the goal is to determine, in a large number of patients with one particular cancer, whether the drug is as active or more active than standard care or in patients not responding to standard care. These are typically the final studies done before FDA approval and often are not open to patients with less common types of cancer.

Information sources

It is often difficult to identify clinical trials for thyroid cancer or more general clinical trials for which thyroid cancer patients would qualify (typically solid or epithelial tumors). Since the trials open and close quickly, most endocrinologists may not have all the accurate or up-to-date information about the nature of the trials to determine whether they would be appropriate for a particular patient. In general, while clinical trials for most cancers are directed and run by research oncologists, research endocrinologists usually will also be involved in a clinical trial for thyroid cancer. Patients interested in participating in a clinical trial are advised to consult with a clinician-researcher in endocrine oncology.

The clinical trials specialist (endocrine oncologist) and his or her staff will likely be members of several large multi-center cooperative study groups and can describe current protocols for which you may qualify. The Internet provides several additional resources for clinical trials. Some provide details of the medication being studied while others describe the protocol, funding agency and participating sites. Some of these sites are provided in appendix C. Further information about participating in clinical trials is noted in chapter 27.

Summary

Thyroid cancer that does not respond to TSH suppression and radioiodine therapy is uncommon, but it can occur and develop into aggressive disease. Currently available options include those used in some centers, such as re-differentiation therapy and chemotherapy. These two alternatives have uncertain benefits, and, in the case of chemotherapy, significant side effects that are probably acceptable only for patients with the most aggressive disease.

However, this is an exciting time as the genetic profiling of thyroid tumors already is being performed in the research setting in an effort to better predict which patients might benefit from more aggressive therapy. New drugs designed to block specific abnormalities known to be involved in thyroid cancer progression are either entering or are already in clinical trials.

CHAPTER 23

Radiofrequency Ablation
Howard Richard, M.D.

Introduction

Ablation—a fancy word meaning the destruction of tissue—can be accomplished in many different ways, such as with radiation, toxic chemicals and freezing temperatures. Heat also can be effective in tissue ablation (destruction), and one type of treatment that uses this method is called radio-frequency.

In brief, radio-frequency uses a fine probe, which is composed of thin "tines" that look and act like an antenna. The interventional radiologist, who is trained in this procedure, places these tines into the tumor, and then the tines disperse electrical waves of energy into the tumor. This energy delivers enough heat to the tumor to raise the temperature of the mass to almost the boiling point, which destroys the tumor.

Indication

Radiofrequency is commonly used for tumors in the liver, kidneys and bones, including the spinal column, and is an option for the treatment of metastatic thyroid disease that cannot be surgically removed.

Pre-procedure evaluation

The interventional radiologist will evaluate the patient's imaging studies to determine whether the site or sites of cancer are suitable for radio-frequency treatment. If so, then the radiologist will meet with the patient and discuss the logistics of the procedure as well as its risks and benefits.

Procedure

On the day of the procedure, the anesthesiologist administers anesthesia to the patient, and then the patient undergoes CT or ultrasound imaging to localize the tumor for the placement of the probe. The probe is inserted inside the tumor, and the CT or ultrasound images are repeated to verify the correct position of the probe.

The probe is then connected to the radio-frequency generator, which monitors the temperature inside the tumor. The tumor is heated to the target temperature, which is discussed further below, for a prescribed length of time. The interventional radiologist is the one who determines the target temperature and length of time based on multiple factors, including the tumor's size and proximity to critical structures. Masses in the bone of the spinal vertebral column, for example, often are several millimeters from the spinal cord and would be treated at lower target temperatures and for shorter times. Small tumors near critical structures generally are heated for no longer than two to three minutes while large tumors can be heated for 15 to 20 minutes provided they are not near critical structures. Once the radio-frequency probe is removed, the patient is taken to the recovery room for monitoring and to awaken from anesthesia. The entire procedure generally lasts less than two hours, and most patients are released the same day.

Recovery from the procedure

Recovery is different for every patient. Some patients report no discomfort after radio-frequency ablation while others may experience pain and bruising at the site where the needle was inserted. Symptoms can last for two to eight weeks.

Follow-up care

Your interventional radiologist and endocrinologist or primary physician will monitor any symptoms you may have, any findings on physical exam, your thyroglobulin blood levels and any diagnostic imaging studies you may undergo, such as CT, MRI, ultrasound or PET. These assessments, if done both before and after the radio-frequency procedure, should give you and your physicians the data you need to assess the success of the treatment. Possibilities include symptoms that improve or even disappear, a decrease in thyroglobulin blood levels, and imaging studies demonstrating a significant reduction in size of the metastasis. Your physician will determine the best follow-up program for you, which typically starts two to eight weeks after the treatment.

Side effects

Bruising, pain and blood clotting can occur when the needle or probe passes through normal tissue overlying the tumor. Additional side effects are possible depending on the type of normal tissue surrounding the tumor that also gets "heated" as well as the sensitivity of that tissue to the heat. For example, if the tumor is in the spinal column, the nerves that exit the spinal cord or the spinal cord at the level of the treatment may be injured. If the tumor is in the neck, the skin overlying the tumor or an adjacent nerve to the tumor could be injured. If the tumor is in the liver, the bile duct system within the liver could be injured. Patients considering radiofrequency should discuss with the interventional radiologist any side effects specific to the area to be treated.

Frequently asked questions

Will there be general or local anesthesia?

Both general and local anesthesia are used in radio-frequency procedures. The interventional radiologist will give you local anesthesia at the time of the procedure, and you also will be under general anesthesia, which you and your anesthesiologists selected before the procedure. Types of general anesthesia include medicine for pain that can make you drowsy or medication that puts you to sleep completely.

Should I stop taking my medications the day of the procedure?

Except for blood thinners and aspirin you should continue to take your medications, with sips of water.

I am on "blood thinners." Should I stop taking them?

Yes, **but you should first obtain permission to stop these medications from the physician who prescribed them.** If possible, blood thinners such as Coumadin® should be stopped three to four days before the procedure and aspirin should be stopped one to two days before the procedure. Discontinuing these medications helps minimize the risk of developing bleeding surrounding the needle path to the tumor. If your physician determines you must continue taking these medications, you should inform the interventional radiologist planning to perform the radio-frequency procedure.

How many tumors can be treated at one time?

While it is possible to treat two or even three tumors simultaneously, physicians generally prefer to work on one tumor at a time. Targeting the tumors can be time consuming and take as long as two hours, particularly if the lesion is near critical structures. Most physicians prefer to have patients under moderate sedation for no longer than three to four hours at a time. Additional tumors can be treated within two to four weeks after the initial procedure. Your interventional radiologist will advise regarding the appropriate schedule for you.

Are there any limitations to the number of times the treatment can be performed?

Additional treatments can be performed depending on previous side effects and the proximity of vital structures to the tumor being treated.

What is the effect of temperature on the tissues in the body?

Temperatures within the body can range from 35 to 40 degrees Celsius (95 to 104 degrees Fahrenheit). When body temperatures are raised to 42 to 45 degrees Celsius (108 to 113 degrees Fahrenheit), it is considered hyperthermia. Irreversible cell damage occurs in most tissues when temperatures hover between 46 and 50 degrees Celsius (115 to 122 degrees Fahrenheit) for at least 45 minutes. The spinal cord, which is particularly sensitive when compared with the rest of the body, can be damaged when temperatures reach 45 degrees Celsius (115 degrees Fahrenheit). Cell death (necrosis) occurs in four to six minutes at temperatures greater than 50 degrees Celsius (122 degrees Fahrenheit) and immediately when temperatures are higher than 60 degrees Celsius (140 degrees Fahrenheit). Tissue vaporizes at temperatures greater than 110 degrees Celsius (230 degrees Fahrenheit).

Does the treatment completely kill the tumor?

High enough temperatures—generally those above 60 degrees Celsius (140 degrees Fahrenheit)—will kill tumor cells within the ablation zone. However, physicians aim to treat tumors adjacent to important and heat-sensitive structures with temperatures near 80 degrees Celsius (176 degrees Fahrenheit) to make sure that the entire treatment zone is raised to a lethal temperature. Temperatures greater than 100 degrees Celsius (212 degrees Fahrenheit) are considered safe to use on tumors that are not surrounded by critical tissue.

Is there anyone who cannot have this procedure?

Radiofrequency would not be possible on patients who have implanted metal prostheses located in places that would block the area to be treated. Implanted metal prostheses may include a spinal cage from spinal reconstruction or metallic rods from repair of fractures of the long bones. Patients with pacemakers may be candidates for treatment if a suitable external pacemaker is available.

Are there alternatives to radio-frequency ablation?

Microwave and directed ultrasound also can be used to destroy tissue through heat. Other methods of ablation include cryotherapy, which freezes tissue, and chemicals such as ethanol, absolute alcohol or acetic acid. Your endocrinologist or primary physician can help you determine which procedure is best for you.

CHAPTER 24

Medullary Thyroid Carcinoma (MTC)

Yasser Ousman, M.D.

Introduction

Earlier discussions in this book have explained how some thyroid cancers are well "differentiated," meaning more like normal thyroid cells, and other types of thyroid cancer are less differentiated or even undifferentiated. The most well differentiated tumors are papillary and follicular thyroid cancer, and the least differentiated tumor is anaplastic carcinoma. Indeed, anaplastic tumors are so undifferentiated that when examined under the microscope the tissue often does not even look like thyroid cells. However, there is a fourth type of thyroid cancer, which is medullary thyroid carcinoma (MTC), and this originates from a completely different cell than either papillary, follicular or anaplastic cancer cells. This chapter presents an overview of this cancer, MTC.

Overview

MTC represents about 5 to 10 percent of all thyroid cancers. Unlike papillary and follicular thyroid cancers, MTC arises from the thyroid parafollicular C cells and not from the thyroid follicular cells. Thyroid parafollicular C cells are different from thyroid follicular cells in that they do not synthesize or produce thyroid hormones or thyroglobulin. Rather, they elaborate a different hormone named calcitonin or thyrocalcitonin, which is involved in the regulation of calcium levels through its effects on bone.

MTC has a prognosis intermediate between well-differentiated thyroid cancer (papillary and follicular cancers) and the un-differentiated anaplastic thyroid cancer. MTC can occur either as a spontaneous or isolated tumor (sporadic) or be inherited. When these MTC tumors occur in the inherited form, other abnormalities will commonly coexist in the same patient at the same time or occur before or after the discovery of the MTC. These coexisting abnormalities taken together constitute a "syndrome." Because the additional abnormalities are usually other tumors (neoplasms), the syndromes are known as Multiple Endocrine Neoplasia

(MEN). MEN results from several genetic mutations, and the two main types of MEN are simply called MEN-1 and MEN-2. MEN-2 is further divided into MEN-2a and MEN-2b. Although MTC occurs in both types of MEN-2, statistically speaking, most patients with MTC have the sporadic, non-inherited form of the condition. However, because of the implications of a hereditary disorder upon the children of a patient with MTC and to facilitate the earliest possible detection of coexisting other tumors, it is recommended that all patients diagnosed with MTC be evaluated for the inherited forms. The evaluation usually involves genetic testing to determine if a patient with MTC carries one of the multiple gene mutations seen in the inherited forms. In the next section, we will discuss in more detail the inherited forms of MTC.

Inherited forms of MTC

Inherited forms of MTC represent about 25 percent of all MTC cases. There are three entities or categories of inherited MTC that have been described and are listed in Table 1.

TABLE 1		
Familial MTC (FMTC)	**MEN-2a**	**MEN-2b**
MTC	MTC	MTC
	Pheochromocytoma	Pheochromocytoma
	Hyperparathyroidism	Marfanoid habitus
		Mucosal neuromas

As seen in the Table 1, MTC is part of all three inherited forms, and several clinically important aspects of MEN-2 should be emphasized. MTC tends to occur at an earlier age in patients with MEN than in patients with sporadic MTC. This is particularly true in the case of patients with MEN-2b where MTC can be detected in infancy. The clinical course of MTC in patients with MEN-2b tends to be more aggressive and to have a worse prognosis than the sporadic MTC and the other inherited forms of MTC. There is a very rare tumor of the adrenal glands called a pheochromocytoma ("pheo" for short) that produces excessive amounts of the adrenalin-like substances known as epinephrine and norepinephrine. High levels in the blood of these hormones cause episodes of high blood pressure (hypertension), often associated with blackout spells. A pheo may frequently, but not always, occur in MEN-2a and MEN-2b. Because of the risks of life-threatening hypertension or heart rhythm abnormalities during thyroid surgery in a patient with a pheo, these latter tumors need to be diagnosed and treated before thyroid surgery is performed for MTC. Even more rarely, pheos can be cancerous and more difficult to treat.

Another tumor that can occur with MTC in the MEN 2a variety involves the parathyroid glands. The parathyroid glands usually consist of four little glands, each the size of a pea, which are located behind and slightly embedded into the back of the thyroid gland. The tumors of the parathyroid gland are almost always benign or non-cancerous and may produce parathyroid hormone. Parathyroid hormone is sometimes called parathormone and is abbreviated as "PTH." This hormone serves to regulate calcium balance in the body, and if a tumor of the parathyroid gland produces too much PTH, a condition known as "hyperparathyroidism" occurs, which causes elevation of serum calcium levels ("hypercalcemia"). The overproduction of PTH is seen in some patients with MEN-2a.

At the cellular level, there is a genetic alteration or "gene mutation" that is responsible for the abnormalities in MEN-2a and 2b, and this gene has been identified as the *ret*-oncogene. As mentioned in the previous section, patients found to have MTC should have genetic testing to determine if they carry a *ret*-oncogene mutation. Because of the danger associated with having an undiagnosed pheochromocytoma, patients in whom a *ret*-oncogene mutation is detected should have diagnostic studies for a pheo to determine if they have all of the tumors and abnormalities of MEN-2a (MTC, pheo and hyperparathyroidism). Close relatives of a patient with the *ret*-oncogene mutation should also be offered genetic testing to determine whether they are a carrier of the mutation. Relatives of a patient with a ret mutation are at high risk themselves for developing MTC. Indeed, depending on the type of mutation, they may develop MTC very early in life. As a consequence of confirming the presence of the *ret*-oncogene mutation in children of a family member with MEN-2b, a thyroidectomy would be recommended on a preventative basis as soon as possible after birth, before MTC develops.

Clinical presentation of MTC

As mentioned above, these hereditary forms of MTC are less common, and approximately 75 percent of patients with MTC have the spontaneous (non-inherited) type. Typically a thyroid nodule may be incidentally discovered in these patients during the course of a routine physical examination. Sometimes the thyroid nodule is incidentally found in the neck through imaging studies such as ultrasound, MRI or CT scan that were done for some other purpose. Generally, an early step in the diagnostic evaluation of patients with thyroid nodules would be a fine needle aspiration (FNA) to obtain cells for examination under the microscope (see chapter 6). If the findings on FNA are suspicious for MTC, the patient should be first tested for the *ret* mutation before thyroid surgery is performed. In such cases, it is important for the surgeon to know what to expect prior to the operation.

Many patients with MTC, in particular patients with MEN-2b, will already have some local spread of the cancer to lymph nodes in the neck and sometimes will even have spread at other locations. In this regard, patients with MEN-2b have the most aggressive forms of MTC, and those with familial MTC (FMTC) have the least aggressive forms. Calcitonin, the hormone produced by the C-cells composing MTC, will be produced in excess by these tumors and levels in the blood can be measured and found to be elevated. Consequently, it is useful to your physician to measure calcitonin in patients with MTC prior to surgery. Postoperatively, after removal of the MTC by the surgeon, measurements of calcitonin serve as a "tumor marker" for any remaining MTC cells. Another tumor marker produced by some but not all MTC tumors is carcinoembryonic antigen (CEA), and physicians may measure this along with calcitonin prior to surgery and at follow up. Undetectable levels generally indicate absence of tumor recurrence, whereas persistently high levels or progressively increasing levels after surgery indicate the persistence or recurrence of the tumor.

Imaging studies to evaluate the extent of the cancer are also typically performed prior to surgery. These studies include ultrasound of the thyroid gland, CT scan and MRI of the neck, chest and abdomen, and bone scan.

Treatment

Surgery is the main treatment for MTC, and because the tumor may be present in multiple areas of the thyroid gland, the initial surgery for MTC is a total thyroidectomy. As with other thyroid cancers, thyroidectomy should be performed by a surgeon with experience in thyroid surgery in order to improve the chances of complete removal of the tumor and reduce the risk of surgical complications. Because of the tendency of MTC to metastasize early during its course to lymph nodes located in the neck, particular attention will be paid by the surgeon to these nodes during the operation. As a result, the surgeon will perform what is called a central neck dissection (identification and removal of lymph nodes located in the front or central area of the neck). Patients in whom the MTC has already spread to the lymph nodes on the sides of the neck usually require more extensive surgery. Because of the high likelihood of spread of MTC to the lymph nodes, some experts recommend dissection of both the central neck area and the sides (lateral neck) for all patients with MTC. In some series of patients so treated, there has been a reduced risk of recurrence of the tumor, although this is somewhat controversial.

Contrary to other types of thyroid cancer, such as papillary and follicular thyroid cancer, postoperative treatment with radioactive iodine is not used. The C-cells of MTC are not truly thyroid cells, and they do not have the ability to trap or collect radioactive iodine.

Course and prognosis

As mentioned above, MTC can metastasize early to lymph nodes in the neck and in the upper part of the chest centrally above the heart, which is known as the "mediastinum." In addition to spreading to these regional neck and mediastinal lymph nodes, MTC can also spread through the blood to distant organs such as liver, lungs and bone.

The long-term outcome or prognosis of patients with MTC depends on the "stage" of the cancer at time of diagnosis. Patients with early stage MTC have a better chance of survival compared with patients who have more advanced stages of the disease. The stage of MTC depends on the size of the tumor, presence or absence of tumor spread to cervical lymph nodes, and presence or absence of distant spread (distant metastasis).

For more information on staging, see Table 2, which shows the staging of MTC based on the commonly used system called the TNM cancer staging system:

TABLE 2
TNM Stage System

Stages:

Stage I	T1, N0, M0
Stage II	T2-4, N0, M0
Stage III	Any T, N1, M0
Stage IV	Any T, any N, M1

Definitions of T, N, M

Primary tumor

T0 = No evidence of primary tumor

T1 = Tumor of 1 cm or less in maximum diameter limited to thyroid

T2 = Tumor more than 1 cm but not more than 4 cm in greatest dimension limited to thyroid

T3 = Tumor greater than 4 cm in greatest dimension limited to thyroid

T4 = Tumor of any size extending beyond the thyroid capsule

Regional lymph nodes (N)

N0 = No regional lymph node metastasis

N1 = Regional lymph node metastasis

Distant metastasis (M)

M0 = No distant metastasis

M1 = Distant metastasis

About one third of patients will have recurrence of MTC after initial surgery and as many as half the patients have elevated calcitonin levels after initial surgery indicating that they have persistent or recurrent disease. Familial MTC (FMTC) tends to have the best prognosis of all MTC. The most aggressive form of MTC is MEN-2b. Sporadic MTC and MTC in MEN-2a have an intermediate prognosis. Patients diagnosed through *ret*-oncogene screening are typically detected earlier in the course of their disease and therefore can have an excellent prognosis if treated early with total thyroidectomy.

For all types of MTC, the five-year survival rate is 80 to 90 percent. The ten-year survival is between 60 to 75 percent. Patients with very high levels of calcitonin prior to surgery are more likely to have persistent or recurrent disease than patients with lower levels. One reason for the relatively good prognosis is that in many cases, MTC has a slowly progressive course in spite of the presence of metastasis.

Post operative follow up and treatment

After initial surgery, patients with MTC are followed periodically with physical examination, measurement of calcitonin and CEA. An elevation or rising level of either of these tumor markers will prompt a search for recurrent disease, which is usually accomplished by use of imaging studies described earlier in the chapter. Most MTC recurrences are located in the neck, mediastinum, lungs, liver or bone. Sometimes no tumor can be identified by these techniques even though the patient has an elevated post-operative calcitonin level. In this case other imaging scans may be of value, and these include radioactive labeled somatostatin, sestamibi, MIBG or CEA. Your physician will determine when these studies may be appropriate.

Patients with elevated post-operative calcitonin and identifiable recurrent disease in the neck generally would be offered repeat surgery. Additional surgery in the neck may also be indicated in patients with elevated post-operative calcitonin levels with no identifiable disease on the various imaging studies. Such surgery is considered "exploratory," and often these patients are found to harbor small, or microscopic, amounts of tumor in the neck.

Other, non-surgical treatments have been used in patients with MTC in whom surgery has failed to achieve cure of the disease. External radiation therapy of the neck is sometimes used to treat patients with bulky disease in the neck. Some types of chemotherapy have also been used in metastatic MTC with limited success. Radioiodinated meta-iodo-benzyl-guanidine (MIBG) and somatostatin are other agents that have limited efficacy.

CHAPTER 25

Anaplastic Thyroid Carcinoma

Nicholaos Stathatos, M.D.

Introduction

Every part of the human body is made up of tissues, each one with its own specialized structure and function. The cells in these tissues develop, or differentiate, from other cells to do a specific function. Normally developed cells are described as *well-differentiated*. With various mutations in cells leading to cancer, the cancer cell may change back to a primitive type of cell, referred to as *dedifferentiated* or *undifferentiated*. Anaplastic cancer refers to a type of cancer that is highly undifferentiated, having lost most or all characteristics of the tissue from which it originated.

Fewer than six percent of all thyroid cancers are anaplastic. The exact number is unknown because it is not always possible to distinguish between anaplastic and certain other types of tumors. Anaplastic cancer is the rarest of all cancers originating in the thyroid gland. It is most often seen in people age 60 or older and is slightly more common in women than in men. In many cases, it is seen together with other forms of thyroid cancer including the more common well-differentiated thyroid cancers. These well-differentiated thyroid cancers, such as papillary and follicular thyroid cancer, maintain some of the characteristics of the thyroid tissue, which has led some scientists to suggest that the development of a cancer progresses from normal tissue to well-differentiated cancer to anaplastic thyroid cancer. On the other hand, the finding of both anaplastic and papillary cancer in the same surgical specimen may simply be the occurrence of two different cancers in the same patient.

As described in the opening chapters of this book, the thyroid gland uses the element iodine to make thyroid hormones. In areas of the world where there is not enough iodine in the diet there appears to be an increased number of anaplastic thyroid cancer. Adding iodine to the diet causes an apparent change in the frequency of this tumor with occurrence of more well-differentiated tumors instead of anaplastic ones.

In contrast with most other thyroid cancers, anaplastic thyroid cancer is more aggressive. While the average survival time for a patient with anaplastic thyroid cancer varies in different medical reports, an average survival time of a patient with anaplastic thyroid cancer is two to 12 months after the diagnosis is made. Currently about 5 percent of these patients survive more than five years. Research is needed and underway to try to improve the survival.

Causes of anaplastic thyroid cancer

The structure and function of each cell in the human body is controlled by the genes within them. Genes also are in charge of cell replication. Cancer cells have typically lost these control mechanisms of cell multiplication and grow uncontrollably. The result is the formation of cancer masses.

Rapid cell replication is a complicated process that requires multiple steps before a cancer forms. The best-described theory for this is called the *multi-hit hypothesis,* which describes multiple changes that must occur in the cell in a specific order and time frame in order for cancer to develop. Even after a cell becomes cancerous, the process may continue. The result will be that such a cell will continue to lose many of the characteristics of the original cell, and it will become "less differentiated." The less differentiated a tumor is, the more aggressively it behaves with more rapid growth, more spread to distant sites in the body and ultimately more rapid death. What causes these changes to occur in the first place is not known. Several factors have been studied and found to contribute, such as exposure to radiation and chemicals such as lead. Each person has a different degree of susceptibility to these agents, and this is highly dependent on their genetic makeup, that is, their specific genes. Intense research is under way to study and understand the factors that cause cancer. With more knowledge and research new approaches should be identified that will allow us to more effectively treat or perhaps even prevent these tumors.

Clinical presentation

A neck mass that grows relatively quickly is the most common presentation of an anaplastic thyroid cancer. It can cause multiple symptoms depending on the speed and location of its growth. It can compress the trachea (wind pipe) and cause difficulty breathing. It can press against the esophagus (gullet or food pipe) and cause difficulty swallowing food, first with solids and later with liquids when the tumor becomes more advanced. It also can cause hoarseness of the voice due to the effect the tumor can have on the nerves of the larynx (voice box), which is located next to the thyroid gland in the neck. Rarely, the anaplastic cancer may directly invade the voice box.

The tumors can grow into the chest and compress the blood vessels that go to and leave from the heart, head, and arms. This condition may lead to a condition called "superior vena cava syndrome," a name that relates to the large vein that returns blood from the head and the arms back to the heart. When compressed by the cancer, blood cannot flow freely through the superior vena cava and back down to the heart. This results in swelling of the head, neck, and arms, flushing, and possible difficulty breathing. The superior vena caval syndrome can occur with other tumors as well, but it is more typical of anaplastic thyroid cancer because of the tendency of this type of cancer to be more aggressive and grow more quickly before it is diagnosed.

Sometimes these anaplastic thyroid cancers are discovered inside a "differentiated" thyroid tumor that grows more slowly. They have also been found inside large goiters, which are thyroid glands that are not cancerous. These goiters are common and can cause some of the same symptoms as cancerous tumors simply due to their extensive volume or mass. As a result, the presence of a cancer hidden within the goiter may not be suspected until it has already spread to other parts of the body.

Indeed, anaplastic thyroid cancer in most cases will already have spread to distant sites of the body ("metastasis") by the time it is diagnosed. These metastases can produce a number of symptoms depending on their location, number, and size. Common sites of metastasis for anaplastic thyroid cancer include the lungs, liver, and bones.

Finally, these tumors can produce a number of substances that are either secreted into the bloodstream or "leak" out in significant excess. The release of these substances is not normal and not recognized by the control mechanisms that the body has in place to produce these substances. As a result, patients end up with excessive amounts of these substances, which can create various other problems. Examples of these substances are parathyroid hormone—related peptides (PTH-RP) and Granulocyte Colony Stimulating Factor (G-CSF). The first one is a protein that is similar to a hormone that the body makes to regulate calcium in the blood. When produced in excess by a tumor, PTH-RP may result in a significant elevation of the serum calcium causing fatigue and constipation. More severe complications such as lethargy and even coma can result if the problem is not brought under control. G-CSF is a protein that the body normally makes to stimulate the production of white blood cells, the cells of the defense system of the body. When G-CSF is produced in excess, it causes a condition called leukocytosis, which means elevated white blood cell count.

Diagnosis

Just like any other cancer, the diagnosis of anaplastic thyroid cancer requires a pathologist to examine a sample of the tumor under the microscope. This can be done in several ways, the most common of which is called fine needle aspiration (FNA) (see chapter 6). A simple and accurate method of diagnosing thyroid cancer, FNA is done by inserting a needle, smaller than those commonly used for drawing blood from the arm, in the area of the thyroid gland suspected of having cancer. Three to four samples are usually collected from each suspicious area of the thyroid, and they are then examined under the microscope using special stains. The characteristics of the cells collected are used to determine the presence and type of cancer. FNA is accurate in more than 90 percent of cases depending on several factors, including the technique used to obtain the aspirate and the experience of the pathologist evaluating the samples. Alternatively, the diagnosis is made from specimens of tissue removed during surgery, again by examination of samples under the microscope.

Because anaplastic thyroid cancer cells have lost most of the original characteristics of normal differentiated thyroid cells, special techniques often are required to distinguish them from other poorly differentiated cancers, such as lymphoma. One such method to do this is called flow cytometry. With this technique, special features of the cancer cells can be assessed and so allow us to distinguish their origin. This distinction is extremely important because the treatment of different cancers can vary quite a bit. Once anaplastic thyroid cancer has been diagnosed, an extensive work-up is necessary to determine the extent of the tumor spread. The degree to which the tumor has metastasized will have a great impact on the treatment options and the prognosis (how well the patient will do).

Several methods are available to learn the extent of the tumor, and this determination allows the physician to make an appropriate therapeutic plan. The neck, where thyroid cancers originate, can be assessed by ultrasound, magnetic resonance imaging (MR) or computerized tomography (CT). These methods allow us to establish how much disease is in the neck and help decide the extent of the surgery needed to remove the tumor. MR and CT also can be used to examine the rest of the body (chest, abdomen, and head). As mentioned earlier, anaplastic thyroid cancer has lost most of the characteristics of normal thyroid tissue, including the ability to concentrate iodine. As a result, scanning techniques that depend on the uptake of radioactive iodine as are used for well-differentiated thyroid cancers are not useful here. On the other hand, because these cells are very active metabolically, that is, they use a lot of energy in order to grow and multiply, scanning by the positron emission tomography (PET) technique is often useful. PET uses glucose (the main fuel for all cells of the body) that is labeled with a radioactive fluorine element. When given to a patient with anaplastic thyroid cancer, most of the glucose and radioactive tag will go the tumor cells because they are the most metabolically active. We can then determine where the radioactivity has localized in the body by using special cameras that detect the radioactive glucose agent that was given.

We also can determine the presence of metastasis to the bones using another nuclear medicine study, a bone scan. This technique utilizes a substance that has the ability to accumulate in areas of the bones that are broken down by cancer growth. Again, a special camera is used to detect the radioactive material in these areas of bone.

Treatment

Because of its unusual cellular nature, the treatment of anaplastic thyroid cancer is different from the other "differentiated" thyroid cancers. The loss of characteristics such as the ability to take up radioactive iodine and respond to the thyroid-stimulating hormone (TSH) makes some treatment options ineffective. As described in chapter 2, TSH is a hormone produced by the pituitary gland to stimulate the production of thyroid hormone. TSH also has the ability to stimulate growth of both normal thyroid cells and well-differentiated thyroid cancer cells. Radioactive iodine treatment and suppression of TSH are thus not viable options for anaplastic thyroid cancer

When possible, the initial approach to treatment for anaplastic thyroid cancer is surgical removal of the primary, original tumor from the neck. This requires complete removal of the thyroid gland. If the tumor has spread to structures around the gland, an effort has to be made to remove as much of the cancer as possible. This often requires removal of lymph nodes, soft tissues, and even muscles and nerves, depending on the extent of the tumor. If the tumor involves the windpipe (trachea) and a partial resection of the windpipe is needed, then a tracheostomy is often done. This procedure involves the creation of an opening at the base of the neck that provides a new connection of the airway with the outside environment, through which the patient will be breathing. Also, if the esophagus (gullet or food pipe) is involved and has to be removed or is obstructed, a tube called a PEG can be inserted through the skin of the abdomen and placed into the stomach pouch to allow feeding. The patient takes in nutrition in liquid form through this PEG tube.

For most thyroid cancers, radioactive iodine would be employed after surgery to destroy any remnant tissue. However, because anaplastic cancer does not take up radioiodine, external beam radiation therapy is usually given after surgery. If surgery is not possible, external beam radiation therapy may be considered by itself. As discussed in chapter 21, radiation causes lethal changes in the genetic material of cells. In general, cells that replicate fast are more susceptible to radiation. Radiation therapy may be most effective at providing relief of local symptoms of pain or obstruction in the neck. This is inferred from the results of therapeutic trials evaluating the effectiveness of radiation treatment. The results noted that the therapy was helpful in controlling the disease at the site where it was applied but that there was not necessarily an improvement in the survival of these patients.

External beam radiation therapy may also be applied to parts of the body other than the neck region and is commonly used for a distant metastasis, such as in bone.

Radiation therapy may involve complications. Normal cells and tissues that are within the part of the body exposed to the radiation are also affected and side effects can develop. Some of these side effects have been discussed in chapter 21.

Another option for the treatment of anaplastic thyroid cancer is chemotherapy. This treatment involves the administration of medications that have the ability to stop the cancer cells from multiplying. One of the most commonly used medications today is doxorubicin, and in one research series, 22 percent of patients had a partial response, meaning there was some decrease in the tumor.

Another medication is Taxol® (paclitaxel), and several trials with this agent are underway. Other medications, either alone or combination, are also being studied, and these chemotherapeutic agents include bleomycin, etoposide, methotrexate, and cisplatin. Some of the chemotherapeutic agents have been combined with radiation therapy. In response to the various treatment regimens, some patients have had partial responses as already discussed above, and some patients have had a complete response, although this does not mean a cure in most cases, only a temporary beneficial result.

Clinical trials are underway to test additional treatment approaches. For example, one clinical trial currently underway involves a drug called combretastatin. Further information is available from the National Cancer Institute (see appendix C).

Conclusions

Anaplastic thyroid cancer is one type of thyroid cancer and is rare. Early diagnosis and aggressive treatment with surgery, external beam radiation therapy, and possibly chemotherapy are the most important means of control. A large effort is under way to better understand this form of cancer and hopefully identify new methods of treatment.

CHAPTER 26

"Living with Thyroid Cancer"

Ron Sall, Dianne Dodd, Ph.D., Joan Shey,

Diane Patching, Jeanne F. Allegra, Ph.D.,

Stephen Peterson, M.D.

Introduction

In this chapter, we have invited several patients as well as a spouse of a patient to share with you their experiences with thyroid cancer, and the chapter concludes with a discussion by a psychologist and psychiatrist. In our opinion, this is the most valuable chapter of the book. It reinforces that you are not alone. Others have gone before you. Your thoughts and emotions are not unique. You do have options. You can live with thyroid cancer.

In order for the patients to tell their stories in their own words, we have minimized changes such as in grammar and content. As a result, some medical information may be incomplete, controversial or possibly incorrect. In these situations, we have italicized in parentheses either comments or referred you to other sections of the book for additional information or clarification.

D. VAN NOSTRAND

"Living with Thyroid Cancer"

Ron Sall

In each of our lives there are many defining moments. Possibly, it is the day that you met your wife or husband, the day you married or the day your first child was born. For some, it may have been the day the planes were crashed into the World Trade Center and Pentagon, September 11, 2001. Certainly, each of these is significant and meaningful, but in my opinion, to the cancer patient, the truly defining moment is the day you first learn of your cancer diagnosis. It is on this day that you realize that you are mortal and all of the issues surrounding possibly dying become a reality.

For me this day was February 12, 1997. I vividly recall waiting for the surgeon whom I had not previously met and having him look at me and say: "You know that you are very sick." Yes, I knew something was wrong, but until that moment I was under the mistaken assumption that the back pain I experienced, coupled with the pressure on my leg, was "merely" a slipped or herniated disk. With MRI in hand, I had painfully driven to his office to meet him and discuss treatment options. I was shocked when he informed me that I had cancer that had metastasized to my fourth and fifth lumbar vertebrae and that I had to enter the hospital immediately for treatment.

That was the start of a process that continues to this day. After a biopsy and the determination that, in fact, I had thyroid cancer, I immediately went on the offensive. This is a key issue, because upon being initially diagnosed with a malignancy there may be a tendency to withdraw because of the fear associated with cancer. In my opinion, this may be the worst approach you can take after being given the diagnosis. The moment this initial diagnosis is made may be the time to admit to a relatively thorough lack of knowledge of your illness. I freely admitted my ignorance and started with the basics—"What is a thyroid, where is it and what does it do?" Needless to say, I learned a lot about the thyroid gland rather quickly.

Upon learning of the diagnosis, there are two areas that may be approached. The clinical, which will be discussed later, and the personal. On the personal side, what you do and how you do it are of great import. How will you function on a daily basis? Do you or should you continue working, and are you able to? What foods should you eat? In essence, are you going to continue to enjoy living or merely withdraw?

I chose to live, to work, to seek balance—fully realizing that I have a serious problem but never letting that problem become the overriding factor controlling my life. I did achieve better balance, but I still work full time, eat well, sleep well, and exercise as much as possible. Frankly, there is no reason not to continue acting normally as long as you fully recognize that you have an illness that needs monitoring. With monitoring and proper and timely medical intervention, you can live with thyroid cancer while still leading a "reasonably normal life."

I was also very fortunate to have a great support system—a loving wife and family and many friends who would and will go out of their way to help whenever asked. How valuable this is can never be adequately measured, but having the knowledge that there are people available to help when needed makes dealing with your illness that much easier.

It is the dealing with the fact that the cancer is always somewhere on your mind that is hard, especially after the initial diagnosis. In your mind, every new ache or pain is a reoccurrence of your cancer. As you learn more about your illness and what to expect from your medical team, you also learn how to deal better with your concerns. Are they ever completely disregarded? Not as far as I am concerned. However, over time you learn to distinguish between that which should be addressed immediately and that which is of a more theoretical concern. Here is where your medical team can be of great help.

I was fortunate to be referred by my surgeon to an endocrinologist who specializes in thyroid tumors and who provided me with a number of books to read on the matter while I recovered from my surgery. Again, this is a matter of considerable import, since without knowledge and inquiry it is difficult to participate really effectively in your treatment. If you fail to participate, you fail to maximize the potential benefits of your treatment and recovery.

Now the real work begins. Diagnosis and initial surgery are merely the beginning. My goal as a cancer survivor is to have my doctor tell me that I am "in remission" (the state where your body has rid itself of cancer cells). Active participation is critical to achieving this goal.

After reading about your illness and how it is treated, you can participate in an informed manner. The learning process is slow. However, as you probe you learn more and more about preferred options, the latest in treatment protocols and the role played by each of your physicians (endocrinologist, surgeon, nuclear medicine specialist, radiation oncologist—yes, I also was treated with external radiation). The more you understand, the more you can participate in your care.

Once the diagnosis is confirmed, the first task is to have your cancerous thyroid removed. A word of caution before proceeding: the trend for care of thyroid cancer patients is a total thyroidectomy of the cancerous thyroid. Clearly, there are many excellent surgeons, but not all surgeons perform thyroid surgery routinely enough to have developed considerable skill at it, and not all are sufficiently experienced and skilled to avoid the risks associated with possible damage to the parathyroid glands or the nerves to the vocal cords. Thus it is important to learn from your surgeon how many thyroid operations he or she has performed, and what has been his or her experience with the patients he or she has treated. The surgeon you choose should be very comfortable discussing this matter with you and also delving into the surgery itself so you will know what to expect and how to deal with what you experience, both routinely and in the event that something is out of the norm.

Upon completion of the thyroidectomy and depending upon the findings at surgery, the next suggested action is generally a post-operative scan and treatment with radioactive iodine (RAI). You have to be hypothyroid to have an adequate scan and RAI therapy *(Editors' comment: see chapters 9 and 10),* which means that thyroid hormone replacement is not started after the surgery, and you are allowed to drift into hypothyroidism, which causes the pituitary hormone, thyrotropin (TSH), to rise in the blood. This high TSH level facilitates the treatment. Possibly at this juncture I was spoiled. Due to a number of factors I was given injections of a synthetic recombinant human TSH (Thyrogen®) to prepare me for my RAI treatment. Let it suffice to say that later when I was made "hypo" in preparation for a second RAI treatment, the effect on me was considerably different in a negative way. The RAI treatment is done to attack any residual cancer cells that the surgeon may not have removed out of fear of damaging your parathyroid and/or nerves to the vocal cords, but the RAI hopefully will also destroy any cancer cells that are outside of the thyroid bed. Other than the preparation (the hypothyroidism), the treatment is not painful. Yes, you will be put into isolation so that the radiation does not affect other patients; and yes, this can be terribly frustrating, but it usually lasts for only 24 hours. Given the benefit to be derived, the isolation pales in comparison. *(Editorial comment: with new NRC rules, some patients may be treated with RAI as an outpatient. See chapter 20.)* It is the preparation of becoming hypothyroid that is the most debilitating.

As noted, you are generally made hypothyroid to maximize the results from the RAI. Hypothyroidism brings with it a slowing of your metabolism such that the most basic of functions seem demonstrably more difficult. It is not the RAI treatment that the thyroid cancer patient generally complains about; rather, it is the period leading up to it and immediately thereafter that are the most difficult. Subsequent to the initial RAI ablation of residual thyroid tissue, you may be given RAI again at a later date when you are taking thyroid medication. At such times, you will be taken off your medication over a period of weeks so that your blood TSH level will rise and stimulate the RAI uptake by any residual thyroid cells. The best way in which I can describe the effect of the RAI is to use the analogy of the old Pac-Man video game. The iodine acts in this same manner—your body stimulates the thyroid cells by the high TSH of hypothyroidism to seek out the bad cells and destroy them.

Upon completion of the RAI treatment, the next step is to determine whether the treatment was successful. This could include a RAI body scan, a PET (positron emission tomography) scan, and/or a simple blood test to look for residual cells *(Editors' comment: see chapter 16)*. The blood test measures thyroglobulin (Tg), a protein derived only from thyroid cells so that its presence indicates the presence of thyroid cells. The desired result is zero "hot spots" and extremely low levels of serum Tg. If these conditions result, you know that your treatment has been successful and you are on your way to remission.

What if, as in my case, these are not the results? Clearly you do not give up. Not going into remission from the first treatment does not mean that subsequent treatments will not be more successful or that there are not other options. As previously addressed, my cancer had spread to the lumbar area of my spine, an area rather distant from the thyroid and somewhat difficult for the RAI to destroy completely. Given that there were residual cells detected through my blood work, and since the RAI treatments had not fully removed them from my body, on the advice on my thyroidologist I agreed to have external radiation on my spine.

External radiation is another approach to combating your cancer once it has spread to a distant site or is specific to a site and can be destroyed. The process itself is not painful but can make you extremely tired since you are treated on a daily basis over an extended period of time. The treatment basically involves focusing a beam of intense external radiation on the affected area. It is less debilitating than surgery and yes, as demonstrated in my case, it can work.

As you can see from the description of my treatment, I am still living with my cancer. I was like many "macho men" who didn't think I needed to visit a doctor unless something clearly was broken and had to be fixed. Interestingly, after my diagnosis I seemed to go full cycle to almost becoming a hypochondriac. The least little pain resulted in a trip to one of my doctors. Is this natural? I don't know. However, given my initial prognosis and failure to eliminate the disease, it certainly seemed the right approach. Slowly but surely, I began to accept more of these little pains and discovered that with proper treatment I can live with my illness. Do I become anxious awaiting the blood test results? Definitely! Do my anxieties preclude me from leading a reasonably normal life? Not to my knowledge. This is another important point to consider. I have learned that my response to my cancer is no different than the response of the person diagnosed with a heart condition or diabetes. We all must respond to our illnesses, but we all can live full and happy lives if we take care of ourselves. Not to preach, but proper diet, exercise and rest will help, and the more we do to help ourselves, the better the chance we have for full recovery.

What can you expect after surgery? You will be given a prescription for thyroid medicine—a pill taken daily on an empty stomach, generally in the morning (I take mine first thing when I awaken). This pill substitutes for your thyroid and helps keep your metabolism in proper balance. When you have your blood work done, not only will your physician measure your thyroglobulin (Tg) levels, but he or she usually also will check your thyroid hormone and TSH levels. Your thyroidologist will work with you to maintain your TSH level at the appropriate and desired range for the type and extent of your cancer. If extensive residual tumor remains, the thyroidologist usually will want to maintain TSH at very low levels. In theory this can make you hyperthyroid, but given the options, this condition is considerably more attractive than the possible growth and spread of your cancer through too much TSH stimulation.

Throughout the process, vigilance, and participation are key: vigilance in the sense of being aware of your body and responding to anything abnormal, participation in terms of your willingness to seek out and try options to eradicate your disease.

Can you live with thyroid cancer? I have, and I have done it reasonably well considering where I was when I started. Can you live with thyroid cancer as a newly diagnosed or recovering cancer patient? Absolutely! Does it ever leave your mind even when "clean"? I doubt it, but I sincerely look forward to the day when my scan is clean and my blood level of thyroglobulin (Tg) cannot be measured because it is so low. On that day I will be able to answer that question. Until then I continue to monitor my illness, seek professional advice, and participate in my recovery. When I am clean, and only then, will I truly know the answer to this question.

There's No Such Thing as a "Good Cancer"*

Dianne Dodd, Ph.D.

*Thanks to the Thyroid Foundation of Canada for permission to reprint these two articles from their newsletter, *thyrobulletin*. I would also like to thank both the ThyCa Association and the Canadian Thyroid Cancer Support Group (Thry'vors) Inc. for their support and inspiration. The many thyroid cancer survivors I met online provided much of the material and the inspiration for this work. My family, Michael, Elizabeth, Kathleen, and Melanie, was just always there.

The first part of this article is the story of my personal experience with thyroid cancer and the second, which constitutes peer advice on surviving the emotional aspects of treatment, is the result of research I did following my cancer journey. It all fits together, however. My experience of treatment—the fear of illness, of the unknown, the grief at losing my health, the lack of information I had to make decisions, the powerlessness I and my family felt—all of this brought me to a important realization. That is, no matter how good the prognosis of any cancer, the support of one's peers, of others who had gone through it and survived, is not only comforting for many patients but essential to full recovery, emotionally, and physically. My search for information and for emotional support led me to a full volunteer commitment to online support groups, first the American ThyCa group, and later the Canadian Thyroid Cancer Support Group (Thyr'vors) Inc. As well I am an active member of the Thyroid Foundation of Canada.

In the summer of 1999, I discovered that I had a lump on my throat. My family doctor assured me that these lumps are usually benign but sent me for an ultrasound just to be sure. I suspected something was wrong when the ultrasound technician left to get the radiologist, and I heard the two of them whispering. They were counting, up to 8 or 10 I think. 8 or 10 what??!! They didn't tell me anything, of course. That gave me something to think about while I waited two months to see an endocrinologist who told me that I had a multi-nodular goiter and that one of the nodules was quite large. He asked if I had ever been exposed to X-ray radiation as a child or teenager, which I hadn't. Later I found out that this is often the cause of thyroid cancer. The endocrinologist told me that I would have to have the left lobe of my thyroid removed and sent me to see a general surgeon to do a fine needle aspiration biopsy. The results indicated "suspicious," and the surgeon set a date for surgery but assured me "this could wait—it's probably benign." Further, he said, even if it is malignant, it's no big deal because "if you have to get cancer, the thyroid is the place to get it." Thyroid cancer is slow growing and relatively easy to treat.

I found out later that there is controversy among physicians as to whether a total thyroidectomy should be done in a case such as mine, as opposed to a partial, or lobectomy. But my surgeon was not a thyroid specialist, seemed nervous about the risks involved in total thyroidectomy and didn't seem to believe that I had thyroid cancer. So he took the conservative route and removed only half.

The surgery wasn't that bad—a little scary but not all that painful as the nerves in your neck are severed and don't grow back for a year or so. We had also been told that there was no lymph node involvement—if the cancer spreads, it usually goes to the lymph nodes first.

When I went back to see the surgeon a week post-surgery, I was devastated to hear the word "carcinoma" as he read the pathology report to me. That's about all I got out of what he said, except that I needed iodine radiation treatment, but before that, another operation to take out the other half of my thyroid. Because the thyroid naturally absorbs iodine, a dose of irradiated iodine is administered to kill all remaining thyroid tissue left after surgery. *(Editors' comment: The irradiated iodine is radioactive iodine. See chapter 17.)*

But at that moment, all I could think about was having to have a second operation. Just the thought of opening up an incision that was not yet healed made me shudder. Sitting alone in his office, I wished I had brought my husband or a friend along for support, but of course they don't tell you ahead of time, "Oh, we're going to tell you that you have cancer, so bring lots of emotional support." That's the insidious thing about having cancer. You feel that they're taking away your health a little bit at a time. The bad news comes in slow increments and undermines your confidence in anyone who says, "Don't worry, it's probably nothing."

My second surgery seemed like deja vu, or perhaps a recurring nightmare, I'm not sure which. Although I had next to no voice left, which worried me greatly at the time, about six months later my voice returned to normal. Still, I hadn't been sick that long and there were visits, phone calls from people I hadn't heard from in years, cards, flowers, etc. I was OK.

All my surgeon could tell me at that point was that I had to become hypothyroid for the treatment and that I would feel really sick, (boy, was he right about that!!!) but he didn't know how long I would have to be off medication. His office made an appointment for me at the Cancer Clinic, but I had to wait three weeks after surgery. I called and tried to find out how long I would need to be off medication before the RAI, but the Cancer Clinic would not tell me anything until I had my initial visit. So I waited, feeling frustrated and scared. I felt I had fallen through the cracks in the medical system.

Finally, I went to the bright shiny offices of the Cancer Clinic at the Ottawa Hospital, General Campus. All the stops were pulled to make me feel warm and fuzzy. My husband was with me, and they even had a partition in the doctors' offices so that patients had privacy when being examined, while one's partner or friend could be there to ask questions or absorb information. This was all based on the theory that patients are stressed out and don't listen well when being told they have cancer. But, by the time I got there, I already knew I had cancer and had absorbed that information at a time when I had least expected it. Now I was being offered counseling! I declined, thinking "Oh, that's just for people with real cancer, people who have to have chemo, lose their hair and worry about dying." And I had no idea then how much I would need help later on.

At three weeks post-surgery, I was so hopeful that I would be admitted to the hospital immediately for my RAI that I had already packed my bag. I wanted to get it over with and get back to my life. I was devastated to find out that it took SIX weeks to become sufficiently hypo to have the treatment. I still had three weeks to go! By the end, I felt like I was dying. I needed to take Gravol® and Tylenol® every day to control the horrible headaches and nausea. I was sleeping a lot of the time and gradually getting more and more depressed. My skin turned gray, my eyes got puffy, and I went through a period of insomnia. My reflexes slowed down so much that, not only could I not drive, but I also could barely speak or even think clearly. By the last week, I couldn't have a conversation with anyone or even concentrate enough to read. I just sat in my recliner and stared out the window, waiting to go to the hospital.

By comparison with the hypo-hell, the RAI was uneventful enough, though 24 hours in isolation was alienating. Everybody was being so careful with the dose of irradiated iodine, yet I had to drink it! Everything in the room was covered in plastic, including the phone, and the floor was covered in paper. The nurses wouldn't come into my room and left food trays outside my closed door. When my husband came to get me they almost wouldn't let him in!

When I came home, I had to be careful not to contaminate my family. My husband took the children away for a few days, and I stayed mostly in my room for a week *(Editors' comment: see chapters 17 and 20)*. The hardest thing was not being able to kiss or hug my youngest child, who was only seven then. My husband was also nervous about me preparing food for a while, so I really felt like a leper. All of these precautions are of course reasonable, but they are hard to handle when you're very sick and depressed. Everything looked so hopeless at that point, and I had withdrawn so much from my husband and kids that I felt like a Martian in my own home.

After three weeks of taking Synthroid®, I began to feel human again, but I knew I would have to go back to hypo-hell for a post-treatment scan to confirm that all the thyroid cells were gone. While the second hypo period was, in some ways, not as bad—it was still awful. By the time I went for the diagnostic scan in November my husband and I were barely speaking to each other.

Fortunately, my diagnostic scan was "clean." I no longer had any thyroid cancer left in my body! But I was much too sick and too sad and worn down by illness to celebrate. I went back on Synthroid®, went back to work and waited to feel normal again. But like most people, it took a year before I was really well. I was tired and felt like I was still hypo even though my TSH was normal. Actually below normal, as thyroid cancer patients need to have a suppressed TSH to prevent recurrence. Some days it felt like I was reliving the nightmare—it would suddenly come back to me—the way I had felt when hypo. I tried a combined dose of Cytomel® and Synthroid® but became so hyperthyroid that I had tremors and couldn't concentrate. Hyper symptoms are surprisingly similar to being hypo, except one feels very anxious and restless while experiencing extreme fatigue, and there can be violent mood swings, insomnia, and other distressing symptoms.

I was still struggling when I found an Internet support group for survivors of thyroid cancer, sponsored by the U.S.-based ThyCa Association. At first, I spent hours on line and soaked up information like a sponge. It was an immense relief to talk to people who understood how I felt. My family had long since lost their patience with the Mom who didn't seem to ever get better and didn't want to hear about it anymore. But I wasn't well enough yet to put it behind me. The amazing thing about the support group was that people could rant and rave and bash their families, or their doctors . . . really just say anything at all, and someone would give them a sympathetic, helpful response.

Finally I realized I was suffering from a lingering depression—a common side effect of thyroid cancer treatment. With help from my family doctor, a psychologist, the support group, as well as some special people in my life, I recovered and regained my energy. Everyone is unique, but for me, part of recovering meant acknowledging my own feelings. While well meaning relatives and physicians took comfort in the treatable nature of thyroid cancer, I felt they dismissed my illness as not very serious. And I still get angry when I hear someone refer to thyroid cancer as the "good cancer." As we say in our support group, there is no such thing as a good cancer. The treatment process is lengthy and stressful for patients as well as families. In one sense, I was very lucky—I had a very treatable form of cancer, only had to have two hypo-hells and one RAI (some people have more), and I'm not likely to have a recurrence. On the other hand, having cancer forced me to confront some scary realities and reevaluate my priorities, values, and relationships.

Though painful, it wasn't all bad. I did learn to take better care of myself. Now I conserve my energy for the important things, I cherish the people who supported me while I was ill and do more fun things. The other thing I learned was the value of support through the treatment process. In my experience, medical personnel, specialists in particular, provide minimal, sporadic information. The patient never gets the big picture, and that makes it harder for individuals, as well as their families/caregivers to cope. Most of the information I got came from books, the Internet and my support group. Having met online, I became president (fall 2003 and am now past-president) of the Canadian Thyroid Cancer Support Group (Thry'vors), which provides support to Canadian thyroid cancer survivors. As well, I am an active member of the Thyroid Foundation of Canada and volunteer with Cancer Connection, a service that matches by telephone newly diagnosed patients with survivors.

As part of my recovery, I did some research not only into thyroid cancer in particular but generally into the burgeoning field of cancer and the family, or the psychosocial aspects of cancer treatment. The following is the result of this research, as well the knowledge gained from personal experience and from talking online and by phone to many others who have walked in the same shoes as I. All of this has made me a firm believer in the importance of peer support from someone who's been there, too.

Surviving the Emotional Turmoil of Thyroid Cancer Treatment

Thyroid cancer affects women three times as often as men, often during their childbearing years, and its impact is often felt on the whole family. Although thyroid cancer is treatable, patients who have thyroid cancer undergo a draining and often lengthy treatment. As with any major illness, patients may face anxiety, anger, depression, reduced self-esteem and even marital and/or family strain. But patients who have thyroid cancer must also cope with hormonal changes. To help thyroid cancer patients, survivors and their families be better prepared, the rest of this article is meant to let patients and caregivers know what to expect through the treatment process and to reassure patients and caregivers, family and friends that they are not alone. There are resources in the community to help families shoulder the burden of a major illness.

Diagnosis and the Waiting Game

Many patients experience long waiting periods leading up to a cancer diagnosis. This can be a real roller coaster ride, with one physician reassuring the patient while the next makes some passing comment that sends her crashing into despair. Some patients research their illness on the Internet or through books; however, until a diagnosis is made, this may only serve to worry rather than empower. It is difficult to make day to day decisions not knowing what the future will bring. Many patients choose to wait until a diagnosis is confirmed before telling family, friends and colleagues, thus facing their anxiety alone. Receiving a diagnosis, whether good or bad, is often a tremendous relief.

Absorbing the reality of a cancer diagnosis initially throws most people into a state of shock, fear, and sometimes denial. Each person must set her own timetable for sharing the diagnosis with others. But remember this: now is not the time to cut yourself off from loved ones. Communicating the news openly with friends and family allows them the chance to share their feelings and to offer help and support. Sometimes parents try to protect their children from the truth. But when a family is turned upside down by cancer, children sense their parents' distress. Not knowing the cause, they will imagine things to be much worse then they really are, or worse, blame themselves for the mysterious upheaval. Explain that "Mommy (or Daddy) will be sick, maybe tired or even sad for a while, but will get better in time." Children have wonderful capacities to help, to understand, and to be warm and nurturing toward a sick parent.

Everyone will need time to absorb the information. Some want to talk about it, others to avoid the topic for a while. Sometimes timetables and approaches differ within a family. For example, a caregiver tries to protect himself or herself or his or her loved ones by engaging in "false cheeriness." This denies the person with cancer the opportunity to discuss real fears and anxieties. Each suffers alone, the patient feeling emotionally deserted while the caregiver feels unappreciated in carrying the extra burden of housekeeping, childcare, and nurturing. Such resentments are difficult to express, however, because "cancer is no one's fault."

Families can avoid such an impasse. While *it is the patients' right to set the agenda,* patients can help by sending clear signals to family or friends that they are ready to talk, or not. Caregivers and friends should be receptive to these clues. Patients can also help by telling friends, family, and colleagues what kind of help and/or support they need. Most people are happy to help if they know what to do. Similar communication approaches will also work with physicians, may of whom believe that cancer patients cannot, or do not want, to absorb all the information at once. They too wait for clues from the patient. Some additional helpful suggestions are noted in the Table 1.

TABLE 1
Other Helpful Suggestions

- Illness causes as much stress to a spouse as to the patient. A worried spouse burdened with extra work could use a "day off," assistance with chauffeuring kids, or maybe some help at mealtimes.
- Listen while she sounds off. There's a lot happening to her and she needs to verbalize without hurting someone's feelings.
- Act normal, and don't try to cheer her up when she's depressed. It's normal to be depressed when things are going badly.
- Children are amazingly resourceful. Coming to understand that when "mommy is hypo, she's going to be sad," and that she still loves her child, can help him or her mature and eventually deal with adult relationships.
- When I'm hypo, don't ask if you should walk the dog, do the laundry or bring dinner over, just do it.
- Invite my family over. Sometimes I need time alone. Even if they're being good, my children can keep me from resting.
- Drive me to appointments until I can drive.
- Handle phone calls, faxes, emails from family, friends, and well-wishers. Sometimes it's just too much.
- Patients are often anxious and distressed when visiting their physician. Take a tape recorder, or better yet, a calm friend or relative to help ask questions, and/or "remember" what the doctor said.

Surgery

Thyroid surgery, whether a partial or total thyroidectomy, invokes fear and anxiety. Many patients report that the thyroid surgery is relatively painless and that their surgery was the easiest part of their treatment. Following surgery, most patients prepare for iodine radiation treatment. It is especially important at this time for patients to preserve their physical and mental health by getting lots of rest, eating healthy foods, and avoiding stress-causing situations. Caregivers and patients may need to relax housekeeping standards for a while or get help with childcare and housework. Patients who accept offers of help will not only keep themselves well rested but will provide friends and family with an opportunity to express their concern.

"Going Hypo"

To prepare for iodine radiation treatment, patients must be off thyroid medication, usually for six weeks *(Editors' comment: see chapter 9),* which induces a state of hypothyroidism. Being hypo can be debilitating, and it is a process that is often repeated for follow-up diagnostic scans. It helps to know what to expect.

Every patient is different. A few lucky thycans breeze through what survivors have affectionately dubbed "hypo-hell." However, most individuals experience considerable discomfort and emotional upset. Hypothyroidism causes a general slowing of metabolism, which may result in indigestion, constipation, nausea, headaches, weight gain, fatigue, muscles aches, slow reflexes, memory loss and cognitive problems, intolerance to cold and puffy eyes.

Thyca patients are especially vulnerable to depression due to the hormonal imbalances caused by rapid hypothyroidism. Rapidly changing, contradictory feelings are not uncommon. Patients may become angry and irritated and exhibit unexplained hatred toward partners, spouses, relatives and friends. Patients may also get confused and forgetful—a phenomenon sometimes called "brain fog." Hypothyroid patients may also become extremely withdrawn and appear not to care about family, friends—even their own children. Patients may also become emotionally dependent.

Remember that, however bizarre your thycan's behaviour may be, it is a normal reaction to withdrawal of hormones. Remind yourself of this, and remind your partner. All of this will pass. Indeed, caregivers play an important role during hypothyroid periods by being supportive, by avoiding negative reactions, and by assessing whether the patient and/or family may need professional help. While it can be very draining to be around a depressed person, it is important to relate to him or her frequently. Even if the patient is withdrawn, try sitting nearby, reading a book or the newspaper if they don't want to talk. Just letting them know that you are there helps. Caregivers may find the thycan's expressions of anger, fear, and inner confusion frightening, especially those who avoid confrontation in their relationships. However, lashing out in anger at the patient will serve only to reinforce the sick person's feeling of worthlessness. Patients need to express negative feelings—indeed, it is part of recovery. Remember, they are not angry with you. They are angry at fate, or God, or whom or whatever they blame for bringing cancer into their lives. Also try to avoid distancing yourself from the patient—another common reaction—as this will leave the patient feeling abandoned. Guard against excluding the thycan from family activities, conversations, and decision-making. Patients are ill; they are not mentally incompetent!! They will recovery more quickly if you make them feel included, loved, and needed.

Thycans themselves can also help, even when in the depths of hypo-hell. Fatigue is a significant contributor to depression and mental distress, so try not to overdo it. Accept offers of help and don't be afraid to tell people what you want or need. If you begin to feel emotionally neglected by your spouse, children, friends or family, ask yourself whether they are ignoring you or whether you have withdrawn from them.

Sexual relations can also be fragile at this time. Although fatigue, depression, illness, loss of self esteem, and changes in both body image and relationships may cause a loss of interest in physical intimacy, illness alone is rarely the cause of infidelity or marital breakdown. Remind the patient that it is not her physical attributes that make her attractive to you, but intangible qualities, like sense of humour, caring and intellect, none of which are lost during illness. Keep talking and don't be afraid to show affection. Hugs work wonders.

Iodine Radiation (RAI)

Once the patient is sufficiently hypothyroid, she undergoes iodine radiation treatment. Perhaps the worst aspect of this phase of treatment is its necessary isolation. Hospital personnel often refuse to come into a patient's room and everything is covered in plastic and cellophane to prevent contamination and for ease of clean up. Upon discharge, and especially if treatment was administered on an outpatient basis, patients are asked to follow a number of precautions to avoid contaminating other people. Being instructed not to touch their own young children for up to a week, nor to be near pregnant women leaves many patients feeling like lepers. Already sick and tired, patients find it incomprehensible that everyone is so fearful of this irradiated iodine, when they have to drink it!! Still, once the treatment is administered patients may begin taking thyroid medication and will feel better within several weeks.

Follow-Up

Following treatment, many physicians recommend diagnostic scans, which require the patient to become hypothyroid once again—each time for six weeks *(Editors' comment: see chapter 9)*. Following each treatment or scan the dose [of thyroid hormone] must be adjusted, a process which takes time and patience. Thycans need to maintain a suppressed TSH in order to reduce the risk of recurrence. That means living with slight hyperthyroidism, which can cause agitation, anxiety, mood swings, insomnia, tremors, weight loss, diarrhea, heart palpitations and intolerance to heat. In the initial phase, many patients experience confusing swings between hypo and hyperthyroid symptoms.

In the period immediately following active treatment, both patients and family members expect everything to go back to the way it was before. They may become angry, resentful and/or depressed when this doesn't happen, or it doesn't happen as quickly as they'd like. But many people take a year, or even longer, after treatment before they feel normal again, and many thycans, like other cancer patients, discover that they must find a different definition of "normal."

After a lengthy absence from work, most thycans find that returning to employment helps them to feel more normal. However, they aren't always sure what or how much to tell co-workers. Again, it is up to the patient to send the right signals. Most people are genuinely concerned, and they will respect your right to privacy or your need to talk. Just as no healthy marriage falters as a result of illness, most employers accommodate illness. However, if you find that ungrounded fears of absenteeism, death or contagion caused by your cancer result in dismissal or unfair treatment at work, there are human rights provisions in place to protect you. Become familiar with them and stand up for your rights.

Don't Be Afraid to Ask for Help

While most people can cope admirably well with a temporary emergency, thyca treatments, which can extend into months and even years of disruption, can add strain to families. A few may find they need professional help. For example, if a patient has a predisposition to depression and/or anxiety disorders, hypothyroidism can trigger onset of these conditions. Depression, co-incident with cancer treatment, is not unusual nor is it "just something one has to suffer through." In fact, suffering through can actually inhibit recovery. During thyca treatment, patients CAN be treated for depression, a very treatable medical condition, usually with a combination of anti-depressants and/or counseling. Because depression causes great lethargy and because there is a stigma attached to being treated for depression, patients often feel they don't deserve to be treated. Caregivers can play an important role in encouraging the patient to seek treatment.

Although it may not fit with our image of families as loving and nurturing groups, the reality is that families, like individuals, are not perfect. They respond to the crisis of illness in ways that reflect their distinctive coping strategies. Some remain open and calm while others react with fear and anger. Thyca treatment may exacerbate existing unresolved psychological, personal, marital or relationship problems within a family. Gender differences in communication and in coping strategies can add further strain. When the patient is a woman and her caregiver a man—often the case with thyroid cancer—our social conventions are challenged. Unaccustomed to performing the social, emotional management work that most women perform in families, a husband may suddenly find himself called upon to sooth children's disputes, keeping dinnertime conversations on an even keel, and just listen.

If you need to ask for help, do so. It does not mean your family is falling apart. On the contrary, asking for help is the first step in strengthening a family or relationship. There are support groups where spouses and close relatives or their partners who have to live with thyroid cancer can talk to each other. Many find this beneficial. As well, many cancer clinics offer psychological counseling and other professional counselors for individuals and families.

No One Forgets: The Years After

Having cancer is something that no one ever forgets. Cancer forces us to face our own mortality, to lose our sense of control and security and to accept a compromised state of health. Aptly compared to grieving the death of a loved one, this loss may be initially greeted with denial, then anger, depression, and eventually acceptance. Most patients find that they must acknowledge all these tumultuous feelings before they can fully recover. All of this takes time. Well meaning relatives and doctors should not dismiss the suffering of thyca patients by telling them they have the "good cancer," leaving patients feeling guilty that their illness is less severe than someone else's. This is not helpful.

The long-term emotional impact of cancer is not all negative. Most people discover hidden strengths and compassion in people they least expected it from, and many relationships are strengthened. Many spouses do learn to nurture, and children may also learn to be more considerate of an ill parent. Sadly, however, some cancer patients have reported the loss of one or more friends. Many people are unsure of how to treat an ill person. They may avoid calling, or even looking at you. If this happens, ask yourself whether you may have withdrawn from them in a period of anger or depression. Then, once you are feeling well enough, try contacting them and letting them know what they can do for you. If this doesn't work, however, it is not your fault. Perhaps your illness reminds them of their own mortality, forces them to relive some particularly painful episode in their past, or they have their own unresolved fears of desertion or rejection. Although it is inescapably sad, many patients have to accept the fact that some people will slip away.

Many patients also report that having faced cancer—that much feared disease—that everything else seems insignificant by comparison. This can have a calming effect. Many find that they worry less over small things and have the vision to see each day as a precious gift. Maybe this means enjoying enhanced relationships or starting a new hobby. For some patients, volunteer work is good therapy, which allows them to put their newfound knowledge and empathy to good use. If you think this might be for you, there are lots of agencies, who would be glad to hear from you.

For me personally, recovery meant involvement in our Canadian support group and doing volunteer work for the Thyroid Foundation and Cancer Connection. In offering support and encouragement to other individuals who are sick with thyroid cancer, I feel I am repaying the countless people who gave me support when I was sick. I also feel I am putting to good use the knowledge and wisdom I gained from my experience of cancer. Good health is much more than physical recovery from illness. It has important social and psychological components, which can best be met through patients taking responsibility for their own health, by supporting each other, and by ensuring everyone has the information they need to make decisions and survive the onslaught of surgery, radiation and hormonal withdrawal.

MY STORY: "Living with thyroid cancer"

Joan Shey

Introduction

(Editors' comment: The following is an interview with Joan Shey, founder and manager of "Light of Life Foundation" (see appendix C) (www.lightoflifefoundation.org). In addition to managing the foundation, Mrs. Shey is a wife and a mother of two children. Mrs. Shey lives in New Jersey. This interview is reprinted from the newsletter, "Thyrogram," Volume 1, Issue Two, pp. 1-3, with permission from the Genzyme company.)

Interviewer: *What happened when you found out that you had thyroid cancer?*

Joan Shey: In 1995, I had gone to a doctor for a completely different, unrelated problem. While he was examining my neck, he found a lump that he said might be a "nodule" on my thyroid. The first thing I did was to go home and look in my family medical dictionary to find out what a thyroid was.

At first the doctors tried just watching the lump to see if it was getting any bigger, but eventually they determined that it was thyroid cancer. I was angry, and I was scared. I was told, "You're lucky, because you have a good cancer." I guess that was supposed to make me feel better, but instead it was hard to take, because I couldn't help feeling that no cancer is a good cancer.

I ended up having an operation in which my whole thyroid and 39 lymph nodes were removed. After my surgery, I was given a thyroid hormone medicine called Synthroid® (levothyroxine sodium tablets, USP) to replace the hormones that my thyroid used to make.

Interviewer: *Did you have to have tests to see if the cancer was gone?*

Joan Shey: Yes, each year for three years. I had to stop taking my Synthroid® to have my checkups done. Each time, I had to go about six weeks from start to finish without the thyroid hormone. Those six weeks each year were very difficult. Without thyroid hormone, I became what doctors call "hypothyroid." Each week it would get harder. I felt depressed. I got bloated and gained weight. Each time, I would gain about 10 pounds even though I was eating the very limited low-iodine diet that was another requirement for testing. I always took the diet really seriously, wanting to do my part to make my test work well. The hardest part of the whole process, though, was how tired I got. Every day, my body felt less energetic than the day before. Just like when the battery in your car goes dead and your car doesn't run anymore, I felt like I couldn't function without my thyroid hormone. It was hard for me to just get through my day, much less to take care of my family. My son was 13 and my daughter was 17 the first year I went through this, so they depended on me to be there for them. They saw the changes in me, and they wondered whether I was ever going to be myself again. Finally, after the test was done, the doctors put me back on my Synthroid®, but even then it took a few weeks for me to feel normal again.

My doctor saw how difficult it was for me to go through being hypothyroid, and he told me that there was a drug being studied that would someday allow patients to keep taking their Synthroid® while they were being tested. So I waited for the day when Thyrogen® (thyrotropin alfa for injection) would be available. In the meantime, I went through two more years of testing without it. Finally, in 1998, Thyrogen® was available to use.

I get tested every year now with Thyrogen®. The Thyrogen® allows me to stay on my Synthroid® throughout the testing process. I'm not tired. I'm not depressed. It just makes it better. I still have the anxiety of going through the testing and having to be on the low-iodine diet, but it makes a tremendous difference in the way I feel.

Interviewer: *How does having had thyroid cancer affect your life today?*

Joan Shey: There's not a day, honestly, that goes by when I don't think about my cancer. I don't think about it as intensely as I did three years ago or two years ago, but there's not a day I don't realize that I'm dealing with it.

At first I had felt very much alone with my condition. I didn't know anyone else who had thyroid cancer, and I couldn't find any support groups in my area that were just for people with thyroid cancer. So I worked with my local hospital to start a foundation to educate people about this disease and help support the ones who have it. Our support group meets once a month, and we get a chance to share our feelings and experiences. It really helps to talk with other people who have been through the same things firsthand. In addition to the support group, our foundation does many other things to help people with thyroid cancer. For example, we have a Web site (www.lightoflifefoundation.org) that provides answers to questions people frequently ask about thyroid cancer, as well as a cookbook with appetizing recipes for the low-iodine diet, a chat room, and message boards.

Interviewer: *What suggestions do you have for the other people who have thyroid cancer?*

Joan Shey: First and foremost, I think it's important to have a positive attitude. And I feel exercise and diet and going out there and enjoying yourself with your friends and your family will help you. The more you do things that you enjoy, the more you eliminate some of the depression and fears and the day-to-day think-ing that "I have cancer."

It allows you to live your life the way you normally would live your life. Also, I try to find a little bit of humor in situations, because that helps me cope.

My son just applied to college this year, and I just found out that he wrote his essay to get into the colleges based on what his mother has shown him in life (that when life throws you a hard one, you can pick yourself up and do the best you can). It was an incredible essay, so I was happy because it made me feel that my posi-tive attitude through all this has taught him a valuable lesson.

Why I Started the Thyroid Cancer Foundation*

Joan Shey

(*Editors' comment:* The following article is printed in toto from "Cancer," Volume 91, Number 4, 15 February 2001, pages 623–624 with permission from the American Cancer Society.)

I have been a thyroid cancer survivor for 5 years now. From the onset, it has been a long, tough journey.

In 1993, I saw my gastroenterologist for an unrelated problem. During the examination he found a lump in my neck that he thought might be a thyroid nod-ule. Tests revealed it to be cold. I knew enough to know what that meant: CAN-CER. But after an ultrasound and a blind needle biopsy, two more physicians reas-sured me it was not cancer after all.

I started Synthroid® (Knoll Pharmaceutical Co., Mount Olive, NJ) and for two years had my thyroid watched. But I couldn't get rid of the worry. After many requests for another ultrasound, my doctor finally agreed. I wasn't on the table for long before I heard that the nodule was suspicious and that lymph nodes seemed to be involved. I left angry and scared. I was 43 years old, married with two children 13 and 17 years of age. I had cancer, and I didn't want to die.

A head and neck surgeon at a major cancer center performed a thyroidectomy and removed 39 lymph nodes in my neck. Each year since that surgery in 1995, I have received 6 weeks of treatment with ^{131}I for metastases that has persisted in my lungs. These 6 weeks each year are very difficult. Without thyroid hormone, I feel depressed, bloated, tired, and worried about the outcome of the tests to come.

My doctor saw how difficult it was for me to be hypothyroid. He told me that a drug soon would be available that would allow me to stay on Synthroid" during the dosimetry scans. So I waited for the day when Thyrogen® (Genzyme Therapeutics, Cambridge MA) would be available. At last, in 1998, it was here, and it has made a tremendous difference in the way I feel. But I still have the stress of the scanning and the low-iodine diet.

Not a day goes by that I don't think about my cancer. For the first two years, I knew no one else with thyroid cancer, and I felt very much alone with it. There were no support groups for patients with thyroid cancer, despite the fact that the disease has increased in incidence over the years. The American Cancer Society's publication, *Cancer Facts & Figures,* estimates that there will be 18,400 new cases of thyroid cancer in 2000.

I tried a general support group for cancer patients, but treatments were so different for each of us that it was of little comfort to me. The next time I saw my doctor, I expressed how alone I felt and said that other patients must feel the same way. At that moment in 1997, the Light of Life Foundation was born.

The missions of the Foundation are to educate, to provide support to patients with thyroid cancer, and to promote public awareness of the disease. Many people, then and now, do not know that thyroid cancer exists or even what the thyroid is. My hope is to change that, so others will not remain undiagnosed or go through treatment alone.

In the past three years, the Light of Life Foundation has made great strides. Oncologists who specialize in thyroid cancer offer their guidance and support as members of the Board of Directors. We hold monthly meetings of support groups, and we have created a video library of entertaining movies to help patients during isolation treatment. The foundation also provides isolation patients with baskets containing lemon candies to keep salivary glands working, and a book. The baskets also contain a glow-worm doll that shines in the dark, the symbol of our Foundation. Reactions to all this have been very moving. Patients feel less alone during this very trying time even when they are isolated and hypothyroid.

With the help of dieticians at my cancer center, I have created a low-iodine cookbook for patient use during periods of scans. Now available in several medical centers, it offers suggestions about how to cook and eat healthfully during this time. I had found the required low iodine diet very difficult, and I was afraid to eat something that might throw my scans off. Most patients take their diet very seriously; it is the one thing they can do to participate actively in getting the best treatment possible. Only a patient can understand this feeling.

An annual educational symposium is also part of our mission. We feel there are great benefits to bringing physicians, patient, and families together to discuss issues of mutual concern and to learn about advances in therapy. Another goal is to raise funds for research devoted to thyroid cancer. The Light of Life Foundation established a fund to help support the development of new methods of diagnosis and management. We will continue to help support this work.

The Light of Life Foundation Medical Advisory Board established an annual award to be given to the most outstanding physician in thyroid cancer research. In 1999, Ernest Mazzaferri, M.D., Professor of Medicine Emeritus at Ohio State University, Columbus, Ohio, received the award. Orlo Clark, M.D., Professor and Chief of Surgery at UCSF, was the year 2000 recipient.

With the continuing support of patients, doctors, hospitals, the Knoll Pharmaceutical, and Genzyme General company, we hope to reach many more patients and institutions in support of patients with thyroid cancer. The Light of Life Foundation has lit up many lives, especially my own. I am no longer alone, and this feeling brings me much comfort. I hope to be able to bring that comfort to others.

Metastatic Thyroid Cancer—Five Years Later

Diane Patching

It is five years since my husband, Wally, was told by his surgeon and endocrinologist that his hemithyroidectomy had indicated thyroid cancer and that the rest of the gland must be removed. This was a complete surprise since none of the previous testing including fine needle biopsy had been positive for cancer.

Both doctors tried to soften the blow by saying that this was the best kind of cancer to have, and after surgery, a little drink of radioiodine would get rid of it, and it wasn't fatal; he'd live to a ripe old age and probably die from a heart attack or stroke. Reassuring words to be sure, but unfortunately these learned gentleman were mistaken in this case. I know that doctors mean well when they tell patients that thyroid cancer is "good," but if only they would add "in most cases" to their little speeches it would go a long way to lessen the feelings of betrayal that occur when their words belie them, and it would also improve the trust necessary between doctors and patients as treatments continue.

However, Wally is no longer seen by these doctors. He was sent to London, Ontario, for his "little drink," and after a dozen or so not so little drinks of radioactive iodine, he still exhibits thyroid cancer and has never had a clean scan. Many people find this hard to believe, since this is so often publicized as the "good cancer," easily treated and cured. Fortunately for many this is true, but not for all.

Wally tolerated the therapy well initially, but as time passed, he found the hypothyroid period, which had to be endured before the treatments were given, increasingly harder to tolerate. At first he made a joke of it and said that he now knew what it felt like to be an old man as his bodily functions slowed down and he stumbled around. It also didn't help that for the last two weeks of being hypo he would be on a low iodine diet, which did not allow for many of the things he preferred to eat. Being hypo helped solve that problem because it suppressed his appetite, and the whole digestive process slowed down resulting in severe constipation. Memory loss was evident at these times, and words and names would be forgotten. I don't know what would have happened if Wally wasn't already retired; he couldn't have performed his job.

The last time Wally was hypo from thyroxine withdrawal was in 2000, and he ran into trouble when his kidneys began to fail and his calcium levels rose. His parathyroids were damaged during surgery, and he has had seesawing calcium levels ever since. Wally was unable to walk straight, and I was afraid of him using the stairs so we opened up the sofa bed and lived downstairs for several months. During this time Wally's vision was affected, and he was unable to focus enough to read the newspaper until late in the day. Of course, he was seen by the ophthalmologist, who blamed the hypo condition. A usually very active person, Wally was bedridden for weeks recovering, and even today he cannot believe how weak he felt, and how he was unable to walk properly.

What would happen next, we wondered. The radioactive iodine (RAI) therapy required a high TSH level obtained by stopping the thyroid hormone, and Wally was told he could not go through this again, his body was too vulnerable. Since this cancer had metastasized to his lungs and several skeletal areas, treatment was vital to help slow down the spread.

He had previously volunteered for a chemotherapy study using an infusion of 5-fluorouracil, epirubicin, and carboplatin as an adjuvant to the radioiodine treatment. It was hoped that there would be a synergistic effect that would kill the cancer cells, but they decided that it might cause perforation of Wally's stomach when he drank the radioiodine. They had believed the iodine was injected not ingested.

Dr. Al Driedger suggested that Wally's TSH be raised by a couple of injections of a new product he was using, a recombinant human thyrotropin, Thyrogen®. This sounded too good to be true. It was hard to comprehend that instead of six miserable weeks of thyroxine withdrawal, plus more weeks of waiting for the TSH to get down to a suitably suppressed level, a couple of injections of Thyrogen® would enable Wally's RAI therapy to continue. Hard to believe, but it worked, and no side effects were noted.

Thyrogen® was not approved for general use by Health Canada at this time but was available via the Special Access Program, and Wally took part in a compassionate use study. Because Thyrogen® acts quickly to raise and lower the TSH, the RAI treatments were planned at three month intervals. This was not always possible since his blood counts were affected, and he has had three rounds of external radiation for bone metastases. The important thing is that his treatments can be continued, thus buying more time. A cure is not expected due to the proliferation of bone involvement, so perhaps you may now understand my aversion to the "best cancer" label. Of course, things could always be much worse. Wally's cancer could be non-avid for iodine and radioiodine would have no effect, which limits treatment considerably.

We are grateful for all the assistance that Wally has received, particularly from Dr. Al Driedger in London who respects his patients and works tirelessly for them.

Another excellent source of support has come from Thry'vors, and I would recommend this group to anyone who has any form of thyroid cancer. There is a wealth of information in the files and many kind, considerate members who are so willing to offer the benefit of their experiences. There is also a more detailed tale of Wally's adventures in thyca land on the listserv there, and he wasn't known as Wally Murphy for nothing: Murphy's Law dogged him along this journey. It has not all been smooth sailing, but as mentioned previously, things could be worse, and we must dwell on the positive aspects of our life and make the most of them.

Wally is now 63 years old. He used to be a long distance runner until his knees told him otherwise, so he has tried to keep fit while on this thyroid cancer trip by using a rowing machine. When a sore shoulder prevented this, he got a treadmill. He retired at an early age, and our retirement project was raising Clydesdale horses, which gave us much satisfaction. We no longer do this but keep a couple of Clyde geldings around; it is hard to give them up, and we'll keep them as long as possible.

Wally and I have been married for more than 40 years and, as you may imagine, I want him around as long as possible, too! We both hope that the aggressive radioiodine treatments enabled by Thyrogen®, backed by external radiation, will provide more years together.

Diane and Wally Patching live on a farm near the village of Dundalk, Ontario. Diane is a member of Thry'vors and is the publicity chair for that organization. Diane is also a member of the Thyroid Foundation of Canada. Wally had external beam radiation to his neck and for a while he was unable to eat or drink, but he refused to go to a hospital so he could be properly hydrated. Wally is doing all right now and waiting for his next radioactive iodine treatment.

Psychological Issues Facing Cancer Survivors

Jeanne F. Allegra, Ph.D.

Editors' Introduction

(Editors' comment: Dr. Allegra writes from her experience as a cancer survivor and as a psychologist offering group and individual psychotherapy for patients

diagnosed with cancer. Dr. Allegra is a survivor of breast cancer, and although many of the specific aspects of chemotherapy and external beam radiation thera-py for breast cancer do not apply to most patients with thyroid carcinoma, she discusses many issues that do apply to patients with thyroid carcinoma. She shares many insights about denial, fear, guilt, loneliness, and depression, to name a few.)

I have reached my seventh year of cancer survivorship . . . seven years of good luck, hard work, and added insight into the dreaded ravages of the disease. When the diagnosis knocked on my door, I had two children ages 8 and 11, a husband of 17 years, a very ill father living with us, a mother who had died of breast cancer six years before and an active clinical psychology practice that never addressed any issues related to cancer. Before being diagnosed, I had resolved to change my diet, increase my level of physical activity, do only "healthy things," and never, never speak of the horrible disease that robbed me of my mother when she was a young, 70-year-old woman. Life had a different plan for me.

Throughout the times following the devastation of my diagnosis, the reality of the breast cancer and reconstructive surgeries, and the feared chemotherapy and its side effects, I felt alone and terribly vulnerable. My shining light had been a wonderful and insightful social worker who helped me put "humpty dumpty together again." It was about two years after the initial diagnosis that I began to focus my energies on helping other cancer patients deal with psychological effects of this disease. That, which had always scared me prior to my own diagnosis, has become my passion and life's work. It's as if the universe had had a plan for me all along. It took a cancer diagnosis of my own to slow me down enough to truly incorporate my understanding of the psychological issues facing others similarly diagnosed. The discussion that follows is based on five years of experience of doing group and individual psychotherapy with the newly diagnosed patient as well as with those who have been living with the disease for up to 10 years.

A common question asked in cancer support groups is "When can I consider myself a 'survivor'"? I often hear myself answering: "From the moment you receive your diagnosis and begin living with the reality of the disease." Other survivors begin to mark their "survivorship" at other points in their experience with the disease. It seems that everyone needs to mark time according to his or her own reality. Each stage of cancer survivorship seems to challenge the person diagnosed to come to grips with major life issues.

The Initial Diagnosis and Surgery

The overwhelming feeling and experience of those newly diagnosed with any type of cancer is that of shock and disbelief. It is very common for cancer survivors to recall very little of the times and discussions immediately following "the news."

They talk of "going blank" and needing to be accompanied on subsequent doctor visits by significant others who can think clearly for them.

Many survivors of the diagnosis have long associated death with the word cancer and may for the first time come face to face with their own mortality. "I had never thought about a time that I would not be here. What would it feel like not to be alive?" are common reactions to the initial diagnosis. Depending on the prognosis given to the patient, the intensity of this reaction will be affected. This primary reaction also seems dependent on other factors: how many others does the patient know with a similar diagnosis/prognosis and what have the outcomes been for these others.

As the reality of the diagnosis seeps into consciousness, shock can become depression. There can be the feeling of lifelessness, lethargy, sleeplessness or extreme sleepiness, and a generalized experience of depression. Questions often arise: "Why me"? "What did I do to deserve this"? "Am I being punished for something I did or failed to do"? "Did I eat the wrong foods"? "Did I smoke too many cigarettes"? "Did I live in the wrong places"? "Did I wait too long to have children"? "Should I have nursed my kids"? "Should I have nursed my children longer"? The questions are endless and represent self-doubt and guilt about the way one has chosen to conduct his or her life.

In actuality there are few known causes for a variety of cancer types. When individuals diagnosed with this disease ask the above questions they are really asking what they could have done differently in order to control their current state of affairs. Most people have come to believe that they are masters of their own destiny. And when they are confronted by circumstances that do not lend themselves to simple cause-and-effect explanations, they are confronted (perhaps for the first time in life) with their true lack of control in this universe of endless possibilities and seemingly random events.

Surprisingly, some people find themselves humiliated and embarrassed. They experience the fear that others will find them pitiable. They fear that the others, whom they considered to be among their friends, will experience a kind of fear and revulsion at their diagnosis and will choose not to associate with them any longer. Unfortunately, this fear of rejection by those once considered to be good friends is real and sometimes actually occurs.

If the diagnosis is followed by surgery, the patient experiences the normal fear associated with any surgical procedure, heightened by the sense of the gravity of the situation. The potential surgical patient often spends sleepless nights asking questions like: "Will they find that the cancer has spread further than they first thought"? "How will I react to the drugs given to me during surgery"? "Will I survive the surgical procedure"? "How will I feel after I wake up"? "What will my recovery be like"? "Who will take care of my family if I don't make it"? The preparation and signing of living wills, etc., at this time often relieve the patient's fear that he or she is unprepared.

The attending physician can be extremely helpful prior to surgery, addressing the patient's pre-surgical questions and concerns. In the event that the patient is unable to put his or her fears into words, it is helpful if the doctor can anticipate the questions. Often patients are reluctant to ask the questions that wear on their minds, with the belief that they shouldn't take their busy doctors' time with foolish concerns. Doctors would be wise to anticipate the concerns because a more knowledgeable surgical patient is usually one who recovers more swiftly.

Post-surgical treatments

Cancer patients often receive post-surgical treatments to halt the spread of their disease. Chemotherapy and/or radiation treatments bring their own set of psychological concerns to the affected person. People in treatment find that they are in conflict between "doing whatever the experts recommend to prolong my life" and dealing with the sometimes devastating effects of the drugs and/or radiation. Throughout the chemotherapy experience, men and women must deal with the physical side effects of the drugs they are receiving. However, the present medical community can provide "an action for every reaction." In other words, there is almost always some treatment to counteract the bad effects of the drugs. The psychological side effects of being on chemotherapy are not always as easily managed.

For almost all women and some men who are told that chemotherapy will be necessary, the concern about hair loss emerges almost immediately. Few are consoled by the information that the hair loss is only temporary. Grieving the loss of hair as one might grieve the loss of any significant part of oneself is critical and leads to acceptance and the ability to deal effectively with this new challenge.

When the patient's only response is to deny that future hair loss is a possibility, he or she can set himself or herself up for a future crushing blow. This loss is particularly poignant for women because they feel that up to this time they could "hide" the fact that they have been cancer patients. One woman in denial about this possibility related that she was sure nothing would happen to her long, thick hair. Soon after her first chemo treatment, she awoke to find large clumps of her hair scattered on her pillow. Another woman, similarly rejecting the possibility of this loss, was sitting beneath a kitchen ceiling fan after having received two chemotherapy treatments. Without warning, long strands of hair flew off her head and were strewn throughout the kitchen.

Many women describe this loss of hair as being robbed of their last vestige of femininity. It strips them naked, while announcing to the world that they have the most dreaded of diseases. Perhaps it's not only that they cannot hide their diagnosis from the rest of the world, but also that they must finally face the diagnosis themselves. One can only imagine the emptiness and, for some, horror when look-ing into a mirror and not recognizing the bald-headed face peering back, sans eye-brows and eyelashes.

During this difficult psychological period, men and women alike find comfort in hats and caps. Women often choose scarves, turbans, and wigs for a time. Some brave souls come to grips with this loss and have so adjusted their self-image they are no longer able to tolerate the discomfort of hats and wigs and decide to face the world with a bald head. This bald, bold move is not for the faint-of-heart. This bare statement to the world is often met with stares, knowing glances, and expressions of pity.

(Editors' comment: patients who have well-differentiated thyroid cancer and are treated with radiation from radioiodine do not lose their hair. Interestingly, some of these patients have stated that they are frequently perceived by others as not being sick because they have not lost their hair. This is despite the patient experi-encing extreme fatigue or other symptoms due to their hypothyroidism, which is associated with testing and treatment.)

Loneliness is another difficult issue that many patients face. They often relate that everyone rallied around at the time of the initial surgery but disappeared when chemotherapy started. That period of time, however, is the easy part in comparison to that which follows. Many times a working adult chooses to suspend his or her professional commitments until "chemo is over." Others, who decide to continue to work, are often happy that they have work "as a distraction from my disease," especially if their organization has granted them a liberal leave policy. Working allows a temporary return to normalcy. As long as the patient is able to perform adequately at work, he or she feels able to forget that cancer has such a prominent hold on life. Despite the patient's decision to work or not work, the experience that family members and friends have scattered and are not as supportive as before seems relatively consistent from person to person.

Radiation, though often described by patients as physically easier to tolerate, presents its own set of challenges. People receiving radiation may not feel differ-ently soon after treatments begin and often experience anxiety about whether any-thing is really happening and whether the growth of their cancer can be stopped by such a benign treatment. Patients, receiving radiation only and not chemotherapy, often question the wisdom of their physician in selecting this treatment. Then, on the other hand, there are those recipients of radiation who fear its somewhat mys-terious effects on their bodies more than the effects of chemotherapy. *(Editors' comment: patients who are treated with radioiodine in the hospital may have the additional challenge of dealing with the isolation and radiation safety procedures associated with radioiodine treatment. See chapter 17.)*

While in general more easily tolerated by cancer patients, radiation treatments take their toll in other ways. External radiation therapy is often offered daily for an extended period of time. Weariness with the treatments and the rigid schedule in which they are offered are among common complaints. One woman continued to work a regular schedule, adjusted to accommodate chemotherapy appointments. However, when she began her radiation, she thought it was time to take a break and did not work for about six weeks. After reevaluating her commitment to the work she had done for a quarter century, she decided to retire and invest her time in pursuits that really interested her. Although she may eventually have decided to do something similar even if she had not had her experience with cancer and cancer treatments, her new appreciation for the meaning of life helped her order her priorities in such a way that this decision was a natural outcome.

The End of Formal Treatments

When the prescribed treatments have come to an end, one might predict that the patient would experience much jubilation and celebration. In fact, experiences quite to the contrary seem to exist. One patient put her uneasiness following the end of treatments into words: "I am so uncomfortable at a time when I expected to be so happy. I feel that I have spent so much time hoping that the end of treatments would come so that I could go back to being normal. Now I feel as if a tether on a balloon has been cut. I'm the balloon, and I'm drifting aimlessly. Something will happen to bring the balloon crashing down to earth, and I'm afraid it won't be a pretty sight." Surprisingly, as long as a patient is in treatment, he or she is reassured that something is being done to keep the cancer in check. When there are no more scheduled chemotherapy or radiation treatments, many experience a depression, an unexpected "let down." One man described the experience saying, "As long as I had a scheduled chemotherapy appointment on my calendar, I knew that I was doing something that would positively affect my future health. Once those ended, I felt as if I had been dropped into a deep, dark hole, never to be found again." Such feelings are predictable and will lessen if the patient continues on a healthy path.

Cancer survivors often report that the medical community seems to view them differently after a cancer diagnosis and treatment. Once a cancer survivor, always a cancer survivor. Normal aches and pains lose their "normalcy." All bumps and bruises are viewed as a potential cancer awaiting screening. One five-year survivor related the following experience: "I began to develop back pain. I had gone to the chiropractor for a number of months without much change. He recommended that I see a medical doctor specializing in spinal problems, which I did. He ordered an MRI of my spine. There was a shadow on the picture, and he feared that it could be a signal of the return of the cancer. Then a bone scan was ordered and done. After many anxious days, accompanied by a belief that the cancer had metastasized to my back, the bone scan returned a negative result." After almost two years and many doctor visits, this man still has great back discomfort and is no further along in the diagnosis of the problem.

Many view the experience with cancer as a totally life-altering event. If given a very favorable prognosis, patients are struck by the real possibility that they may actually survive. It is then that they begin to reassess their life's choices and reevaluate marital status, partners, their role as parents and career choices. Major changes often follow and represent new commitments to different, and perhaps more fulfilling, lives.

Managing Life after a Cancer Diagnosis

A sage cancer survivor put it this way, "No matter how you cut it, life after a cancer diagnosis is never the same. It can actually be better in some ways, but it is never the same." So, what are survivors to do?

Individual insight therapy can be helpful, especially if the therapist is no stranger to the "cancer experience" and is able to relate to the stages of acceptance that the patient endures. A support group may even prove more beneficial to the patient, family members and caregivers. It is only in support groups that patients find others who are struggling with the same issues. This type of support is helpful because it demystifies many of the cancer patient's struggles and experiences. Meeting and listening to people with similar diagnoses is very validating. It also frees the affected person to admit concerns among those who may truly understand because they have been there.

Whatever the vehicle—a caring nurse, a special hospital-based social worker, a clergy person, an individual therapist, a support group—one thing is clear: the cancer survivor needs an outlet for his or her concerns.

Psychiatric Considerations for the Patient with Thyroid Cancer

Stephen Peterson, M.D.

When a person learns he or she has cancer of the thyroid gland, "something bad has happened" and there are fears that more bad things might follow. When something bad has happened or is about to, Dr. Charles Brenner says that this often results in depression, which is our emotional reaction to bad events, and anxiety, which is our feeling when we fear that bad things are about to happen. Depression worsens when we feel that we are hopeless and helpless to do anything about it, that it's not going to get any better. Anxiety is intensified, depending on the degree of danger and how soon in time it might occur. Hence, it isn't hard to understand that someone diagnosed with thyroid cancer might become depressed and anxious.

But even before a person learns of the problem, he or she may become anxious or depressed. This is because the thyroid gland secretes a hormone that regulates metabolic rate in the body. Too much hormone can produce anxiety, irritability, sleeplessness, loss of temper and confusion. Too little can produce weakness, fatigue, feeling blue, down in the dumps with little energy. In other words, thyroid is like the carburetor determining how fast we metabolize fuel. It directly impacts brain function.

Disorders of the thyroid gland, especially cancer, pack a double effect because both the body and the mind are directly influenced. For this reason, people with thyroid cancer are especially vulnerable to mixed states of depression, anxiety, and various combinations of these.

When someone has anxiety and/or depression, there are, fortunately, two effective routes to deal with the problem, physical and psychological. In the case of thyroid hormone abnormalities, both of these approaches are essential. Normalization of the thyroid hormone level in the body is essential. One must have optimal thyroid hormone available to foster appropriate coping and function. Therefore, the first step must be to work with your medical doctor to assure that your thyroid hormone levels are appropriate, and this usually means receiving replacement hormone.

Once a more normal thyroid function is achieved, depression and anxiety may still be present. There are many reasons someone develops anxiety and/or depression; after all, these are normal reactions to life in the course of everyday routine. Clearly a series of mishaps can lead to either problem. And the onset of a serious medical illness can bring on a sustained and intense mood disorder. Indeed, in seniors, the biggest reason for more severe depression or anxiety is the onset of a new physical illness and all that it implies for the person. Lesser problems result in milder depression or anxiety. There are two approaches to treat these disorders of mood—learning and medication. The learning referred to is a specialized type called psychotherapy. Such therapy enables the person to work on his or her reactions to loss such as when we perceive a loss of health. This technique also helps us identify and reduce stressors and put our feelings into perspective so that sadness and fear can be sorted out and become manageable. Imaging studies of the brain confirm that psychotherapy has direct effects on improving function in those areas of the brain directly responsible for depression and anxiety. We now know that psychotherapy is the best treatment we have for emotional illness, especially in the hands of a competent psychotherapist.

But also, the physician must consider medicine for some patients as a way to improve mood disorders. In the past 40 years, psychotropic medications have evolved that directly improve mood and reduce anxiety as a function of their effects on neurotransmitters. These medications can help even the most severely depressed and anxious person and have enormously improved the quality of life for many. It's no surprise that one of the biggest drugs in America is the antidepressant, Prozac®.

Many antidepressants and anti-anxiety medicines have been developed since the 1960's, and second and third generation agents may be even more effective with fewer side effects. More studies need to be done to prove these things, but clinical trials already prove that the combination of antidepressants and psychotherapy boosts the effectiveness of each treatment alone beyond monotherapy from 60 to 85 percent. The decision regarding appropriate treatment, including the possibility of medicines, should be based on a thorough assessment by a qualified health professional who is experienced in this area.

Since the ancient Greeks we have known the therapeutic effects of a caring support group and the value of the doctor-patient relationship. The therapeutic interactions at the Temple of Asclepius, the ancient Greek god of medicine, involved ritual purification by telling one's dreams and discussing life's stresses. The ancient Romans noted therapeutic effects of seizures on the depressed. In the last century, the birth of psychoanalysis and the discovery of psychotropic drugs have revolutionized treatment of the medically ill. Increasingly, studies show how careful attention to our emotional health and well-being is enabling those with physical illnesses to cope better and get along.

There is much hope when it comes to the diagnosis of thyroid cancer, especially nowadays when a good outcome is highly likely. But you may be feeling overwhelmed, pessimistic or have other signs typical of depression or anxiety such as a loss of interest in ordinary life events, feelings of fear or sadness, tendency to dwell on problems and worry, less energy, increased pain and preoccupation with one's body. If you are having trouble coping, talk with your doctor. Reassurance can go a long way. But if this is not enough, or if you are still troubled, then it would be important to see a psychologist or psychiatrist. Effective help is available for you and can be enormously beneficial for the troubled person with the diagnosis of thyroid cancer. You'll be glad you did.

CHAPTER 27

Participation in Research Studies

Shari Thomas, C.R.C.

So you have been asked to participate in a research study?

The reasons people choose to participate in clinical research are as varied as there are research studies. Also known as clinical trials, research studies are ongoing for almost every type of cancer. Trials may involve chemotherapy, radiation therapy, surgery, new experimental therapies or any combination of these treatments.

Clinical research trials are extremely important in expanding treatment options in all cancers. Most of the treatments that are available today are due to the participation of other cancer patients in clinical research trials. The research field is constantly trying to identify better treatments to cure cancer.

Why should I volunteer?

By taking part in a clinical trial, you can play a more active role in your own health care. You can gain access to new treatments before they are available, help others by contributing to medical research or try a new treatment that may or may not be better than those already available. You also can contribute to a better understanding of how the treatment works in people of different ethnic backgrounds and genders.

Where do the ideas for trials come from?

Ideas for clinical trials usually come from researchers. After researchers test new therapies or procedures in the laboratory and in animal studies, they move treatments with the most promising laboratory results into clinical trials.

During a trial, researchers gain more and more information about a new treatment, its risks and how well it may or may not work. Carefully conducted clinical trials are the fastest and safest way to find treatments that work in people.

What is a protocol?

A protocol is a study plan with a set of rules. The plan is carefully designed to safeguard the health of the participants as well as answer specific research questions. A protocol describes the types of people who may participate in the trial, the schedule of tests, procedures, medications, and dosages, and the length of the study. While in a clinical trial, participants following a protocol are seen regularly by the research team to monitor their health and to determine the safety and effectiveness of their treatment.

Who pays for clinical research?

Clinical trials are sponsored or funded by a variety of organizations or individuals such as physicians, medical institutions, foundations, voluntary groups, pharmaceutical companies, and federal agencies. The research sponsor "hires" physicians, who may work in a wide variety of health-care settings, to conduct the trials. Physicians typically are paid on a per-patient basis. The medical care often is provided free to the patient.

What should I consider before participating in a trial?

Choosing to participate in a clinical trial is an important personal decision. It often is helpful to talk to your physician, family members or friends about deciding to join a trial. You also should seek to understand the credentials and experience of the individuals and the facility involved in conducting the study. After identifying some trial options, the next step is to contact the study research team and ask questions about specific trials. Questions to ask should include:

- How long will the trial last?
- Where is the trial being conducted?
- What treatments will be used and how?
- What is the main purpose of the trial?
- How will patient safety be monitored?
- Are there any risks involved?
- What are the possible benefits?
- What are the alternative treatments besides the one being tested in the trial?
- Who is sponsoring the trial?
- Do I have to pay for any part of the trial?
- What happens if I am harmed by the trial?

How do I know if I can participate in a clinical trial?

All clinical trials have guidelines about who can participate. The criteria that allow someone to participate in a clinical trial are called "inclusion criteria," and those that disallow someone from participating are called "exclusion criteria."

These criteria are based on such factors as age, gender, the type and stage of a disease, previous treatment history, and other medical conditions.

Before joining a clinical trial:
- You must have the disease that is being studied or be at risk for it.
- You must be able to take the treatment that is being studied, if treatment is part of the study.
- You must be able to follow the study rules.
- Before you enter the study, members of the medical team will make sure that you can participate. They may ask you questions about your health, give you a physical exam, and draw some blood or obtain other specimens for lab tests.

Study visits

After you enter a trial, you will need to attend regularly scheduled study visits. If you are taking a drug as part of the study, you will be checked by a doctor or treatment research team member for side effects and signs of whether the drug is working. Studies that do not involve drugs also typically require regular visits. Some studies can last several years. However, you may stop at any time if you decide that you no longer want to take a study treatment or take part in other study activities. Just be sure that your doctor knows about your decision. Your doctor will stop your study treatment if it is not working for you or if it causes harmful side effects. However, even if you stop study treatment or take part in other study activities, you still will be in the study, and you will be asked to continue your clinic visits until the study ends. Of course you are free to withdraw from the study at any time. If you get sick from taking a study drug, the research team will make sure that you get any necessary treatment.

Patient information

Patients' rights and safety are protected in two important ways during clinical trials. First, any physician awarded a research grant by a company must obtain approval to conduct the study from an Institutional Review Board. The review board, which usually is composed of physicians and lay people, is charged with examining the study's protocol to ensure that patients' rights are protected and that the study does not present an unnecessary risk to the patients. Second, anyone participating in a clinical trial in the United States is required to sign an informed consent form. The informed consent is the process of learning the key facts about a clinical trial before deciding whether to participate. It is a continuing process throughout the study. The study doctors and research team must tell you everything that would affect whether you would want to be in or continue in the trial. The form details the nature of the study, the risks involved, and what may happen to a patient in the study. The informed consent tells patients that they have a right to leave the study at any time. Before you enter a trial, the research staff must have your agreement in writing that you have been given this information and that you are willing to take part in the study.

Will I continue to work with my primary health care provider while in a trial?

Yes. Most clinical trials provide short-term treatments related to a designated illness or condition but do not provide extended or complete primary health care.

By having the health care provider work with the research team, you can ensure that other medications or treatments will not conflict with the clinical trial.

What are side effects and adverse reactions?

Side effects are any undesired actions or effects of a drug or treatment. Negative or adverse effects may include headache, nausea, hair loss, skin irritation or other physical problems. Experimental treatments must be evaluated for both immediate and long-term side effects.

Are there other risks?

Yes.
- There may be unpleasant, serious or even life-threatening side effects to treatment.
- The treatment may not be effective for the participant.
- The protocol may require more of your time and attention than a non-protocol treatment, including trips to the study site, more treatments, hospital stays or complex dosage requirements.

Can I leave a clinical trial after it has begun?

Yes. A participant can leave a clinical trial at any time. When withdrawing from the trial, you should let the research team know about it and the reasons for leaving the study.

Frequently Asked Questions

About Well-Differentiated Thyroid Cancer

What is radiation?

Radiation is energy that moves from one location to another. Sunshine, microwaves, gamma rays, and X-rays are all examples of radiation. Some types of radiation deposit energy in material and produce heat (sunshine and microwave). Other types of radiation remove electrons from material and produce direct chemical changes (gamma and X-rays). Radiation is in every part of our lives.

On a more scientific level, radiation is energy emitted as electromagnetic waves such as those of visible light, infrared rays, ultraviolet rays, X-rays, gamma rays or alpha, beta, and other streams of particles. Sources of radiation include natural, or "background," radiation such as cosmic rays from outer space, naturally occurring substances found on Earth and man-made substances such as some X-rays.

Since light, radio waves, TV waves, ultrasound, etc., are all forms of radiation, why is the hazard from these forms of radiation so much less than that from radioactive sources?

The answer largely has to do with the amount of energy carried by the waves or particles. This in turn affects the size of the objects that the radiation tends to interact with. In the case of the beta particles and gamma rays released by ^{131}I, the interactions are often with the electrons of individual atoms. As a consequence, electrons are knocked out of the atom, a process referred to as ionization. In some cases these are the very electrons that are responsible for holding atoms together in a molecule or molecules in a complex structure such as DNA. It is this type of damage to critical components on a cellular level from ionizing radiation that can often lead to the death of that cell.

What is radioactivity?

Radioactivity is the characteristic of a material to emit particles or waves. These waves are called ionizing radiation. Gamma rays produced from radioiodine are an example of ionizing radiation.

What is radioiodine?

Iodine is a naturally occurring element like oxygen, nitrogen, and carbon. Your thyroid gland needs iodine to make thyroid hormone. Because of this, many foods such as bread and table salt are fortified with iodine. Radioiodine is identical to iodine except that the radioiodine is radioactive.

Are there different types of radioiodine?

There are different types of radioiodine, and they are called isotopes of iodine. The number next to the "I," the abbreviation for iodine, represents the specific isotope, such as ^{123}I and ^{131}I. Both ^{123}I and ^{131}I are used for imaging, but presently only ^{131}I is used for therapies.

How do these radioisotopes of radioiodine allow you to image (see) my thyroid tissue?

After the oral administration of the radioiodine, the radioiodine is absorbed through your gastrointestinal tract into your blood. Because thyroid tissue needs iodine to make its thyroid hormone, the thyroid tissue will pull the iodine out of the blood and into the thyroid cell. This is called "uptake" of radioiodine. Once the radioiodine is in the thyroid cell, it emits a small amount energy. Although our eye cannot see it, a special camera can "see" this energy and obtain an image of your functioning thyroid tissue.

Why does my physician want a radioiodine whole body scan?

Radioiodine whole body scanning is performed to help image both normal and abnormal thyroid tissue in patients who have well-differentiated thyroid cancer. It is important for your physician in planning your treatment to be aware of any normal thyroid tissue remaining in your thyroid bed or whether your thyroid cancer has spread (metastasized).

Who performs radioiodine whole body scanning?

Radioiodine whole body scanning is widely available in most hospitals and outpatient nuclear medicine and radiology facilities.

How often do I need a scan?

Your endocrinologist will evaluate you to determine how often you need a scan. But in general, individuals who have a small, single, initial site of well-localized cancer may have just one scan. Other patients may have scans performed from six months to one year after the first scan, and still other patients may have a follow-up scan only if their blood thyroglobulin level increases.

How does radioiodine allow you to eliminate thyroid tissue?

Once the radioiodine is in the thyroid cell (see above question), it delivers energy to the thyroid tissue. This energy (radiation) destroys the cells.

What is ^{131}I radioiodine ablation or treatment?

^{131}I radioiodine ablation or treatment is therapy in which radioactive iodine is administered to ablate normal thyroid tissue or well-differentiated thyroid cancer by irradiating that tissue.

What is the difference between ablation and treatment?

Many physicians use "ablation" and "treatment" interchangeably. Other physicians use "ablation" to mean the administration of radioiodine to eliminate any normal thyroid tissue remaining in the neck after initial surgery and "treatment" to mean the administration of radioiodine for the elimination of metastatic disease in the neck or elsewhere. Although we believe the terms can be interchanged, we will use the above definitions to avoid confusion.

Why do I have any thyroid tissue left after my surgery? I thought my surgeon took it all out.

Although your surgeon removed your thyroid gland, most surgeons leave behind small amounts of thyroid tissue to minimize any damage to the nerve that controls your voice box. This nerve is called the recurrent laryngeal nerve and runs next to, in or behind your thyroid tissue. Your surgeon may also leave some thyroid tissue behind to make sure some or all of your parathyroid glands remain in tact. These glands control your body's calcium levels and are usually located behind your thyroid tissue.

Why do I need an initial radioiodine ablation when my physician believes he or she has removed all of my thyroid carcinoma?

Most physicians will recommend that patients with well-differentiated thyroid cancer undergo at least one ablation therapy with radioiodine. Research suggests that the combination of surgery, radioiodine ablation, and thyroid hormone replacement can reduce the chances of your thyroid carcinoma recurring. There are some situations, however, in which your physicians may not recommend an initial ablation with radioiodine. A brief overview of these special situations is discussed below and in chapter 4 and 6.

What happens to me if all of my thyroid tissue is destroyed?

The goal is to destroy all of your thyroid tissue, but you will be fine. Your physician will place you on thyroid hormone medication, which you will take by mouth. This medication is identical to the hormone that your thyroid produced and will meet your body's needs.

What are the criteria for not receiving an ablation with radioiodine?

Radioiodine ablation may not be recommended depending on several factors. These include the size of the original thyroid cancer, the number of sites involved, any involvement of the borders of the thyroid or adjacent tissues, and a lack of evidence that the cancer has spread. Your physician will review all of your medical information to decide whether radioiodine ablation is necessary for you.

If radioiodine ablation is recommended, what is its benefit?

Radioiodine ablation has three goals.

First, and for most patients with well-differentiated thyroid cancer, it will reduce the chance of the thyroid cancer recurring. Although the exact reason is not known, one possibility is that the radioiodine helps kill any thyroid cancer cells that may be present in the remaining thyroid tissue.

Second, destroying the remaining thyroid tissue will improve the ability of the radioiodine whole body scan and thyroglobulin blood levels to monitor you for evidence of any recurrence of the cancer. If any healthy thyroid tissue remains in your neck, that tissue may take up a significant amount of the radioiodine, making it difficult to detect any cancerous tissue. If the healthy thyroid tissue is destroyed, a radioiodine whole body scan will be better able to detect any spread of thyroid cancer in this area. Likewise, destroying any remaining thyroid tissue also will improve the ability of your thyroglobulin blood levels to monitor you for metastasis. Normal thyroid tissue also produces thyroglobulin, and thus in the presence of normal thyroid tissue, changes in your blood thyroglobulin levels are not as reliable for indicating spread of your cancer. The use of the thyroglobulin blood test as a marker for cancer has been discussed in more detail in chapter 2. Thus, the ablation of any remaining normal thyroid tissue improves the ability of future radioiodine whole body scans and thyroglobulin blood tests to detect spread of your cancer.

The third goal is to enhance the effectiveness of future radioiodine treatments, if needed, by allowing you to receive a higher dosage of radioiodine, which has the potential to deliver more radiation to your cancer cells. Any significant normal thyroid tissue remaining may restrict the amount of radioiodine that could be used for your treatments.

If I had only one lobe of my thyroid removed, do I need to have the other lobe removed also? If so, should it be removed by surgery or radioiodine treatment?

The decision to remove the other lobe will depend on many factors: the size of your original primary tumor, any spread into the walls of the thyroid, adjacent tissue or lymph nodes, your age, and your health. Your physician will advise you based on your clinical situation.

Surgery or radioiodine treatment may be used if the decision is to remove the other lobe. The advantages and disadvantages of each are controversial. Supporters of surgery argue that there is a chance of cancer being present in the remaining lobe and that removal of this lobe improves the prognosis. Supporters of radioiodine treatment argue that surgery does not affect the overall prognosis and that the risks of surgery should be avoided whenever possible.

Physicians who recommend radioiodine treatment also say that the dosage of radioiodine needed to destroy the remaining lobe is usually smaller than that needed to destroy any small area of thyroid tissue left after removal of that lobe. While we prefer surgery to radioiodine, you should discuss these options with your physicians.

What dosage of radioiodine should I receive for ablation?

The dosage for your first-time ablation will typically range from 29 mCi up to 150 mCi. You should speak with your endocrinologist, nuclear medicine physician or nuclear radiologist if your planned treatment dosage is not in this range.

In deciding what dosage between 29 and 150 mCi should be administered, there are many factors to consider and many advantages and disadvantages that must be weighed. These factors include federal or state radiation regulations, insurance coverage, your physicians' treatment objectives and your clinical situation. Patients who have a small, single site of cancer and no evidence of spread may not even receive a radioiodine treatment. Patients who have a large amount of thyroid tissue that takes up a lot radioiodine may—paradoxically—receive smaller dosages. Patients and physicians who wish to avoid hospitalization may also use lower dosages while those who want to reduce the chance of a repeat ablation or treatment may use higher dosages. Some facilities may use dosimetry (see chapter 15) to determine the dosage, which will deliver an estimated, pre-determined amount of radiation exposure to the tissue.

What is an mCi?

An mCi is an abbreviation for millicuries, which is a unit of measurement of radioactivity. Typically 1 to 10 mCi's of radioiodine are used for scanning. Thirty to 150 mCi's of radioiodine are used for your initial ablation. High amounts of radioiodine may be used for subsequent treatments.

What is a Becquerel?

"What is a Becquerel?"
One Becquerel equals one nuclear disintegration per second. f radioactivity, and it is typi-
1 mCi equals 37 MBq. A megabecquerel (MBq) is 1,000,000)0 Bq, and a gigabecquerel
Becquerels (Bq), and a gigabecquerel (GBq) is 1000 es.
megabecquerels (MBq).

In what ways should I prepare before arriving for my scan or treatment?

The preparation prior to your scan or possible ablation is very important. Please see chapters 14 and 17 for a detailed discussion.

Why am I admitted to the hospital?

You are not admitted to the hospital because the radiation will make you ill. You are admitted to the hospital to minimize any radiation exposure to other people. The treatment you will receive is radioactive, and you will be radioactive for a short period of time. Although this radioactivity is beneficial to you, there is no benefit to other people. You are admitted to the hospital to minimize their exposure.

Once your radiation decreases to an acceptable level, you will be discharged. Radiation precautions to follow at home are discussed in chapters 14 and 20.

Will I be admitted to the hospital for my treatment?

This will depend on the dose of radioiodine for your treatment and the regulations of your hospital. Your nuclear medicine physician, endocrinologist or radiation safety technologist will inform you regarding whether you must be admitted to the hospital.

If I have to be admitted to the hospital, what physician or endocrinologist will admit me?

This will depend again on the regulations of your hospital as well as the arrangements between your endocrinologist, nuclear medicine physician or nuclear radiologist.

How is the radioiodine administered?

The radioiodine comes in either liquid or capsule form. One dose of liquid iodine is typically 2 to 6 tablespoons. This is followed by water. If you prefer one form to another, please let your nuclear medicine physician know before treatment. Usually, the institution can obtain the form you desire; however, some institutions have contracts only for one form or the other. The liquid radioiodine has a slight "tin-can-like" taste. This is the same taste as the water that campers drink after purifying it with iodine tablets.

If I am admitted to the hospital, am I allowed visitors?

You will not be allowed visitors in your room. Depending on the regulations of the institutions, you may be allowed adult visitors, who must remain behind a pre-established line. The duration of visiting is usually limited.

What items should I bring to the hospital?

You should bring selected items and leave most other items at home. These are discussed in chapter 14.

What can I expect about my hospital room?

Typically, your room will be a standard private hospital room with a private bath, television, telephone, and closets. Your room will be specially prepared. Because the radioiodine comes out in your saliva, perspiration, and urine, and because your physician wishes to control the spread of that radioactivity to other individuals, the floor and other furniture items will be covered such as with plastic or paper. The doorknobs, telephone, and other items may also be covered in plastic like Saran wrap. All of this helps prevent the spread of any radioactivity and should expedite the cleaning of your room after you are released. However, again the items covered will depend on the regulations of your hospital.

Will I be in a private room? Yes.
Will I have a telephone? Yes.
Will I have a TV? Yes.

If I am on a low iodine diet, when will I be able to go back on my regular diet?

Your physician will instruct you regarding when you may re-initiate your regular diet. This may be as early as the second meal in the hospital or upon discharge.

What should I do about my medications?

You should follow the instructions of your admitting physician. Some physicians recommend that you bring a two- to three-day supply of all medications except thyroid hormone, and then administer the medicines to yourself. This helps minimize the nursing staff from entering your room. However, some hospitals' procedures and regulations prohibit this. Again, your physician will instruct you.

Should I take my medications the morning I am admitted?

Yes. But do not take any thyroid hormone medication.

What radiation safety precautions do I need to follow after my dose for my scan?

The radiation safety precautions will depend on how much radioiodine you receive, whether it is administered in the hospital, and with whom you live and come in contact. Sample radiation safety instructions are presented in chapters 14, 17, and 20. Your endocrinologist, nuclear medicine physician, nuclear radiologist or radiation safety technologist will review the radiation safety precautions that apply to you.

Why do I have to follow radiation safety precautions?

The radiation that you will receive is given to help treat your thyroid cancer. However, the radiation you receive does not help anyone else. The measures taken to minimize the radiation exposure to those you live, work or socialize with are called "Radiation Safety Precautions." The radiation safety precautions will depend on the amount of radioiodine you receive, the type of people you come in contact with, and the policies and regulations of the institution where you are being treated.

What is Health Physics?

Health Physics is the study of certain aspects of physics that apply to your health. This may include many areas of physics, however; in regard to your thyroid cancer, this involved the physics of radiation as it affects your health. Some larger institutions have a dedicated department for this, and this department may be called the Department of Health Physics.

How much radioiodine will I receive?

Doses are determined on an individual basis. However, if this is your first treatment, the standard dose is typically 30 to 150 mCi.

Am I required to take laxatives?

This will depend upon the amount of your dose and your policy and procedure of your physician. However, unless there is a reason not to administer a laxative, we encourage you to take a laxative or stool softener to help ensure regular bowel movements. The radioactivity accumulates in the stool, and it is beneficial to have regular stools to minimize radiation exposure to your gastrointestinal tract.

Will I be awakened during the night?

Whether you are admitted to the hospital or are allowed to go directly home, we encourage you to wake up several times and preferably multiple times during the night. This will allow you to empty your urinary bladder, to drink fluids, and to eat hard candies, which make you salivate. Emptying your urinary bladder will reduce radiation exposure to your bladder. Drinking fluids will help hydrate you to clear the radioiodine from your body, thereby reducing the total radiation exposure to your whole body. Eating a candy will make you salivate, and this will help reduce the radiation exposure to your salivary glands. We also encourage you to massage your salivary glands. This may help reduce the radioiodine in your salivary glands, which then also helps reduce the radiation exposure to your salivary glands. Further information and instructions are in chapter 18.

Are there special precautions for diabetics?

Yes. If you are diabetic, you should notify your physician for additional instructions.

If I am admitted to the hospital, how long will I be in the hospital?

This will depend on how much radioiodine you receive and on the policies and regulations of the facility where you are being treated. This can also depend on what country you are in. If you are receiving an initial treatment in the hospital, typically you should anticipate being in the hospital for at least one night. If for some reason it takes longer to clear the radioiodine from your body, you may be required to stay additional nights.

How will I know when I can be discharged?

Your physician, nuclear medicine technologist or a radiation safety technologist will monitor you with a special meter shortly after administration of the radioiodine and then again one or several times that day and the next day. When you have cleared the required amount of radioactivity, you will be released.

Does radiation cause cancer?

It is important to know the type of radiation and the amount of radiation before one can estimate whether there is any significant increased risk of cancer. In the dose range for your initial ablation (treatment), there is no significant increased risk of developing another cancer. This does not mean that you cannot develop another cancer, but it means the radiation will probably not increase your risk of developing another cancer.

What are the short-term side effects of radioiodine?

In regard to your initial dose of radioiodine, most patients will have no side effects. However, some patients do have short-term side effects. These include pain in the thyroid area, pain in the salivary glands, nausea, and occasionally a change in taste. There are other side effects, and these are discussed in more detail in the chapter 18.

I have a tendency to get easily sick to my stomach. Is there anything that can be done?

Notify your physician that you get sick to your stomach easily. Medication is available to eliminate or minimize any nausea or vomiting.

What are the side effects from *many* doses of radioiodine?

If you receive multiple doses of radioiodine, the frequency and severity of side effects can increase, and this is discussed in greater detail in chapter 18.

What are the long-term effects of radioiodine?

See chapter 18.

Can I get pregnant?

Yes, but we recommend you do not become pregnant until six months and preferably one year after your treatment. You should not be pregnant at the time of treatment, and all women of childbearing age are required to take a pregnancy test before receiving any radioiodine treatment. Birth control is recommended, and you should talk with your physician, endocrinologist, nuclear medicine physician or nuclear radiologist for more information and recommendations (see chapter 18).

Will the radioiodine affect my sperm count?

Radioiodine can reduce sperm count. If you plan on future children and especially if you have had infertility problems, you should discuss this further with your physician, endocrinologist, nuclear medicine physician or nuclear radiologists. Although "banking" of sperm has not been routinely performed, it may be an appropriate option in certain individuals (see chapter 18).

Does radioiodine increase the risk of congenital abnormalities in any future children I have?

The initial dose of radioiodine for ablation does not significantly increase the risk of congenital abnormalities in future children.

What is dosimetry?

Dosimetry is a method used to help select radioiodine treatment dosages. In general, there are two types of dosimetry. The first type of dosimetry is called "lesion" dosimetry and the second is "blood" or "bone marrow" dosimetry. These are discussed in more detail in chapter 15. In brief, dosimetry is a method to attempt to calculate the radiation exposure to thyroid tissue or cancer (lesion dosimetry) or to the bone marrow (blood dosimetry). With this information and with other factors specific to your situation, your physician will selected the dosage of radioiodine for ablation or treatment.

Glossary

Ablation: Elimination of remaining normal thyroid tissue.

Activity: The amount or quantity of radioactivity. One of the units used for activity is called the becquerel in honor of Henri Becquerel who discovered radioactivity in 1896. One becquerel of any radioactive material would be that quantity from which there is on the average 1 disintegration occurring during a period of time equal to 1 second. This corresponds to a very, very small amount of radioactivity. Within the United States a different unit is also used, which is the millicurie (mCi) in honor of Marie Curie (the discoverer of Radium). For comparison, 1 millicurie represents an amount of radioactivity equal to 37 million becquerels. Radioiodine therapies for thyroid cancer generally involve the administration of 30 to 600 mCi of I-131.

Anaplastic thyroid carcinoma: Thyroid carcinoma is divided into several different types of cancer. These types are based upon several factors such as what type of thyroid cell the cancer came from and how the cell looks under the microscopic. If the cell appears very similar to normal cells, then the cancer cell is called *"well-differentiated."* If the cells have lost most of the appearance, organization or function of normal cells, then the cancer cell is called *de-differentiated*. Based upon factors such as these, the thyroid cancer is categorized. Accordingly, one type of thyroid cancer is anaplastic thyroid carcinoma, which has lost most of the appearance, organization, and function of normal thyroid cells. By knowing the type of thyroid cancer, the physician has a better understanding regarding the best treatment options presently available (see chapter 25).

Beta particles: A form of radiation that might be released during radioactive decay. This particle is, in fact, identical to the electrons that are normally found in matter and comprise what we refer to as electricity. What makes these electrons (beta particles) so dangerous is that they are very energetic projectiles that are "fired" out by the unstable radioactive atom as it transforms. One of the radioactive forms of iodine (indicated as ^{131}I) that is used extensively in the treatment of thyroid cancer emits both beta particles and electromagnetic radiation (called gamma radiation).

Brand name: The trademark name that a commercial company gives its product. For example, Kleenex® is the brand name for facial tissue made by the company of Kimberly Clark. Synthroid®, Levoxyl®, and Levothroid® are brand names for thyroid hormone made by the companies of Abbott Laboratories Pharmaceuticals, Jones Medical Industries, and Forest, respectively.

CAT Scan: See computerized axial tomography.

Chemotherapy: The use of chemicals for the treatment of cancer. See chapter 22.

Computerized Axial Tomography: This valuable imaging test, abbreviated as CT or CAT scan, uses low-level X-rays to obtain images of the internal organs. CT typically is used for evaluation of the chest. See chapter 16.

CT: See Computerized Axial Tomography.

Cytology: The scientific study of cells including the evaluation of cells under a microscope that were obtained from fine needle aspiration. See chapter 6.

Cytomel®: The brand name for the drug liothyronine (also known as LT-3 and L-triiodothyronine). Jones Pharmaceuticals makes Cytomel®. This is a short acting thyroid hormone. This is frequently used during withdrawal of the long acting thyroid hormone, levothyroxine.

Dietitian: A person who plans diet programs for proper nutrition. These individuals are usually called nutritionists.

Differentiated: There are different types of thyroid cancer: well-differentiated, medullary, and anaplastic.. These are discussed in more detail in chapter 4. The use of the word "differentiated" refers to the type of thyroid cancer that is "well-differentiated," and these include papillary and follicular thyroid cancer.

Dose: This term is used in two different contexts: (1) as a measure of the dosage or activity administered, namely a certain number of mCi's or becquerels, and (2) as a measure of the energy absorbed from the ionizing radiation in a certain mass of tissue. Every time a radioactive atom decays it releases energy in various forms. Beta particles, for example, travel very short distances (typically less than 1/4th of an inch) before they have expended all of their energy. Gamma radiation on the other hand can travel much larger distances through the body (several inches to several feet) without losing any of its energy. The biological effects of the radiation are directly related to the amount of energy that is deposited in each unit mass of tissue (see the glossary for the definitions of "rad" or "grey").

Dosimetrist: A person who helps plan and calculates the proper radiation dose for treatment.

Dosimetry: The calculation of radiation exposure to a specific organ.

Echo: See ultrasound.

Endocrinologist: A physician who has completed specific training in the subspecialty of endocrinology, which includes the diagnosis and management of thyroid carcinoma. An endocrinologist also has training in internal medicine.

Exposure: Frequently, just being in the presence of radiation is referred to as having been "exposed." However, there is also another meaning. The early devices, which are still commonly used today to measure the presence of ionizing radiation, are based on the effects produced within air itself, namely ionization (see definition above). Exposure is defined in terms of the amount of ions that are produced in a certain volume of air. This is similar to radiation dose, except that this refers only to effects that occur in air and not tissue.

External radiotherapy: The use of radiation that originates from outside of the body for the treatment of cancer.

Family practitioner: A physician who has completed specific training in the specialty of family practice.

Fine needle aspiration: The use of a small needle to obtain samples of thyroid or lymph node tissue. This is discussed in detail in chapter 6.

Follicular thyroid carcinoma: See well-differentiated thyroid carcinoma and chapter 4.

Free T-4: As discussed in chapter 3, a portion of levothyroxine hormone (T-4) produced by the thyroid is attached to protein in your blood and another portion is not attached to anything in the blood (free). The portion of levothyroxine not attached to anything is called "free T-4." This can be measured, and the laboratory test is also called a "free T-4."

Generic name: This is the scientific name of a medication. The trade name that the commercial company gives to the medication is the brand name.

Grey: A unit dose of radiation abbreviated "Gy." One Gy = 100 cGy. "Rad" is an older term for dose of radiation, and one rad equals 1 cGy. One hundred rads equal 100cGy, which equals 1Gy.

Half-life: As the radioactive material releases radiation it transforms into another element. Consequently over time there is less and less of the original radioactive material remaining. How quickly it disappears depends on the radioactive element we are observing, but the rate is a constant for any particular element. The half-life of a radioactive element is the time required for half of the radioactive material to be transformed. In the case of ^{131}I, this is about 8 days.

Hypothyroid: This condition occurs when your levels of thyroid hormone are too low for your normal body needs. Hypothyroidism is associated with various symptoms such as fatigue, intolerance to cold, and emotional changes. Hypothyroidism also can cause weight gain, slowing of the heart, and soft tissue swelling. See chapter 9.

Internal medicine physician: A physician who has completed specific training in the specialty of internal medicine and is frequently known as an internist.

Ionizing radiation: Since light, radio waves, TV waves, ultrasound, etc. are all forms of radiation, why is the hazard from these forms of radiation so much less than that from radioactive sources? The answer largely has to do with the amount of energy carried by the waves or particles. This in turn affects the size of the objects that the radiation tends to interact with. In the case of the beta particles and gamma rays released by ^{131}I, the interactions are often with the electrons of individual atoms. As a consequence, electrons are knocked out of the atom, a process referred to as ionization. In some cases these are the very electrons that are responsible for holding atoms together in a molecule or molecules in a complex structure such as DNA. It is this type of damage to critical components on a cellular level from ionizing radiation that can often lead to the death of a cell.

Levothyroxine: Levothyroxine is the name for one of the two main hormones that your thyroid makes. The other main thyroid hormone is tri-iodothyronine. Levothyroxine is known by many names including T-4, L-T4, LT4, L-thyroxine, and brand names such as Synthroid®. In patients who have had their thyroid gland removed, levothyroxine is given orally to supply the body with the necessary thyroid hormone.

L-T4: See levothyroxine.

LT4: See levothyroxine.

Lymphadenopathy: Enlarged lymph nodes.

Malignancy: Cancer

Magnetic Resonance Imaging: This valuable imaging test, known as MR or MRI, is used to obtain exquisite images. MR uses the property of radio signals that are emitted after a magnetic field has been removed. MR is very useful in the evaluation of the neck region as well as many other organs of the body (see chapter 16).

Metastasis: An area of spread of the cancer outside of its original site.

Millicurie: A unit to measure radioactivity. One millicurie represents 37 million radioactive atoms disintegrating every second.

Millirem: A unit to measure the effective absorbed radiation energy in a volume of tissue. One millirem is a very small amount of energy in tissue. One millirem is approximately equal to the warming effect of a one-watt flashlight bulb lit for one hundred-thousandth of a second in a quart of water.

MR: See Magnetic Resonance Imaging.

Near total thyroidectomy: The nearly complete removal of the thyroid gland.

Neutrophil: One of the types of white blood cells, which are in your blood. White blood cells, and specifically neutrophil, fight infection.

Nuclear medicine physician: A physician who has completed specific training in the subspecialty of nuclear medicine, which includes training in the use of radioisotopes for the diagnosis and treatment of thyroid cancer. A nuclear medicine physician may have additional training in radiology, internal medicine or pathology.

Nutritionist: A person who plans diet programs for proper nutrition.

Oncologist: A physician who has completed specific training in the subspecialty of oncology, which includes the use of chemotherapy and other treatment approaches for many types of cancers. An oncologist has additional training in internal medicine.

Papillary thyroid carcinoma: See well-differentiated thyroid carcinoma.

Parathyroid gland: A gland that controls calcium levels in your body. There are typically four parathyroid glands, which are located on the back side of the thyroid gland.

PET scan: PET stands for Positron Emission Tomography, an imaging study that uses low-level radioactivity to assess metabolic activity in various organs such as in lymph nodes. See chapter 16.

Positron Emission Tomography: See PET scan.

Rad: A measure of the amount of radiation dose absorbed in tissue or an organ and representing a certain amount of energy that is absorbed by each gram of tissue. It is this energy that contributes to the breakdown of chemical bonds, which in turn can result in the permanent impairment or death of cells in an organ. The more energy that is deposited, the larger the dose in rads and the more damage to the tissue.

Radiation: The movement or passage through space or objects of energy that has been released or emitted from some source. There are many different forms that this energy or radiation might assume. Frequently, it is in the form of electromagnetic waves, but it can also include extremely small particles (the same ones that represent the building blocks of atoms). We encounter electromagnetic radiation in many different forms every day. The light from the sun or a lamp that is reflecting off this page (thereby allowing you to read this material) is in fact "radiation." More importantly, however, radiation is often released in conjunction with radioactive decay. See chapter 19.

Radiation nurse: A nurse who specializes in caring for people who are undergoing radiation therapy.

Radiation oncologist: A doctor who has completed special training in the subspecialty of radiation oncology, which includes the use of radiation for the treatment of cancer and other diseases.

Radiation treatment physicist: A person who makes sure that the radiation machine delivers the right amount of radiation to the treatment site. In consultation with the radiation oncologist and dosimetrist, the physicist also ensures that the plan and calculations for your treatment are correct.

Radiation therapist: A person who runs the equipment that delivers the radiation.

Radiation safety technologist: Specialist in the area of radiation safety management who is responsible for overseeing all aspects regarding the safe use of radiation in the hospital.

Radio-ablation: The use of radioiodine to eliminate (ablate) thyroid tissue remaining after surgery.

Radioactivity: The world is comprised of 92 naturally occurring elements. These elements are frequently found in a variety of forms called isotopes. Scientists have devised several methods to artificially transform these isotopes into different forms, which are unstable. Over time all of these unstable atoms will undergo a transformation into a different element entirely. It is this process of change or transformation that is referred to as "radioactivity" or "radioactive decay". The term itself was coined about 100 years ago by Pierre and Marie Curie, both pioneers in the study of radiation and radium. See chapter 19.

Radioiodine: The element iodine can exist in many different forms called isotopes. Chemically and biologically all of these forms behave the same. In fact, of the 25 different isotopes of iodine that have been discovered, only one is stable. The other 24 are radioactive. The term radioiodine is used to indicate that we are referring to one of these radioactive forms. The most common types of radioiodine used for the evaluation and treatment of thyroid cancer are: ^{123}I (imaging and uptake), ^{131}I (imaging, uptake, and treatment), and ^{124}I (imaging using a PET scanner). See chapter 13.

Radioiodine scan: Images obtained of selected or all areas of your body after the administration of radioiodine.

Radioiodine treatment: The use of radioiodine to eliminate (treat) any thyroid cancer occurring after radio-ablation.

Radiologist: A physician who has completed specific training in the specialty of radiology, which includes the use of radiation and other methods for diagnosing by imaging. Radiologists may also perform various types of treatment. Accordingly, a radiologist interprets CT scans, MRIs, ultrasounds, and nuclear medicine studies as well as performs radiofrequency treatments. Radiologists have a minimum of four months of training in nuclear medicine. Some radiologists have additional training in nuclear medicine with a certificate of "Special Competence in Nuclear

Medicine." These nuclear radiologists typically have had a minimum of 12 months of training in nuclear medicine.

Radiotherapy: The treatment of diseases by radiation.

Radiotracer: A radioactive element or chemical that allows the physician to trace and image the metabolism or function of specific cells or organs of your body.

Recurrent external laryngeal nerve: The nerve that controls your voice box, which enables you to speak. This nerve runs behind the thyroid.

Secondary cancer: A cancer that is a result of the treatment for the first cancer.

Sialadenitis: Inflammation of the salivary glands.

Sonogram: See ultrasound.

Subtotal thyroidectomy: A subtotal thyroidectomy is less than the total removal of the thyroid gland by the surgeon. This is frequently assumed to be the same thing as a near total thyroidectomy. Although some physicians use these terms interchangeably, in a strict sense they are not the same thing. Although a near total thyroidectomy is always a subtotal thyroidectomy, it is possible that a subtotal thyroidectomy is not a near-total thyroidectomy. An example of a subtotal thyroidectomy that is not a near-total thyroidectomy is when the surgeon removes 60 percent of the total thyroid.

A near total thyroidectomy is typically what the surgeon performs. A complete total thyroidectomy is rare for reasons discussed elsewhere.

Synthroid®: The Abbott Laboratories' brand name for the hormone levothyroxine (see levothyroxine).

T-3: See tri-iodothyronine.

Thyroidectomy: The surgical removal of the thyroid gland

Thyroid stimulating hormone: See TSH.

Thyrogen®: The brand name of the form of synthetic TSH made by recombinant technology (abbreviated rhTSH) that, once injected into the body, stimulates the thyroid tissue to take up radioiodine and release thyroglobulin.

Thyrogen® scan: This whole body survey or scan is performed after the injection of Thyrogen®. Thyrogen® is typically injected each day for two or three sequential days prior to the administration of radioiodine for the radioiodine whole body survey or scan.

Thyroglobulin: A chemical produced by thyroid tissue, which can be measured in the blood system. If all thyroid tissue or thyroid cancer cells have been eliminated, then this chemical should not be present in the blood. Presence of this chemical in the blood is evidence of residual or recurrent thyroid cancer. Thyroglobulin is frequently called a "tumor marker."

Thyroid gland: A gland typically located in the front lower aspect of the neck. This gland makes thyroid hormone.

Thyroxine: One of the hormones made by the thyroid gland.

Tri-iodothyronine: Tri-iodothyronine is the name for one of the two main hormones that your thyroid makes. Tri-iodothyronine is known by many names including T-3 and the brand name product Cytomel®.

TSH: Thyroid Stimulating Hormone or thyrotropin (TSH) is made by the pituitary gland, which is located in the middle of your head. This gland monitors how well your thyroid gland is making thyroid hormone. If there is not enough thyroid hormone, then the pituitary gland secretes more TSH to try to stimulate your thyroid tissue to make more. If there is too much thyroid hormone, then the pituitary secretes less TSH. TSH is very important for you for many reasons. In the long term, TSH needs to be low so that it does not stimulate any thyroid cancer cells. In the short term, your TSH needs to be high to allow us to image or treat any thyroid tissue.

ug/dl: Micrograms per deci-liter.

uU/dl: Microunits per deci-liter.

uU/ml: Microunits per milliliter.

Ultrasound: An imaging test that uses sound waves that echos back from the various tissues in your body. By listening to these waves, we can obtain excellent images of many different organs and structures. Ultrasound is frequently used to evaluate your neck region. See chapter 3 and 16.

Well-differentiated thyroid carcinoma: Thyroid carcinoma is divided into several different types of cancer. These types are based upon several factors such as what type of thyroid cell the cancer came from and how the cell looks under the microscope. If the cell appears very similar to normal cells, then the cancer cell is called *"well-differentiated."* If the cells have lost most of the appearance, organization or function of normal cells, then the cancer cell is called *"de-differentiated."* Based upon factors such as these, the thyroid cancer is categorized. Accordingly, one type of thyroid cancer is well-differentiated thyroid carcinoma, which has similar appearance, organization and function to normal cells. Well-differentiated thyroid carcinoma can be divided into multiple other classifications. The two most frequent classifications are "papillary" and "follicular." These represent the type of cells that the cancer came from. By knowing the type of thyroid cancer, the physician has a better understanding regarding the best treatment options presently available.

Whole body survey or scan: This scan is performed with a special nuclear medicine camera that images most of your body. It is performed after the administration of radioiodine and after the radioiodine has accumulated in any thyroid tissue. See chapter 13.

Withdrawal scan: This whole body survey or scan is performed after the withdrawal of your thyroid hormone. See chapter 13.

Additional Sources of Information

Gary Bloom

This appendix presents sources of additional information from organizations, Web sites, and books. Every effort has been made to identify these sites and to minimize errors. If you have identified additional sources of information or errors, please e-mail these to the *keystonepress@aol.com*.

Caution: With any organization, Web site or reading material, the information you obtain may or may not apply to you, and frequently this may result in misunderstandings, unnecessary concerns and in some cases incorrect care for your specific situation. Always talk with your physician to determine whether the information you obtained from the Internet applies to your particular health situation.

Patient Support Groups and Informational Sources:

ThyCa: Thyroid Cancer Survivors' Association, Inc. (ThyCa): All volunteer, national, nonprofit organization of thyroid cancer survivors, family members, and health professionals advised by nationally recognized leaders in the field of thyroid cancer, dedicated to education, communication, and support for thyroid cancer survivors, families, and friends.

Address:
  P.O. Box 1545
  New York, NY 10159-1545
Communication data:
  1-877-588-7904 (toll free)
  Fax 1-630-604-6078
  E-mail: *thyca@thyca.org*
  Web site: *www.thyca.org*
Services (more information available through the Web site or the above communication data)
• Local support groups coast to coast.

- Seven E-mail discussion groups.
- Person-to-person support with toll-free survivors' telephone line.
- Web site with over 300 pages plus extensive links list.
- Low iodine diet cookbook (free) and other free publications.
- Newsletter, which is free online.
- National and regional conferences and workshops
- Thyroid cancer awareness materials.
- Thyroid Cancer Awareness Week and Month
- Thyroid Cancer Research Funds

States with local ThyCa support groups are: Alabama, Arizona, California, Colorado, Connecticut, Delaware, District of Columbia, Florida, Georgia, Hawaii, Idaho, Illinois, Iowa, Kentucky, Maryland, Massachusetts, Michigan, Minnesota, Missouri, Nebraska, New Hampshire, New Jersey, New York, North Carolina, Ohio, Pennsylvania, Rhode Island, Texas, Vermont, Virginia, and Wisconsin.

Canadian Thyroid Cancer Support Group (Thry'vors) Inc.

Formed by a group of Canadian thyroid cancer patients, who came together in a common search for information and support in dealing with treatment, recovery, and long-term monitoring of thyroid cancer. Thry'vors offers information and support to those affected by thyroid cancer through our Web site at www.thryvors.org, and through an Internet-based listserv. The listserv, available through yahoo.groups (full address below), allows thyroid cancer patients, regardless of whether they are newly diagnosed, on the road to recovery or long-term survivors, as well as their caregivers, friends or family, to give and receive emotional support. Here, they can post messages, listen, ask questions and/or exchange experiences and information with those who have "been there." Access to our listserv is through: http://groups.yahoo.com/group/Thryvors.

Address:
P.O. Box 23007
550 Eglinton Ave. W.
Toronto, ON M5N 3A8
Communication data:
Telephone: 416-487-8267 (during office hours only)
E-mail: *thryvors@sympatico.ca*
Web site: *www.thryvors.org*
http://groups.yahoo.com/group/Thryvors.

Light of Life Foundation: This foundation improves the quality of life and promotes research and education about thyroid cancer.

Address:
   32 Marc Drive
   Englishtown, NJ 07726
Communication data:
   Telephone 732-972-0461
   Fax 732-536-4824
   E-mail: *info@lightoflifefoundation.org*
   Web site: *http://www.lightoflifefoundation.org*

Thyroid Foundation of American: Provides health education and support to thyroid patients.
   Address:
   410 Stuart Street
   Boston, MA 02116
Communication data:
   Telephone: 800-832-8321
   Fax: 617-534-1515
   E-mail: *info@allthyroid.org*
   Web site: *www.allthyroid.org*

Thyroid Foundation of Canada (TFC)
La Fondation canadiennne de la Thyroide
The Thyroid Foundation of Canada is the oldest North American patient education association. The TFC promotes awareness and education about thyroid disease including thyroid cancer.
   Address:
   Box/CP 1919 STN MAIN
   Kingston, Ontario K7L J7l
Communication data:
   Office: 613-544-8364
         1-800-267-8822
   Fax: 613-544-9731
   Web site: *www.thryoid.ca*

Thyroid Federation International: A worldwide network of affiliated thyroid patient organizations.
   Address:
   96 Mack Street
   Kingston, Ontario
   Canada K7L 1N9

Communication data:

Telephone +1 613 554-8364

Fax +1 613 544-9731

E-mail: *tfi@on.aibn.com*

Web site: *http://www.thryoid-fed.org*

American Cancer Society

Communication data:

1-800-ACS-2345

Web site: *www.cancer.org*

Enter type of cancer or other. On next page click on thyroid carcinoma.

Thyroid Cancer Web Site:

www3.cancer.org/cancerinfo/load_cont.asp?ct:43&lanuag+English

Services:

Information on cancer, your job, insurance, the law, the American with Disabilities Act, diet, vitamins/supplements, complementary treatment approaches.

National Cancer Institute at the National Institutes of Health

Address:

31 Center Drive, MSC 2580

Bethesda, MD 20892-2580

Communication data:

Telephone: 800-4-Cancer (800-422-6237)

Web Site: *www.cancer.gov/cancerinfo*

Click on "Types of Cancer." Under alphabetical list of cancers, click on "T." Then click on thyroid cancer.

Radiation Therapy Web site:

http://www.nci.nih.gov/ cancerinfo/radiation-therapy-and-you.

Services:

Information on types of cancers, treatment, clinical trials, and research.

National Coalition for Cancer Survivorship: The only survivor-led advocacy organization working exclusively on behalf of people with all types of cancer and their families, is dedicated to assuring quality cancer care for all Americans

Address:

1010 Wayne Avenue

Suite 770

Silver Spring, MD 20910

Communication data:
    Office: 301-650-9127
    Fax: 301-565-9670
    E-mail: *info@canceradvocacy.org*
    Web site: *www.canceradvocacy.org*

The Hormone Foundation (c/o The Endocrine Society):
Address:
    8401 Connecticut Avenue, Suite 900
    Chevy Chase, MD 20815-5817
Communication data:
    Office: 301-941-0200
    Fax: 301-941-0259
    E-mail: *endostaff@end-soc.org*
    Web Site: *www.endo-society.org*

THYROID AND/OR CANCER PROFESSIONAL ORGANIZATIONS:

American Thyroid Association, Inc.: A professional medical society of physicians and scientists dedicated to treating and researching thyroid disease.
Address:
    6066 Leesburg Pike, Suite 650
    Falls Church, VA 22041
Communication data:
    Office: 703-998-8890
    Fax: 703-998-8893
    E-mail: *admin@thyroid.org*
    Web site: *www.thyroid.org*
Services:
    For general endocrinologist referrals and general thyroid information. *Patient education materials on the web site.*

American Association of Clinical Endocrinologists: This is a professional medical organization of more than 2500 clinical endocrinologists. The mission of the AACE is to (1) improve the care given to the endocrine patient, (2) increase the public's understanding of the function of an clinical endocrinologist, (3) increase the awareness of endocrine disease, and (4) to make available to patients the choice of care by a specialist trained in the treatment of endocrine disorders.
Address:
    1000 Riverside Ave., Suite 205
    Jacksonville, Florida 32204

Communication data:
    Telephone: 904-353-7878
    Fax: 904-353-8185
    Web site: *www.aace.com*
    To find an endocrinologist, got to *www.aace.com/memsearch.php*
    Clinical guidelines: *www.aace.com/clin/guidelines/*
    Radiation related terms and radiation risk: *www.physics.isu.edu/radinf*
Services:
- Find an endocrinologist
- Clinical guidelines
- Information on radiation related terms and radiation risk

Thyroid Disease Manager: An up-to-date analysis of thyrotoxicosis, hypothyroidism, thyroid nodules, and cancer, thyroiditis, and all aspects of human thyroid disease and thyroid physiology. It provides physicians, researchers, and trainees (as well as patients) around the world with an authoritative, current, complete, objective, free, and down-loadable source on the thyroid. This web site contains a newly revised version of the textbook "The Thyroid and Its Diseases," and much supplementary information, all directed toward helping physicians care for their patients with thyroid problems. WWW.THYROIDMANAGER.ORG is updated continually with important new information, and major revisions are done annually.
    Web Site: *www.thyroidmanager.org*
Services:
    As noted above.

Johns Hopkins Thyroid Tumor Center
    Communication data
    Web site: *www.thyroid-cancer.net*
Services:
- Find a thyroid cancer specialist near you
- Frequently asked questions

COMMERICIAL ORGANIZATIONS:

Genzyme Corporation (manufacturers of Thyrogen®)
    Address:
        500 Kendall Street
        Cambridge, MA 02142

Communication data

Resource "Hot-Line": 800-745-4447

Telephone: 800-326-7002

Web site: *www.thyrogen.com/global/p_hp_homepage.asp*

Information about Thyrogen:

- Genzyme's Patient Information Kit provides understanding about Thyrogen.

Abbott Laboratories (manufacturers of Synthroid®)

Address:

Abbott Laboratories

Abbott Park, Illinois

Communication data

Telephone for customer service (800) 255-5162.

Web sites: *www.abbott.com* (general web site for Abbot Laboratories)

www.synthroid.com

- The latter web site has excellent information on Synthroid®.

www.abbottdiagnostics.com/medical_conditions/thyroid/index.htm

- This web site has excellent addition information

ORGANIZATIONS INVOLVED WITH INSURANCE, BILLING, JOB DISCRIMINATION

Patient Advocate Foundation

Address:

700 Thimble Shoals Boulevard

Suite 200

Newport News, VA 23606

Communication data:

Telephone: 1-800-532-5274

Fax: 757-873-8999

E-mail: *info@patientadvocate.org*

Web site: *http:\\patientadvocate.org*

Services:

From the Foundation's mission statement, the nonprofit organization is ". . . serves as an active liaison between the patient and their insurers, employer and/or creditors to resolve insurance, job discrimination and/or debt crisis matters relative to their diagnosis through case managers, doctors, and attorneys."

Association of Community Cancer Centers
Address:

11600 Nebel Street, Suite 201

Rockville, MD 20852.

Communication data:

Telephone number: 1-301-984-9496

Web Site: *www.accc-cancer.org/publications/patientbrochure.asp*

Services:

This organization offers an eight-page brochure, which describes standard and investigational treatments that should be covered and what to do if reimbursement is denied. The brochure is available only online through the Web site noted above. This is a brochure of the American Cancer Society.

U.S. Equal Employment Opportunity Commission
Address:

1801 L Street, N.W.

Washington, D.C. 20507

Communication:

Telephone: 202-663-4900

Telephone number for EEOC-Basic Information System: 1-800-669-3362

Web site: *www.eeoc.gov/teledir.htmlin*

Services:

• EEOC-Basic Information System

• Information on job retention

• List of all EEOC field offices

Debt Crisis Intervention
See Patient Advocate Foundation above and go to section entitled Debt Crisis Intervention:

Web site: *www.patientadovate.org/resources*

Services:

• On this site, the Patient Advocate Foundation lists companies that will convert a life insurance policy into cash and discusses other options for raising money.

INFORMATION REGARDING CLINICAL TRIALS

National Institutes of Health (Developed by the National Library of Medicine): ClinicalTrials.gov provides regularly updated information about federally and privately supported clinical research in human volunteers. ClinicalTrials.gov gives you information about a trial's purpose, who may participate, locations, and phone numbers for more details

Web site: *www.clinicaltrials.gov*

National Cancer Institute:

Web site: *www.cancer.gov/search/clinical_trials/*

Books and Manuals

The books should be available at libraries or through book stores such as Borders, Barnes and Noble, and Amazon.com. Smaller book stores may also be able to obtain these books by special order.

If a book is out of print, frequently the book is available used at a reasonable price through Amazon.com and its affiliated used books stores. These used books will be listed immediately under the new book prices.

Publication intended for patients, family, and friends

Collection of Low-Iodine Recipes, Leah Guljord, ed., ThyCa: Thyroid Cancer Survivors' Association, Inc. (4th edition, 2003) Free and downloadable from the ThyCa Web site *(www.thyca.org)*.

Light of Life Foundation Cookbook, *contact Light of Life Foundation (information above)*.

Thyroid for Dummies, Alan Rubin, M.D., Hungry Minds, Inc., New York, 2001.

Your Thyroid: A Home Reference, Lawrence C. Wood, M.D., David S. Cooper, M.D., E. Chester Ridgeway, M. D., Ballantine Books, 1996.

Could It Be My Thyroid? Sheldon Rubenfeld, M.D., Sheldon Rubenfeld Publisher, 2003. (3rd edition to be published in 2004 by M. Evans & Co.)

The Thyroid Guide, Beth Ann Ditkoff, M.D., & Paul Lo Gerfo, M.D., Harper Perennial, 2000.

The Thyroid Gland: A Book for Thyroid Patients, Joel Hamburger, M.D., Privately Published, 1991.

The Washington Hospital Center Nuclear Medicine Thyroid Cancer Information Manual. The Washington Hospital Center Nuclear Medicine Thyroid

Cancer Information Manual is the informational manual for a six-step process of scheduling, preparation, logistics, and education for the patients who are scheduled for radioiodine scanning, ablation and/or therapy at Washington Hospital Center, Washington, D.C. The manual is a professionally published three-ring notebook. The manual is available in the United States and Canada for purchase for $20 dollars ($30 Canadian dollars) plus $5 dollars ($7.50 Canadian dollars) shipping and handling. The manual is printed in low volumes in order to keep the manual as current as possible for our patients, and the manual is typically updated every three months in order to incorporate our changes in preparations, instructions and procedures. Checks or money orders should be made out to Washington Hospital Center. Send checks or money order to *Nuclear Medicine Senior Administrative Assistant, Division of Nuclear Medicine, Washington Hospital Center, 110 Irving Street, NW, Washington D.C., 20010.* For international rates, please call 202-877-0348. Sorry, orders will not be taken by telephone, and no credit cards are accepted. Prices are subject to change without notice. Please allow four to six weeks for delivery. All revenues go toward the production costs and improvement of this manual. No one receives any profits from the sale of this manual.

Please note that this information manual is specifically for radioiodine scans, ablations, and/or therapies performed by the Division of Nuclear Medicine at Washington Hospital Center. The instructions from your physician and or medical facility may vary, and you should follow the instructions of your physician. This manual does not dictate the only appropriate approach. The purchase of this manual is for general information only.

Publications intended for physicians

Thyroid Cancer, A Comprehensive Guide to Clinical Management, L. Wartofsky, M.D., Humana Press, Totowa, New Jersey, 2000. (2nd edition to be published in later 2004 or early 2005.)

Thyroid Cancer: H.J. Biersack, M.D., F. Grunwald, M.D., Springer Verlag, New York, 2001.

Werner and Ingbar's The Thyroid: A Fundamental and Clinical Text, Lewis E. Braverman, M.D., and Robert D. Utiger., M.D., J. B. Lippincott, Philadelphia, 2000.

Thyroid Disease: The facts, W.M.G. Tunbridge, M.D., R.I.S. Bayliss, M.D., Oxford University Press, 1999.

Radiation Oncology, J. Cox, M.D., K. Ang., M.D., C.B. Mosby, St Louis, 2003.

Cancer: Principles and Practice of Oncology, V. T. DeVita, Jr., M.D., S. Hellman, M.D., S. A. Rosenberg, M.D., Lippincott Williams & Wilkins, Philadelphia, 2001. (7th edition to be published in later 2004 or early 2005).

Form for Potential "Early Release" from Hospital

Please read, complete, sign, and bring this form with you to your hospital room after you are admitted.

The Nuclear Regulatory Commission has concluded that the radioactive iodine that you receive for therapeutic purposes will cause only small radiation exposures to others if you are released from the hospital in accordance with Nuclear Regulatory Commission guidelines. Exposures occur mainly if other people remain close to you (less than 3 feet) for long periods of time (at least one hour) during the first few days after you leave the hospital. The Radiation Safety Department will make measurements with a radiation detector to confirm that you meet Nuclear Regulatory Commission guidelines prior to leaving the hospital.

Often these measurements indicate that a patient may be released less than 24 hours after receiving the dose of radioactive iodine. Thus you may need to remain in the hospital for only one night or even less. Sometimes the measurements indicate that a patient does not meet the Nuclear Regulatory Commission's guidelines assuming normal contact and activities with other people. In those circumstances, you may need to remain for a second or third night. To be eligible for early release, you must answer the following questions and agree to follow these instructions.

1. Are you nursing a small child or infant?

Yes _____   No _____

NOTE: Nursing after receiving radioactive iodine will cause radioiodine to pass from the mother to the child through the milk. Radioactive iodine ingested by the child will expose the child's thyroid to potentially harmful levels of radiation. Lifelong medication may be required to prevent serious effects both mentally and physically if the child's thyroid receives a high dose of radiation. If you are nursing a child, inform your treating physician or technologist. We must reschedule your treatment at a later date after you have permanently ceased nursing this child.

2. Can you take care of yourself except for brief visits and not be in the same room with another person for more than three hours total during each of the first two days at home?

Yes _____   No _____

If no, briefly explain circumstances:

_____

_____

_____

3. Will you be able to maintain distance from other people, including:
   • Sleeping alone for at least one night or, preferably, three nights?
   • Avoiding kissing and sexual intercourse for at least three days?
   • Staying at least 3 feet away from people if you will be involved with them for more than an hour a day in the first three days?

Yes _____   No _____
If no, briefly explain circumstances:

_____

_____

_____

4. Will you avoid traveling by airplane or mass transit for the first day?

Yes _____   No _____
If no, briefly explain circumstances:

_____

_____

_____

5. Will you avoid traveling in an automobile with others for longer than 1 hour for at least the first two days?

Yes _____   No _____
If no, briefly explain circumstances:

_____

_____

_____

6. Will you have sole use of a bathroom for at least the first two days?

Yes _____   No _____
If no, briefly explain circumstances:

_____

_____

_____

I have read these guidelines, understand the instructions and agree to avoid contacts in accordance with my answers to items 2 through 6. [Note: If you cannot comply with the above and cannot avoid close contact with others, it may be necessary for you to remain in the hospital up to an additional 24 hours.]

Signature: _____

Date: _____

(Patient or other person in accordance with practices of the hospital)

Patient Bill of Rights and Responsibilities

**Reproduced with permission
from Washington Hospital Center, Washington, D.C.**

RESPECT

Your Rights

- To be treated with respect and courtesy
- To receive safe, considerate, ethical, and cost-effective medical care
- To have your individual cultural, spiritual, and psychosocial needs respected
- To have your privacy and personal dignity maintained
- To expect that information regarding your care will be treated as confidential

Your Responsibilities

- To respect hospital personnel
- To respect caregivers' efforts to provide care for other patients
- To respect hospital property
- To be considerate of other patients and to see that your visitors do the same

TREATMENT

Your Rights

- To receive treatment regardless of race, religion or any other discrimination prohibited by law
- To receive emergency treatment regardless of ability to pay
- To expect reasonable continuity of care and to be informed of available and realistic care options when hospital care is no longer appropriate
- To have your needs for pain management addressed and treated

Your Responsibilities

- To follow your caregivers' instructions and help them in their efforts to return you to health

- To inform your caregivers if you think there may be problems in following their instructions
- To participate in decision-making about your medical care
- To recognize the impact of lifestyle on your personal health

INFORMATION

Your Rights

- To understand your diagnosis and treatment, as well as the possible outcomes, risks and benefits of your care
- To have information regarding your medical treatment explained to a family member or other appropriate individual when you are unable to participate in decision about your care
- To access foreign language or American Sign Language interpreter and/or adaptive equipment (including TDDs) if necessary
- To be advised of hospital policies, procedures, rules, and regulations that may affect your care
- To be aware of any proposed hospital research in which you may be involved
- To be aware that the hospital's bioethics committee is available to you to discuss ethical issues related to your care

Your Responsibilities

- To understand that your caregivers may be both teachers and students
- To know the names/titles of your caregivers
- To see your medical records (in accordance with hospital policy and/or the laws)
- To review your bill and to have any questions or concerns your have adequately addressed

INVOLVEMENT

Your Rights

- To be involved in decisions concerning your care
- To have your family members and/or other involved in decisions about your care
- To exclude your family members and/or other from participating in decisions about your care
- To discuss any treatment planned for you
- To give your informed consent or informed refusal for treatment
- To leave the hospital or request a transfer (in accordance with the hospital policy and/or law)

- To refuse to be treated by a student
- To consent or decline to participate in proposed clinical research

Your Responsibilities

- To abide by hospital rules and regulations
- To keep your appointment
- To pay your bills on time
- To inform the hospital if you believe your rights have been violated

D

E

S

T

U

V

Any corrections in the medical information
in this book will be posted on the web site of
ThyCa: Thyroid Cancer Survivors' Association, Inc.
www.thyca.org

If you do not have Internet connectivity, please
send a stamped, self-addressed envelope to:
ThyCa, Inc., Corrections Sheet,
P.O. Box 1360, Germantown, MD 20875
and we'll send the sheet to you.